BROCHERT'S
CRUSH STEP 2

BROCHERT'S
CRUSH STEP 2
THE ULTIMATE USMLE STEP 2 REVIEW
FOURTH EDITION

Theodore X. O'Connell, MD
Program Director, Family Medicine Residency Program
Kaiser Permanente Woodland Hills, California
Assistant Clinical Professor, Department of Family Medicine
David Geffen School of Medicine at UCLA, Los Angeles, California
Partner Physician, Southern California Permanente Medical Group
Woodland Hills, California

Mayur K. Movalia, MD
Hematopathologist
Dahl-Chase Pathology Associates
Bangor, Maine

ELSEVIER
SAUNDERS

ELSEVIER
SAUNDERS

1600 John F. Kennedy Blvd.
Ste 1800
Philadelphia, PA 19103-2899

Brochert's Crush Step 2: The Ultimate USMLE Step 2 Review   ISBN: 9781455703111

Notices

Knowledge and best practice in this field are constantly changing. As new research and experience broaden our understanding, changes in research methods, professional practices, or medical treatment may become necessary.

Practitioners and researchers must always rely on their own experience and knowledge in evaluating and using any information, methods, compounds, or experiments described herein. In using such information or methods they should be mindful of their own safety and the safety of others, including parties for whom they have a professional responsibility.

With respect to any drug or pharmaceutical products identified, readers are advised to check the most current information provided (i) on procedures featured or (ii) by the manufacturer of each product to be administered, to verify the recommended dose or formula, the method and duration of administration, and contraindications. It is the responsibility of practitioners, relying on their own experience and knowledge of their patients, to make diagnoses, to determine dosages and the best treatment for each individual patient, and to take all appropriate safety precautions.

To the fullest extent of the law, neither the Publisher nor the authors, contributors, or editors, assume any liability for any injury and/or damage to persons or property as a matter of products liability, negligence or otherwise, or from any use or operation of any methods, products, instructions, or ideas contained in the material herein.

Previous editions copyrighted 2007, 2003

Library of Congress Cataloging-in-Publication Data
O'Connell, Theodore X.
    Brochert's crush step 2 : the ultimate USMLE step 2 review / Theodore
X. O'Connell, Mayur Movalia. – Ed. 4.
        p. ; cm.
    Brochert's crush step two
    Crush step 2
    Rev. ed. of: Crush step 2 / Adam Brochert. 3rd ed. c2007.
    Includes bibliographical references and index.
    ISBN 978-1-4557-0311-1 (pbk. : alk. paper)
    I. Movalia, Mayur. II. Brochert, Adam, 1971- Crush step 2. III. Title.
IV. Title: Brochert's crush step two. V. Title: Crush step 2.
    [DNLM: 1. Clinical Medicine–Examination Questions. WB 18.2]
    616.0076–dc23
                                                                    2011043807

Acquisitions Editor: James Merritt
Developmental Editor: Christine Abshire
Publishing Services Manager: Peggy Fagen
Project Manager: Deepthi Unni
Design Direction: Steven Stave

Printed in the United States of America

Last digit is the print number: 9 8 7 6 5 4 3 2 1

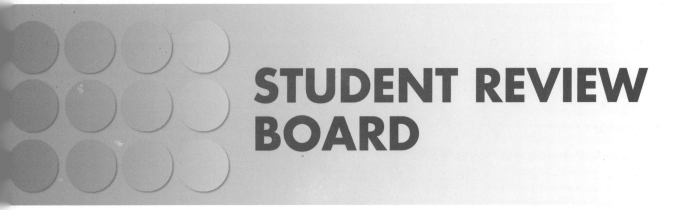

STUDENT REVIEW BOARD

CONTENTS

INTRODUCTION

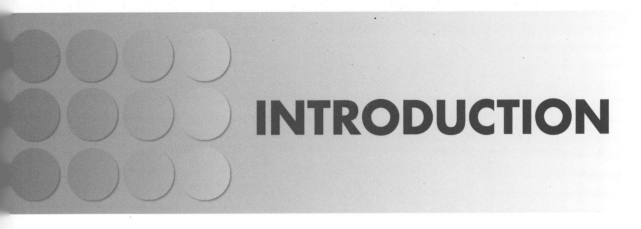

This fourth edition of Crush Step 2 attempts to incorporate the many changes that have occurred in medicine and the exam since 2007, as well as suggestions from readers based on material they encountered on their exams. For this edition, we have created a student review board composed of recent students who each scored in the 99th percentile on Step 2. Their input and suggestions have been invaluable in helping this book reflect the content and structure of the recent USMLE Step 2 exams. Though the format of the exam is constantly changing, many of the basic concepts you need to know to be a successful house officer have not changed in decades. If you understand the concepts in this book, you should do much better than pass: you should *Crush Step 2!*

Though Step 2 is the same level of difficulty as Step 1, the focus is more clinical and the questions are more relevant to the everyday practice of medicine. Knowing how to recognize, diagnose, manage, and treat common conditions is stressed. The exam tests not just theory but practice—in other words, what you should *do next*. Treatable emergency conditions are also tested, because you will soon be asked to take care of patients in the middle of the night, some of whom may require heroic measures if they are to survive until morning rounds.

Some information from Step 1 is still relevant and high yield for Step 2. Epidemiology and biostatistics, pharmacology, and microbiology are all tested with a slightly more clinical slant. Cardiac physiology and pathophysiology and behavioral science are also retested and are high yield. Overall, though, Step 2 has a different focus, and that focus is clinical. If a patient presented with chest pain, what would you do? What kinds of questions would you ask him or her? Which tests would you order? How would you select medications or treatments?

Here are some general tips to keep you focused while studying for and taking the test:

1. Always get more history when it is an option, unless the patient is unstable and you think immediate action is needed.
2. Know the cutoff values for the treatment of common conditions (e.g., at what numbers do you treat hypertension, diabetes, and hypercholesterolemia; below what CD4 count should you institute chemoprophylaxis in HIV patients).
3. A presentation might be normal, especially in psychiatry and pediatrics, and require no treatment!
4. Don't forget to study your subspecialties. Just because you never took an ophthalmology or dermatology rotation doesn't mean there won't be any basic questions on these topics. You don't have to be an expert, but knowing common and life-threatening diseases in the subspecialties can significantly increase your score.
5. Time management during the exam is critical. Make sure you are prepared to answer all of the questions in the allotted time.

Residency programs generally only see those magic two- and three-digit scores, not the breakdown. Don't skip studying a subject because you know you aren't going into it—you might miss out on easy points.

Studying for Step 2 can seem like an overwhelming task. Given the time constraints of medical students in their clinical years, most need a concise, high-yield review of the tested topics. It is our hope that *Crush Step 2*, fourth edition, will meet your needs in this regard.

Theodore X. O'Connell, MD
Mayur K. Movalia, MD

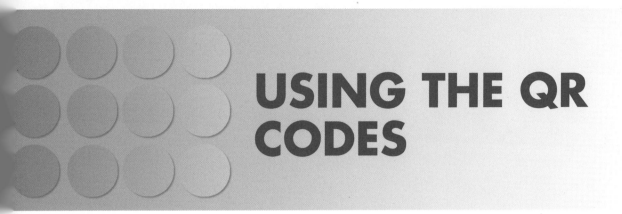

USING THE QR CODES

The QR codes in this book correspond to USMLE-style questions and images. For fast and easy access, right from your mobile device, follow these instructions.

What You Need
- A mobile device, such as a Smartphone or tablet, equipped with a camera and Internet access
- A QR code reader application (If you do not already have a reader installed on your mobile device, look for free versions in your app store.)

How It Works
- Open the QR code reader application on your mobile device.
- Point the device's camera at the code and scan.
- Each code opens questions or images for instant viewing—no log-on is required.

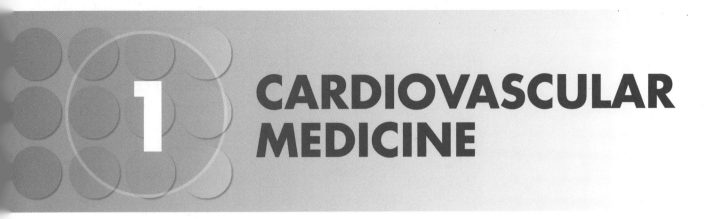

CARDIOVASCULAR MEDICINE

CHEST PAIN, MYOCARDIAL INFARCTION, AND ACUTE CORONARY SYNDROME

When a patient presents with chest pain, your job is to make sure that the cause is not life threatening, which usually means that you investigate the possibility of a myocardial infarction (MI).

Findings that make MI unlikely:

○ **Wrong age:** In the absence of known heart disease, a strong family history, or risk factors for coronary artery disease (CAD), a patient younger than 40 years of age is extremely unlikely to have had an MI.

○ **Risk factors:** A 50-year-old marathon runner who eats well and has a high high-density lipoprotein level without other risk factors for coronary heart disease is unlikely to have had an MI. A long-term smoker with a positive family history and chronic hypertension, diabetes, and hypercholesterolemia has had an MI until you prove otherwise!

○ **Physical characteristics of pain:** If the pain is reproducible by palpation, its source is the chest wall and is not an MI. Pain should *not* be sharp and well localized or related to certain foods.

Findings that elevate suspicion of MI:

○ **EKG:** After an MI, you should see flipped or flattened T waves, ST-segment elevation (depression means ischemia; elevation means injury), or Q waves in a segmental distribution (e.g., leads II, III, and aV_F for an inferior infarct) as shown in Figure 1-1.

○ **Pain characteristics:** Usually described as an intense pressure or crushing sensation that may be poorly localized or in the substernal region. The pain may radiate to the shoulder, arm, or jaw; it is not reproducible on palpation. The pain usually does not resolve with nitroglycerin (as it often does with angina) and generally lasts at least a half hour.

○ **Laboratory values:** A patient with a possible MI should have serial determinations of troponin I or T (usually drawn every 8 hours three times before MI is ruled out). Creatine kinase (the MB isoenzyme) is now less commonly used but results also can be positive. *Late patient presentation (>24 hours):* Troponin I or T can be used because both are still elevated several days after an MI (CK-MB begins to decrease 24 hours after an MI and might give a false-negative test result; if the CK-MB is elevated 2–3 days after an MI, think recurrent infarction). Lactate dehydrogenase (LDH) elevation and flip ($LDH_1 > LDH_2$) is now rarely used, and results take 24 hours to become positive. Aspartate aminotransferase is also elevated in those who have had an MI but is not used clinically. Radiography might show cardiomegaly or pulmonary congestion; brain natriuretic peptide (BNP) may be elevated; echocardiography might show ventricular wall motion abnormalities.

○ **History:** Patients with MI often have a history of angina or previous chest pain, murmurs, arrhythmias, or risk factors for CAD. Some are taking cardiovascular medications (digoxin, furosemide, antihypertensives, cholesterol medications).

○ **Physical examination:** Patients are often diaphoretic, dyspneic, tachycardic, and pale; nausea and vomiting may be present. Bilateral pulmonary rales in the absence of other pneumonia-like symptoms, distended neck veins, S_3 or S_4, new murmurs, hypotension, or shock should make you think along the lines of a large MI. Remember that right ventricle infarcts present with clear lung fields, increased jugular venous pressure (JVP), and decreased blood pressure.

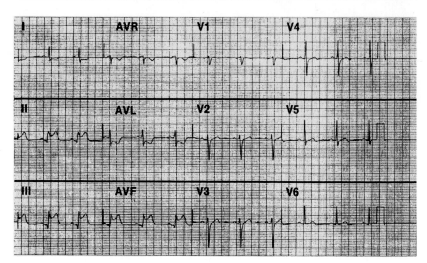

FIGURE 1-1 Acute myocardial infarction localized to inferior leads (II, III, and aV$_F$). The electrocardiogram (EKG) shows ST-segment elevation with hyperacute peaked T waves and early development of significant Q waves. Reciprocal ST depression is also seen (leads I and aV$_L$). *(From Seelig CB: Simplified EKG Analysis. Philadelphia, Hanley & Belfus, 1992.)*

 Twenty-five percent of MIs are silent, meaning that they manifest without chest pain (especially in patients with diabetes who have neuropathy). Such patients present with CHF, shock, or confusion and delirium (especially elderly patients).

Treatment for an MI involves hospital admission to the intensive care unit (ICU) or cardiac care unit with adherence to several basic principles:

○ **Early thrombolysis** (generally ≤12 hours from pain onset) is appropriate if the patient meets strict criteria for use. Early thrombolysis (<4–6 hours) is preferred to try to salvage myocardium. Reperfusion therapy is defined by patient and medical center criteria and may be accomplished by thrombolysis or coronary angiography with percutaneous transluminal coronary angioplasty (PTCA). Coronary artery bypass grafting (CABG) may be required if thrombolysis is contraindicated (or in combination with it).

○ **Electrocardiographic (EKG) monitoring:** If ventricular tachycardia develops, use amiodarone. A common cause of death from an acute MI is reentry arrhythmia such as ventricular fibrillation.

○ **Give O$_2$** by nasal cannula or face mask (maintain O$_2$ saturation >90%).

○ **Pain control** with morphine (which can help with pulmonary edema if present)

○ **Nitroglycerin** causes venodilation that leads to increased pooling the systemic venous circulation and decreased preload.

○ **β-Blocker** (which the patient should take for life if no contraindications are present; proven to reduce the mortality rate of MI as well as the incidence of second MI)

○ Administer **aspirin** (and possibly low-dose heparin or other newer antiplatelet agents)

○ Administer **clopidogrel** if the patient has undergone percutaneous coronary intervention or has unstable angina or non–ST-elevation MI.

○ Administer **unfractionated heparin (UFH) or low-molecular-weight heparin (LMWH).**

○ **Heparin** should be started if unstable angina is diagnosed, if the patient has a cardiac thrombus, a large area of dyskinetic ventricle, or if severe CHF is seen on EKG. The Step 2 examination will not ask about other indications, which are not as clear cut. Do not give heparin to patients with contraindications such as active bleeding.

○ An **angiotensin-converting enzyme (ACE) inhibitor** or **angiotensin receptor blocker (ARB)** should be started within 24 hours. ACE inhibitors are also indicated for patients with CHF because they have been shown to reduce mortality in this setting.

○ Administer an **HMG-CoA reductase inhibitor (statin).**

 Keep post-MI complications in mind. Ventricular rupture and papillary muscle rupture occur approximately 1 week after an MI. Ventricular aneurysms can occur days to months after an MI (may present with akinesis, arrhythmia, or systemic emboli). Post-MI pericarditis (Dressler syndrome) occurs a few weeks after an MI (treat with nonsteroidal antiinflammatory drugs [NSAIDs]; do not give anticoagulation or the patient may develop a hemorrhagic pericardial effusion).

Remember that calcium channel blockers (CCBs) are contraindicated for acute coronary syndrome.

Other causes of chest pain and clues to diagnosis:

○ **Gastroesophageal reflux disease and peptic ulcer disease (PUD):** Pain is related to certain foods (spicy, chocolate), smoking, caffeine and lying down and is relieved by antacids or acid-reducing medications. The most common causes of PUD are *Helicobacter pylori* infection and NSAIDs.

○ **Stable angina:** Pain begins with exertion or stress and remits with rest or calming down. The pain is described as a pressure or squeezing pain in the substernal area and may radiate to the shoulders, neck, or jaw. It often is accompanied by shortness of breath, diaphoresis, or nausea. The pain usually is relieved by nitroglycerin. EKG shows ST-segment depression with pain and then reverts to normal when pain stops. The pain should last less than 20 minutes or be relieved by nitroglycerin; otherwise, there may be progression to unstable angina or MI.

○ In strict terms, **unstable angina** is defined as a change from previous stable angina; thus, if a patient who used to get angina once a week now gets it once a day, he or she has unstable angina. Unstable angina classically manifests with normal cardiac enzymes and EKG changes (ST-segment depression) with prolonged chest pain that does not respond to nitroglycerin initially (e.g., MI). Pain often begins at rest. Treatment is similar to that for MI. The patient is admitted to the coronary or ICU. Initial treatment begins with oxygen, aspirin, and nitroglycerin. The patient should be given a β-blocker, clopidogrel, heparin (UFH or LMWH) and a glycoprotein IIb/IIIa receptor inhibitor. An ACE inhibitor or ARB should be given as well. Consider emergent PTCA if the pain does not resolve. Almost all patients have a history of stable angina and CAD risk factors.

○ **Chest wall pain** (costochondritis, bruised or broken ribs): reproducible on palpation and well localized

○ **Esophageal problems** (achalasia, nutcracker esophagus, or esophageal spasm): Difficult differential diagnosis. The question will probably mention a negative workup for MI or mention the lack of atherosclerosis risk factors. Look for abnormalities with barium swallow (achalasia) or esophageal manometry. Treat patients with achalasia with pneumatic dilation or botulinum toxin injection; treat those with nutcracker esophagus or esophageal spasm with CCBs and then with myotomy if CCBs are ineffective

○ **Pericarditis:** Look for viral upper respiratory infection prodrome. EKG (Fig. 1-2) shows diffuse ST-segment elevation. Other signs include an elevated erythrocyte sedimentation rate and low-grade fever. Classically, the pain is relieved by sitting forward. The most common cause is viral (coxsackievirus); others include tuberculosis, uremia, malignancy, and lupus or other autoimmune diseases. Patients might have a pericardial effusion (Fig. 1-3).

○ **Pneumonia:** Chest pain caused by pleuritis. Patients also have cough, fever, or sputum production with possible sick contacts.

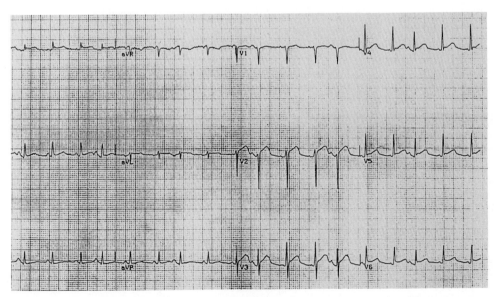

FIGURE 1-2 Electrocardiogram showing pericarditis with diffuse ST elevation most evident in the precordial leads. *(From Silver RM, Smith EA: Rheumatology Pearls. Philadelphia, Hanley & Belfus, 1997.)*

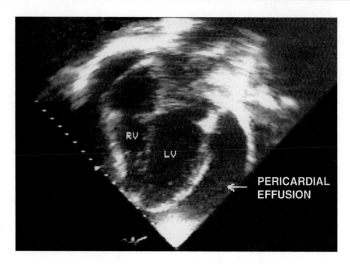

FIGURE 1-3 Echocardiogram revealing a significant pericardial effusion *(arrow)*. LV, left ventricle; RV, right ventricle.

○ **Variant (Prinzmetal) angina** is rare and is associated with anginal pain at rest with **ST-segment elevation;** cardiac enzymes, however, are normal. The cause is coronary artery spasm. Patients with Prinzmetal angina usually responds to nitroglycerin; long-term treatment usually is with CCBs, which reduce arterial spasm.

VALVULAR HEART DISEASE

Characteristics of murmurs are shown in Table 1-1.

An understanding of the pathophysiologic changes associated with long-standing valvular disease (Figs. 1-4 and 1-5) is high yield on Step 2. For example, do you understand why mitral stenosis or regurgitation can cause right heart failure?

Recommendations regarding **endocarditis prophylaxis** have changed. The 2008 American Heart Association recommendations conclude that only an extremely small number of cases of infective endocarditis might be prevented by antibiotic prophylaxis for dental procedures. Cardiac conditions for which prophylaxis with dental procedures is recommended include prosthetic cardiac valve, previous infectious endocarditis, congenital heart disease, and cardiac transplant recipients who develop valvulopathy. Antibiotic prophylaxis is no longer recommended for genitourinary or gastro-intestinal procedures.

An antibiotic for prophylaxis should be administered in a single dose before the procedure. Amoxicillin is the preferred choice for oral therapy. Cephalexin, clindamycin, azithromycin, or clarithromycin may be used in patients with penicillin allergy. Ampicillin, cefazolin, ceftriaxone, or clindamycin may be used for patients unable to take oral medication.

TABLE 1-1 Murmur Characteristics

VALVE PROBLEM	PHYSICAL CHARACTERISTICS (BEST HEARD HERE)	OTHER FINDINGS
Mitral stenosis	Late-diastolic blowing murmur (best heard at apex)	Opening snap, loud S1, atrial fibrillation, LAE, PH
Mitral regurgitation	Holosystolic murmur (radiates to axilla)	Soft S1, LAE, PH, LVH
Aortic stenosis	Harsh systolic ejection murmurs (best heard in aortic area; radiates to carotids)	Slow pulse upstroke, S3/S4, ejection click, LVH, cardiomegaly, syncope, angina, and CHF
Aortic regurgitation	Early-diastolic decrescendo murmur (best heard at apex)	Widened pulse pressure, LVH, LV dilation, S3, intensity increases with increased peripheral vascular resistance
Mitral prolapse	Mid-systolic click or late-systolic murmur	Panic disorder

CHF, congestive heart failure; LAE, left atrial enlargement; LV, left ventricle; LVH, left ventricular hypertrophy; PH, pulmonary hypertension.

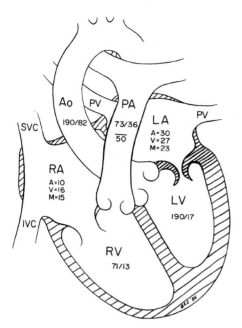

FIGURE 1-4 Mitral stenosis. The mitral valve orifice is narrowed, resulting in obstruction to flow out of the atrium and an increase in pressure in the left atrium and pulmonary veins. Pulmonary hypertension develops secondarily. Systolic and diastolic pressures are shown in arteries and ventricles (in mm Hg). A, A wave; Ao, aorta; IVC, inferior vena cava; LA, left atrium; LV, left ventricle; M, mean pressure; PA, pulmonary artery; PV, pulmonary vein; RA, right atrium; RV, right ventricle; SVC, superior vena cava; V, V wave. *(From James EC, Corry RJ, Perry JF: Principles of Basic Surgical Practice. Philadelphia, Hanley & Belfus, 1987.)*

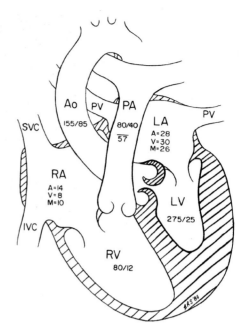

FIGURE 1-5 Aortic stenosis. The narrowed aortic valve results in high pressures in the left ventricle, which are transmitted to the left atrium and ultimately result in pulmonary hypertension. The left ventricle is hypertrophied because of the chronic pressure overload. Systolic and diastolic pressures are shown in arteries and ventricles (in mm Hg). A, A wave; Ao, aorta; IVC, inferior vena cava; LA, left atrium; LV, left ventricle; M, mean pressure; PA, pulmonary artery; PV, pulmonary vein; RA, right atrium; RV, right ventricle; SVC, superior vena cava; V, V wave. *(From James EC, Corry RJ, Perry JF: Principles of Basic Surgical Practice. Philadelphia, Hanley & Belfus, 1987.)*

DEEP VEIN THROMBOSIS, PULMONARY EMBOLISM, ANTICOAGULATION

IMPORTANT POINTS

1. Remember Virchow's triad (endothelial damage, stasis, and hypercoagulable state) as a clue to the diagnosis of deep vein thrombosis (DVT).

2. Common causes or situations in which DVT occurs include surgery (especially orthopedic, pelvic, abdominal, or neurosurgery); malignancy; trauma; immobilization; pregnancy; oral contraceptives; disseminated intravascular coagulation; and hypercoagulable states such as lupus anticoagulant, factor V Leiden, antithrombin III deficiency, protein S deficiency, protein C deficiency, prothrombin *G20210A* gene mutation, hyperhomocysteinemia, and antiphospholipid antibodies.

3. DVTs commonly manifest with unilateral leg swelling, pain or tenderness, or Homan sign (present in 30% of patients and unreliable but classic).

4. The best way to diagnose DVT is Doppler compression ultrasonography. Other acceptable tests include impedance plethysmography, computed tomography (CT), and magnetic resonance venography. Traditional venography is the gold standard but is invasive and reserved for settings in which the diagnosis is not clear.

5. D-dimer is sometimes used in the outpatient setting to help rule out DVT. If the suspicion for DVT is high, lower extremity Doppler ultrasonography should be performed. If the suspicion is low, check a D-dimer. If the D-dimer results are negative, DVT can be ruled out. If D-dimer results are positive, lower extremity Doppler ultrasonography should be performed.

(Continued)

6. The most common source of pulmonary embolism (PE) is vessels above the knee (iliac, femoral, popliteal veins). Calf vein thrombi rarely cause symptomatic PE.

7. Superficial thrombophlebitis (erythema, tenderness, edema, and palpable clot or cord in the distribution of a superficial vein) is *not* a risk factor for PE and generally is considered a benign condition. Treat with NSAIDs or aspirin. Recurrent superficial thrombophlebitis can be a marker for underlying malignancy (e.g., Trousseau syndrome, or migratory thrombophlebitis, is a classic marker for pancreatic cancer).

8. In patients with DVT or PE, systemic anticoagulation is necessary. Use parenteral heparin or LMWH followed by gradual crossover to oral warfarin. Patients are maintained on warfarin for at least 3 to 6 months, possibly permanently if they experience more than one episode of clotting. If clots recur on anticoagulation or the patient has contraindications to anticoagulation, use an inferior vena cava filter (e.g., Greenfield filter).

9. Prophylactic measures for patients undergoing surgery depend on the risk for developing DVT or PE. Early ambulation is recommended for low-risk patients. LMWH, low-dose UFH, or fondaparinux is recommended for patients at moderate risk. High-risk patients should be given LMWH, fondaparinux, or an oral vitamin K antagonist. Pneumatic compression stockings should be used instead if the patient is at moderate risk or higher and is at high risk of bleeding.

10. Pulmonary embolus follows DVT, delivery of an infant (amniotic fluid embolus), or fractures (fat emboli). The classic patient recently went on a long car ride or took a long airplane flight. A massive PE can cause right heart strain leading to a new onset right bundle branch block, hypotension, increased JVP, and tachycardia. Symptoms include tachypnea; dyspnea; chest pain; hemoptysis (if a lung infarct has occurred); and hypotension, syncope, and death in severe cases. Rarely, on chest radiography, a wedge-shaped defect will be seen because of a pulmonary infarct.

11. Left-sided heart clots (from atrial fibrillation, ventricular wall aneurysm, severe congestive heart failure, or endocarditis) that embolize cause arterial-sided infarcts (stroke and renal, gastrointestinal, and extremity infarcts), *not* PEs. Right-sided clots that embolize DVTs cause PEs, *not* arterial emboli. The exception is a patent foramen ovale or other abnormal right-to-left shunt, in which the clot can cross over to the left side of the circulation and cause an arterial "paradoxical" infarct. This event is quite rare.

12. Use CT pulmonary angiography (or nuclear medicine ventilation/perfusion scan if contrast is contraindicated) to screen for PE. Invasive traditional pulmonary angiogram is reserved for unclear cases and treatment of massive PE (i.e., catheter-based thrombolysis). If PE is suspected and the patient is unstable or has respiratory distress, treat with heparin immediately and then perform diagnostic tests.

13. Heparin can cause thrombocytopenia (heparin-induced thrombocytopenia [HIT]) and result in arterial thrombosis in some patients who develop antibodies to heparin bound to platelet factor 4 (PF4). Measure complete blood counts to monitor for this side effect, which usually occurs on day 3 to day 7 of heparin administration. The PF4 antibody test can be used as a screening test but can have false-positive results. The serotonin release assay can be used to confirm the diagnosis. If HIT is suspected or confirmed, *discontinue heparin and LMWH immediately!* Use argatroban or lepirudin instead.

14. Heparin is monitored by determining the partial thromboplastin time (PTT) (internal coagulation pathway). Warfarin is followed by determining the prothrombin time (PT) (external coagulation pathway). Aspirin prolongs the bleeding time, a measure of platelet function. In emergencies, reverse heparin and LMWH with protamine; reverse warfarin with fresh-frozen plasma, vitamin K, or both; and reverse aspirin with platelet transfusion. LMW heparins are *not followed by testing except in rare circumstances* when an anti–factor Xa assay can be measured (PT, PTT, and bleeding time are all unaffected). Table 1-2 lists other factors that affect coagulation tests.

TABLE 1-2 Other Factors Affecting Coagulation Tests

DISEASE	PROLONGED TEST	OTHER AIDS TO DIAGNOSIS
Hemophilia A	PTT	Low levels of factor VIII; normal PT and bleeding time; X-linked
Hemophilia B	PTT	Low levels of factor IX; normal PT and bleeding time; X-linked
vWF deficiency	Bleeding time and PTT	Normal or low levels of factor VIII; normal PT; autosomal dominant
DIC	PT, PTT, bleeding time	Positive D-dimer or FDPs; postpartum, infection, malignancy; schistocytes and fragmented cells on peripheral smear
Liver disease	PT	PTT normal or prolonged; all factors but factor VIII are low; stigmata of liver disease; no correction with vitamin K
Vitamin K deficiency	PT, PTT (slight)	Normal bleeding time; low levels of factors II, VII, IX, and X, as well as proteins C and S; look for neonate who did not receive prophylactic vitamin K, malabsorption, alcoholism, or prolonged antibiotic use (which kills vitamin K–producing bowel flora)

DIC, disseminated intravascular coagulation; FDP, fibrin degradation product; PT, prothrombin time; PTT, partial thromboplastin time; vWF, von Willebrand factor.

 Uremia causes a qualitative platelet defect. Platelet count, PT, and PTT are normal; bleeding time is increased. Treat with desmopressin.

 Vitamin C deficiency and chronic corticosteroid therapy can cause a bleeding tendency with normal coagulation tests.

CONGESTIVE HEART FAILURE AND ARRHYTHMIAS

Symptoms and signs of CHF are shown in Table 1-3.

Elevated BNP levels help make the diagnosis easier in many cases. If the BNP level is less than 100 pg/mL, heart failure is highly unlikely; if the BNP level is 100 to 500 pg/mL, the results are uncertain but suspicious; if BNP is greater than 500 pg/mL, heart failure (or another acute and serious cardiovascular disorder) is highly likely. False-positive test results for CHF diagnosis include other diseases that cause right or left ventricular stretching, such as PE, pulmonary hypertension, cor pulmonale, renal failure, acute coronary syndrome, and cirrhosis. Treatment includes:

○ Sodium restriction
○ ACE inhibitor (first-line agents; proved to reduce mortality in CHF)
○ β-Blockers (also reduce mortality; give only in stable CHF)

TABLE 1-3 Symptoms and Signs of Congestive Heart Failure*

LEFT-SIDED FAILURE	RIGHT-SIDED FAILURE
Cardiomegaly, fatigue, dyspnea	Fatigue, dyspnea, cardiomegaly
Left-sided S3/S4	Right-sided S3/S4
Chest radiography abnormalities (cardiomegaly, Kerley B lines, pulmonary vascular congestion, and bilateral pleural effusions)	Chest radiography abnormalities (cardiomegaly)
Pulmonary congestion, rales	Pulmonary congestion
Orthopnea (shortness of breath when lying down; the patient sleeps on more than one pillow or even sleeps sitting up)	Peripheral edema
Paroxysmal nocturnal dyspnea	Jugular venous distention
Ventricular hypertrophy on EKG	Hepatomegaly, ascites

*Note: both ventricles are commonly affected, so a mixed pattern is commonly seen.
EKG, electrocardiography.

○ Diuretics, including furosemide and spironolactone
○ Digoxin (not in hypertrophic obstructive cardiomyopathy, atrioventricular conduction blocks, or diastolic dysfunction; usually reserved for moderate to severe CHF with low ejection fraction)
○ Vasodilators (arterial and venous)
○ Intravenous sympathomimetics (dobutamine, dopamine, amrinone) or nesiritide (recombinant BNP) for inpatients with severe CHF

IMPORTANT POINTS

1. Many factors can precipitate **exacerbation of CHF** in a previously stable cardiac patient. Common causes are medication or diet noncompliance, MI, significant hypertension, arrhythmias, infections or fever, PE, anemia, thyrotoxicosis, and myocarditis.

2. Cor pulmonale is right ventricular enlargement, hypertrophy, or failure caused by primary lung disease. Common causes are chronic obstructive pulmonary disease and PE. In a young woman (ages 20–40 years) with no other medical history or risk factors, think of idiopathic pulmonary artery hypertension (after excluding PE and other more common causes). Treat with pulmonary vasodilators such as prostacyclins (parenteral epoprostenol), antiendothelins (bosentan), phosphodiesterase 5 inhibitors (sildenafil), and/or CCBs while the patient awaits heart–lung transplant. Sleep apnea also can cause cor pulmonale (look for an obese snorer who is sleepy during the day). Patients with cor pulmonale have tachypnea, cyanosis, clubbing, parasternal heave, loud P_2, and right-sided S_4 in addition to signs and symptoms of pulmonary disease.

3. Restrictive cardiomyopathy usually results from amyloidosis, sarcoidosis, hemochromatosis, or myocardial fibroelastosis (ventricular biopsy is abnormal in all of these conditions). You will usually see normal left ventricular volume, symmetrically thickened ventricles, and right-sided heart failure. **Constrictive pericarditis** acts similarly clinically but has a pericardial knock on examination, calcification of the pericardium, and normal ventricular biopsy results; it can be treated by removing the pericardium. Watch for an S4 (which indicates stiff ventricles) and signs of right-sided heart failure (JVD and peripheral edema) in both conditions.

4. Dilated cardiomyopathy is commonly caused by CAD or ischemia, alcohol abuse, myocarditis, or doxorubicin. Remember the ABCD mnemonic: alcohol, beriberi, Coxsackie virus or Chagas disease, doxorubicin.

5. The most common cause of right heart failure is left heart failure.

Table 1-4 shows treatments and warnings for various arrhythmias.

IMPORTANT POINTS

1. Sinus tachycardia and atrial fibrillation are common presentations for hyperthyroidism. Check level of thyroid-stimulating hormone.

2. Pulseless electrical activity can be caused by the 6 Hs and 6 Ts: hypovolemia, hypoxia, hypoglycemia, H+ (acidosis), hypothermia, hyper- or hypovolemia and tamponade, thrombus (MI or PE), trauma (hypovolemia), tablets (drugs), toxins, and tension pneumothorax.

3. Wolff-Parkinson-White syndrome commonly appears in childhood. The patient becomes dizzy or dyspneic, passes out after playing, and then recovers with no other symptoms. The cause is an arrhythmia via accessory pathway). Look for the infamous delta wave on EKG.

TABLE 1-4 Treatment of Arrhythmia

ARRHYTHMIA	TREATMENT	WARNINGS	ILLUSTRATION
Heart Block			
First degree (benign)	None	Avoid β-blockers and CCBs (both slow conduction)	
Second degree	Pacemaker or atropine only if symptomatic in Mobitz type I		*Mobitz type I second degree heart block*
Second degree	Use pacemaker for all Mobitz type II		*Mobitz type II second degree heart block*
Third degree (complete heart block)	Pacemaker		
OTHER CAUSES			
A-Fib	Anticoagulation (prevent embolic phenomenon); control rate: β-blocker, CCB, or digoxin. If acute (onset <24 hr), cardiovert with amiodarone, procainamide, or electrical cardioversion. If chronic, first anticoagulate and then cardiovert. If this approach fails or A-Fib recurs, leave the patient on rate control medications (β-blocker or CCBs) and warfarin.*		
PVCs	Usually not treated. If severe and symptomatic, consider β-blocker or amiodarone.		Lead 2 15 yrs.
PACs	Usually not treated.	Can be caused by anxiety, CHF, hypoxia, caffeine, electrolyte abnormalities.	Lead 2 17 yrs.

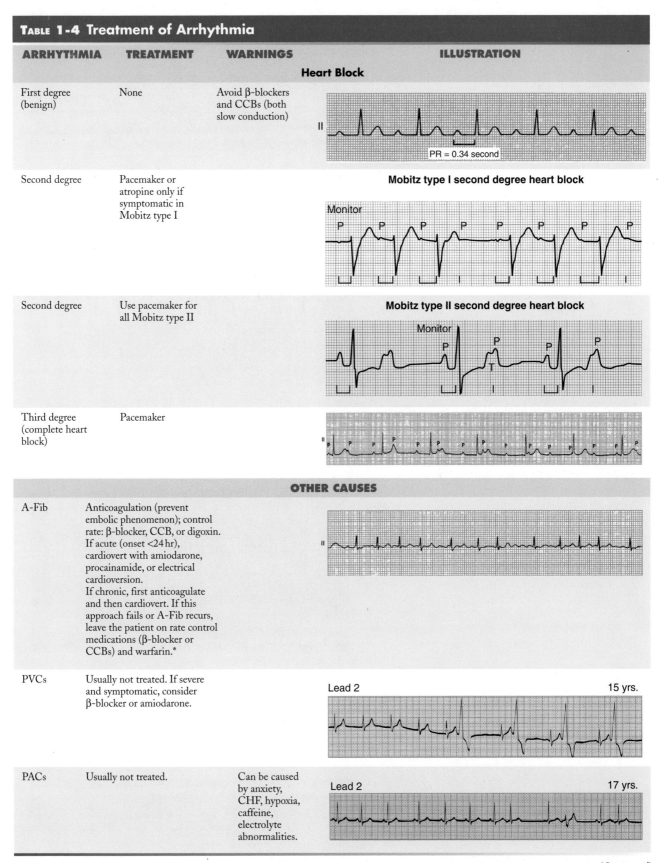

(Continued)

TABLE 1-4 Treatment of Arrhythmia—Cont'd			
OTHER CAUSES			
Sinus bradycardia	Usually not treated; use atropine if severe and symptomatic (post-MI)	Avoid β-blockers, CCBs, and other conduction slowers	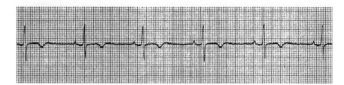
Sinus tachycardia	Usually none; correct underlying cause; use β-blocker if symptomatic		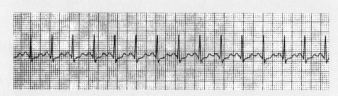
AVNRT	If unstable, cardiovert. If stable, try vagal maneuvers, IV adenosine, metoprolol, or verapamil.		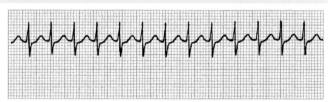
V-Fib	If pulseless, treat with immediate defibrillation followed by epinephrine, vasopressin, amiodarone, or lidocaine. If a pulse is present, treat with amiodarone and synchronized cardioversion.		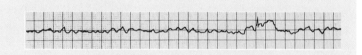
V-Tach	Amiodarone or lidocaine		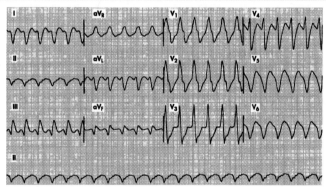
WPW syndrome	Use procainamide or quinidine	Avoid drugs that affect the AV node (digoxin, adenosine, metoprolol, and verapamil)	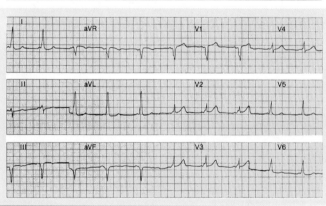

*See Table 1-5 for a discussion of the CHADS$_2$ score.

A-Fib, atrial fibrillation; AVNRT, atrioventricular node reentrant tachycardia; CCB, calcium channel blocker; IV, intravenous; PVCs, premature ventricular contractions; V-Fib, ventricular fibrillation; V-Tach, ventricular tachycardia; WPW, Wolff–Parkinson–White syndrome.

Images 1, 4, 5, 10, and 12 from Goldberger AL: *Clinical Electrocardiography: A Simplified Approach*, 7th ed. Philadelphia, Mosby, 2006; images 2 and 3 from Ferri FF: *Practical Guide to the Care of the Medical Patient*, 8th ed. Philadelphia, Mosby, 2011; and images 6 and 7 from Kliegman RM: *Nelson Textbook of Pediatrics*, 18th ed. Philadelphia, Saunders, 2007.

Table 1-5 CHADS₂ Score

The CHADS$_2$ score is used to estimate the risk of stroke in patients with nonrheumatic atrial fibrillation. The score is used to determine whether treatment is required with warfarin or aspirin.
The points in the table below are added to determine the CHADS$_2$ score.
A score of 0 is low risk for stroke, so aspirin can be used.
A score of 1 is moderate risk, so aspirin or warfarin can be used.
A score of 2 or greater is moderate or high risk, so warfarin should be used unless contraindicated.

	CONDITION	POINTS
C	Congestive heart failure	1
H	Hypertension: blood pressure consistently >140/90 mm Hg (or treated hypertension on medication)	1
A	Age older than 75 years	1
D	Diabetes mellitus	1
S$_2$	Prior stroke or TIA	2

TIA, transient ischemic attack.

QR CODE

The QR code includes three USMLE-style questions and answers. For more questions, redeem the PIN code on the inside cover for the Crush Step 2 question bank powered by USMLE Consult.
   Please see the Introduction for instructions on how to access content using the QR codes.

Question

A 24-year-old man presents with a chief complaint of chest pain. He states that this retrosternal, sharp pain began last night, is fairly constant, and is aggravated by lying down or coughing and relieved by sitting up. The patient had "a cold" roughly 1 week ago with a runny nose, sore throat, and dry cough. He has no significant medical history but notes that his father had a heart attack at the age of 62 years, and his grandmother died of a heart attack around age 70 years. He is not currently taking any medications and has never used drugs or alcohol. Vital signs are as follows:

Temperature	99.8°F
Blood pressure	128/86 mm Hg
Pulse rate	90 beats/min
Respirations	18 breaths/min

The patient is athletic appearing and in no apparent distress. He has mild pharyngeal erythema without exudate, no lymphadenopathy, and no jugular venous distension. His lungs sound clear to auscultation, although the patient is unable to inspire deeply secondary to pain. On cardiac examination, the rate and rhythm are regular, but you hear a scratchy, scraping noise throughout most of the cardiac cycle in the left parasternal area. Which of the following is true?
(A) The patient needs a cardiac stress test given his strong family history.
(B) Nonsteroidal antiinflammatory drugs such as indomethacin are the treatment of choice.
(C) The most likely cause of this patient's symptoms is a streptococcal infection.
(D) The patient most likely had a previously damaged heart valve.
(E) You would expect Q waves in the precordial leads on an electrocardiogram.

2 DERMATOLOGY

Table 2-1 shows common skin lesions.

ACNE

Know the description of acne: comedones (whiteheads, blackheads), papules, pustules, inflamed nodules, and superficial pus-filled cysts with possible inflammatory skin changes (Fig. 2-1). *Propionibacterium acnes* is thought to be partially involved in the pathogenesis as well as blockage of pilosebaceous glands. Acne is associated with changes in androgen levels and is found primarily during puberty. Acne has *not* been proven to be related to food (but if the patient relates it to a food, you can try discontinuing it), exercise, or sex or masturbation, but cosmetics can aggravate it.

Treatment options are numerous. Start with topical benzoyl peroxide and then try topical clindamycin, oral tetracycline, oral erythromycin (for *P. acnes* eradication), and topical tretinoin. The *last resort* is oral isotretinoin. Oral isotretinoin is highly effective, but it is teratogenic (pregnancy testing before and during therapy is mandatory), and it can cause dry skin and mucosae, muscle and joint pain, and liver function abnormalities.

ATOPIC DERMATITIS

Look for family and personal history of allergies (e.g., hay fever) and asthma. This chronic condition begins in the first year of life with red, itchy, weeping skin on the head, upper extremities, and sometimes around the diaper area (Fig. 2-2). The biggest problem is scratching, which leads to skin breaks and possible bacterial infection, as well as lichenification. Treatment involves antihistamines, topical steroids, and avoidance of drying soaps. As a result of skin breakdown, patients with atopic dermatitis are susceptible to eczema herpeticum, a severe herpes simplex virus 1 infection of affected areas.

BALDNESS

Watch out for trichotillomania (psychiatric patients pulling out their hair) and alopecia areata (idiopathic and associated with antimicrosomal and other autoantibodies, lupus, syphilis, or chemotherapy) as exotic causes of irregular, patchy baldness. Typical male-pattern baldness is considered a genetic disorder that requires androgens to be expressed.

BASAL CELL CANCER

Basal cell cancer begins as a pearly papule and slowly enlarges and develops an umbilicated center (which later might ulcerate) with peripheral telangiectasias. Basal cell cancer rarely metastasizes. As with all skin cancer, sunlight exposure increases risk. It is more common in light-skinned people. Treat with excision. Perform a biopsy of all suspicious skin lesions in elderly patients.

TABLE 2-1 Common Terms to Describe Skin Findings

PRIMARY LESION	DEFINITION	MORPHOLOGY	EXAMPLES
Macule	Flat, circumscribed skin discoloration that lacks surface elevation or depression	Macule	Café-au-lait spot Vitiligo Freckle Junctional nevi Ink tattoo
Papule	Elevated, solid lesion <0.5 cm in diameter	Papule	Acrochordon (skin tag) Basal cell carcinoma Molluscum contagiosum Intradermal nevi Lichen planus
Plaque	Elevated, solid "confluence of papules" (>0.5 cm in diameter) that lacks a deep component	Plaque	Bowen disease Mycosis fungoides Psoriasis Eczema Tinea corporis
Patch	Flat, circumscribed skin discoloration; a very large macule >1 cm in diameter	Patch	Nevus flammeus Vitiligo Tinea corporis
Nodule	Elevated, solid lesion >0.5 cm in diameter; a larger, deeper papule	Nodule	Rheumatoid nodule Tendon xanthoma Erythema nodosum Lipoma Metastatic carcinoma
Wheal	Firm, edematous plaque that is evanescent and pruritic; a hive	Wheal	Urticaria Dermographism Urticaria pigmentosa
Vesicle	Papule that contains clear fluid; a blister	Vesicle	Herpes simplex Herpes zoster Dyshidrotic eczema Contact dermatitis
Bulla	Localized fluid collection >0.5 cm in diameter; a large vesicle	Bulla	Pemphigus vulgaris Bullous pemphigoid Bullous impetigo
Pustule	Papule that contains purulent material	Pustule	Folliculitis Impetigo Acne Pustular psoriasis

(Continued)

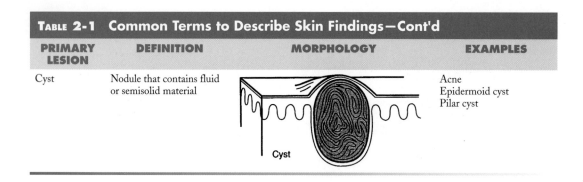

TABLE 2-1	Common Terms to Describe Skin Findings—Cont'd		
PRIMARY LESION	**DEFINITION**	**MORPHOLOGY**	**EXAMPLES**
Cyst	Nodule that contains fluid or semisolid material		Acne Epidermoid cyst Pilar cyst

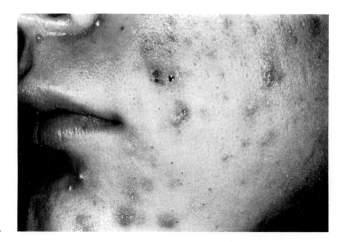

FIGURE 2-1 Acne.

BULLOUS PEMPHIGOID

Bullous pemphigoid is similar to pemphigus vulgaris but is a milder condition that results in a linear immunofluorescence pattern. Treat with corticosteroids.

CANDIDIASIS

Thrush (creamy white patches on the tongue or buccal mucosa that can be scraped off) may be seen in normal children, and candidal vulvovaginitis is seen in normal women, especially when they are pregnant or after taking antibiotics. However, at other times and in different patients, candidal infections are a classic sign of diabetes mellitus or immunodeficiency. For example, thrush in a man should make you think about the possibility of HIV/AIDS.

Treat with local or topical nystatin or imidazoles (e.g., miconazole, clotrimazole). Oral therapy (e.g., fluconazole, itraconazole) is used for extensive or resistant disease.

CONTACT DERMATITIS

Contact dermatitis is often caused by a type IV hypersensitivity reaction; it also may be caused by an irritating or toxic substance. On Step 2, look for a question that mentions new exposure to a classic offending agent (e.g., poison ivy, nickel earrings, deodorant). The rash is well circumscribed and found only in the area of exposure; the skin is red and itchy and often has vesicles or bullae. Avoidance of the agent is required; patch testing can be done, if needed, to determine the antigen. Treatment includes cool compresses, oatmeal preparations, antihistamines, and topical steroids.

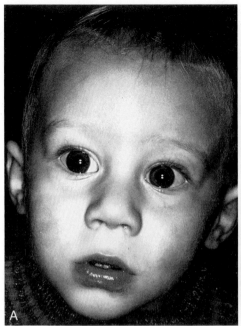

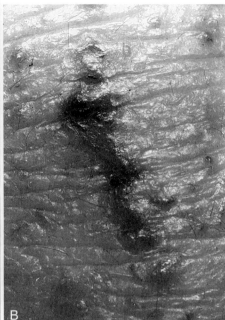

FIGURE **2-2 Phases of atopic dermatitis. A,** Infantile phase. Typical erythematous, oozing, and crusted plaques seen on the cheek of an infant with atopic dermatitis. **B,** Childhood phase. Close-up view of a lichenified, excoriated, crusted, and secondarily infected plaque on the right knee of a 4-year-old girl. **C,** Adolescent or young adult phase with chronic, symmetric, pigmented, and erythematous skin changes. *(From Fitzpatrick JE, Aeling JL: Dermatology Secrets. Philadelphia, Hanley & Belfus, 1996.)*

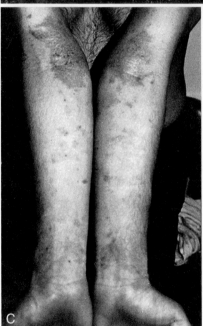

DERMATITIS HERPETIFORMIS

Dermatitis herpetiformis should alert you to the presence of gluten sensitivity (celiac disease); look for diarrhea and weight loss. Skin has immunoglobulin A (IgA) deposits even in unaffected areas. Patients present with intensely pruritic vesicles, papules, and wheals on the extensor aspects of the elbows and knees, possibly on the face and neck. Treat with a gluten-free diet.

DECUBITUS ULCERS

Decubitus ulcers (bedsores or pressure sores) are caused by prolonged pressure against the skin. The best treatment is prophylaxis. Periodic turning of paralyzed, bedridden, or debilitated patients prevents bedsores, as do special dynamic air mattresses. Cleanliness and dryness also help to prevent this condition, and performing periodic skin inspections ensures that you catch the problem early. When missed, the lesions can ulcerate down to the bone and become infected, possibly leading to sepsis and death. Treat major skin breaks with aggressive surgical debridement and antibiotics if signs of infection are present.

DRUG REACTIONS

Penicillin, cephalosporins, and sulfa drugs commonly cause rashes; tetracycline and phenothiazines commonly cause photosensitivity.

ERYTHEMA MULTIFORME

Erythema multiforme (EM) is on a continuum with Stevens-Johnson syndrome (SJS) and toxic epidermal necrolysis (TEN) (Fig. 2-3). Whereas EM usually is limited to the skin, SJS and TEN involve the mucosa. Look for classic target (iris) lesions. These are usually caused by drugs (classically sulfa drugs or penicillins) or infections (e.g., herpes, mycoplasma). Discontinue the inciting agent. EM usually resolves on its own, and treatment is supportive care. Severe cases (SJS and TEN) may require intravenous immunoglobulin.

ERYTHEMA NODOSUM

Erythema nodosum is inflammation of the subcutaneous tissue and skin, classically over the shins (pretibial). Tender, red nodules are present. Look for "exotic" diseases such as sarcoidosis, coccidioidomycosis, and ulcerative colitis as the cause, although more commonly the cause is infection (e.g., streptococcal, tuberculosis), drugs (e.g., sulfonamides), or unknown.

EXCESSIVE PERSPIRATION (HYPERHIDROSIS)

Think of hyperthyroidism and pheochromocytoma. Also consider myocardial infarction and tuberculosis.

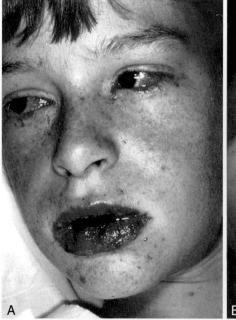 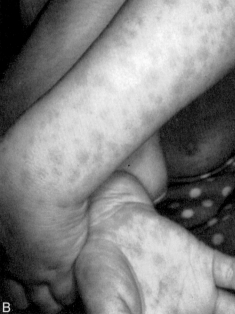

FIGURE 2-3 A, Stevens–Johnson syndrome (SJS). Typical mucosal inflammation of the mouth, lips, and conjunctiva. **B,** Erythema multiforme or SJS. The eruption consists of annular and papular erythema over the acral areas. *(From Fitzpatrick JE, Aeling JL: Dermatology Secrets. Philadelphia, Hanley & Belfus, 1996.)*

FUNGAL SKIN INFECTIONS

Fungal skin infections include dermatophyte infections and ringworm. Depending on the location, fungal skin infections are known as:

○ **Tinea corporis** (body and trunk): Look for red ring-shaped lesions that have raised borders and tend to clear centrally while they expand peripherally.

○ **Tinea pedis** (athlete's foot): Look for macerated, scaling web spaces between the toes that often itch and for thickened, distorted toenails (onychomycosis). Good foot hygiene is part of treatment.

○ **Tinea unguium** (onychomycosis): Thickened, distorted nails with debris under the nail edges

○ **Tinea capitis** (scalp): Mainly affects children (highly contagious), who have scaly patches of hair loss and might have an inflamed, boggy granuloma of the scalp (known as a kerion), which usually resolves on its own

○ **Tinea cruris** (jock itch): More common in obese male patients, usually in the crural folds of the upper inner thighs

Most fungal skin infections are caused by *Trichophyton* species. Infections are diagnosed by scraping the lesion and doing a potassium hydroxide (KOH) preparation to visualize the fungus (Fig. 2-4) or a culture.

Oral agents (e.g., terbinafine, fluconazole, itraconazole, griseofulvin) should be used to treat tinea capitis and onychomycosis. The other infections can be treated with topical antifungals (e.g., miconazole, clotrimazole, ketoconazole) or oral agents for severe or persistent infections. In tinea capitis, if the hair fluoresces under Wood's lamp (Fig. 2-5), *Microsporum* spp. is the cause; if it does not, the probable cause is *Trichophyton* spp.

HIRSUTISM

Hirsutism is most commonly idiopathic, but classic causes include corticosteroid administration, Cushing syndrome, polycystic ovary syndrome (Stein-Leventhal syndrome), and drugs (minoxidil and phenytoin). If other signs of virilization (deepening voice, clitoromegaly, frontal balding) are present, suspect an androgen-secreting ovarian tumor.

KAPOSI SARCOMA

Kaposi sarcoma is seen in patients with AIDS. Look for classic mucosal lesions or an expanding, strange rash or skin lesion that does not respond to multiple treatments (Fig. 2-6).

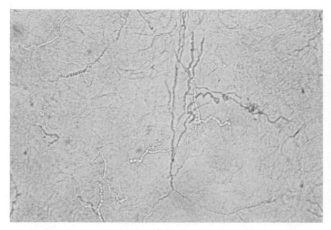

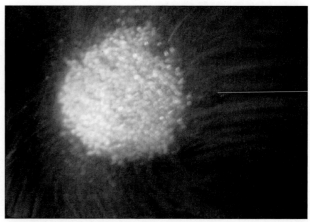

FIGURE 2-4 Potassium hydroxide preparation revealing cylindrical, regularly shaped, branching fungal hyphae typical of tinea infections.

FIGURE 2-5 Wood's light–positive tinea capitis.

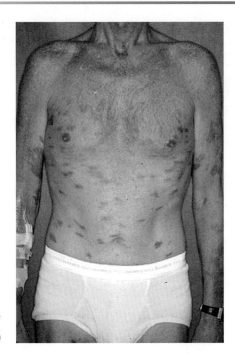

FIGURE **2-6 Kaposi sarcoma.** Multiple violaceous plaques are seen on the trunk of an HIV-positive patient. *(From Fitzpatrick JE, Aeling JL:* Dermatology Secrets. *Philadelphia, Hanley & Belfus, 1996.)*

KERATOACANTHOMA

Keratoacanthoma is mainly important because it mimics skin cancer (especially squamous cell cancer). This flesh-colored lesion with a central crater contains keratinous material and is classically found on the face. The best way to differentiate it from cancer is that a keratoacanthoma has a *very* rapid onset and grows to full size in 1 to 2 months. Such rapid growth almost never occurs with squamous cell cancer. The lesion involutes spontaneously in a few months and requires no treatment. If you are unsure, the best option is a biopsy, but on Step 2, choose observation if the history is classic for keratoacanthoma.

KELOID

A keloid is an overgrowth of scar tissue after an injury and is most often seen in blacks (Fig. 2-7A). Keloids are usually slightly pink and classically are found on the upper back, chest, and deltoid area. Also look for keloids to develop after ear piercing (Fig. 2-7B).

LICE (PEDICULOSIS)

Lice can infect the head (*Pediculus capitis*, which is common in school-aged children), body (*Pediculus corporis*, which is unusual in people with good hygiene), and pubic area (crabs—*Phthirus pubis*, which is transmitted sexually). Infected areas tend to itch, and diagnosis is made by seeing the lice on hair shafts. Treat with permethrin cream (preferred over lindane because of lindane's neurotoxicity) and decontaminate sources of reinfection (wash or sterilize combs, hats, bed sheets, and clothing).

LICHEN PLANUS

Look for the four Ps—pruritic; purple; polygonal papules; and for oral mucosal lesions, whitish with a lace-like pattern. Lichen planus is commonly associated with drugs and hepatitis C virus. Treatment involves steroids and oral antihistamines. More severe cases may require cyclosporine, prednisone, and oral retinoids.

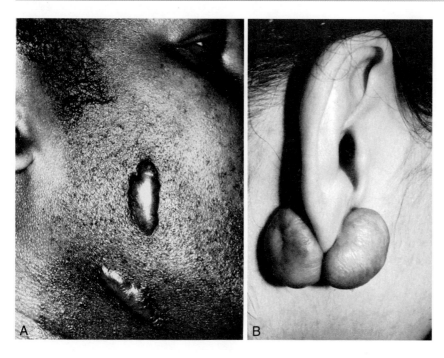

FIGURE 2-7 **A,** Scar tissue overgrowth after an injury. **B,** Keloid after ear piercing.

MALIGNANT MELANOMA

Malignant melanoma usually arises from preexisting moles. Remember your **ABCDs: a**symmetry, irregular **b**orders, **c**olor change, and increasing **d**iameter. The prognosis is directly related to the depth of vertical invasion. Superficial spreading melanoma is the most common type, tends to stay superficial, and has the best prognosis. Nodular melanoma is the worst because it tends to grow downward first. Although uncommon in blacks, melanoma tends to be of the acrolentiginous type; look for black dots on the palms and soles or under the fingernails. Treat with surgery; if surgery fails, the prognosis is poor, though interferon α-2b might help. Systemic chemotherapy is used for metastatic disease.

MOLES

Moles are common and benign, but malignant transformation is possible. *Excise any mole* (or do a biopsy if the lesion is very large) if it enlarges suddenly, develops irregular borders, darkens or becomes inflamed, changes color (even if only one small area of the mole changes color), begins to bleed, begins to itch, or becomes painful. Dysplastic nevus syndrome is a genetic condition (look for family history) with multiple dysplastic-appearing nevi (usually >100). Treat with careful follow-up and excision and biopsy of any suspicious-looking lesions as well as sun avoidance and sunscreen use.

MOLLUSCUM CONTAGIOSUM

Molluscum contagiosum is a poxvirus infection that is common in children but also may be transmitted sexually. A child who has genital molluscum may or may not have contracted the infection from sexual contact; autoinoculation is possible. *Do not* automatically assume child abuse, although it must be ruled out. Diagnosis is made by the characteristic appearance of the lesions (skin-colored, smooth, waxy papules with a central depression [umbilicated] that are roughly 0.5 cm) or by looking at contents of the lesion, which include cells with characteristic inclusion bodies. It is usually treated with freezing or curettage.

PAGET DISEASE OF THE NIPPLE

Watch for a unilateral red, oozing, and crusting nipple in a woman. An underlying breast cancer with extension to the skin must be ruled out.

PEMPHIGUS

Pemphigus vulgaris is a potentially life-threatening autoimmune disease of middle-aged and elderly adults that manifests with multiple bullae, starting in the oral mucosa and spreading to the skin of the rest of the body. Biopsy shows acantholysis and can be stained for antibody and shows a fish-net or lace-like immunofluorescence pattern. Treat with corticosteroids. Patients might have an underlying malignancy (often non-Hodgkin lymphoma) as the trigger.

PITYRIASIS ROSEA

A popular topic for dermatology questions on Step 2. Pityriasis rosea is an idiopathic rash (although some evidence points to a viral cause) seen in older children and young adults. Look for a herald patch (slightly erythematous, ring-shaped or oval, and scaly patch classically seen on the trunk) followed 1 week later by many similar lesions that tend to itch. Look for lesions on the back with a long axis that parallels the Langerhans skin cleavage lines, typically in a "Christmas tree" pattern. Pityriasis rosea usually remits spontaneously in 1 month. Think about syphilis and tinea-type infection in the differential diagnosis. Treat with reassurance.

PRURITUS

Pruritus may be a clue to diagnosis of serious conditions. It is seen in obstructive biliary disease, uremia, and polycythemia rubra vera (classically after a warm shower or bath). Pruritus also may be caused by contact or atopic dermatitis, scabies, and lichen planus.

PSORIASIS

Know what classic lesions look like (Fig. 2-8) and how they are described (dry, *not* pruritic, well-circumscribed, silvery, scaling papules and plaques). Family history is often positive. Psoriasis occurs mostly in whites with an onset in early adulthood. Classic lesions are found on the scalp and extensor surfaces of the elbows and knees. Patients might have pitting of the nails and arthritis that resembles rheumatoid arthritis but is rheumatoid factor negative. Diagnosis is made by appearance; biopsy can be used for doubtful cases. Treatment is complex, involving exposure to ultraviolet light (e.g. sunlight), lubricants, topical corticosteroids, and keratolytics (coal tar, salicylic acid, anthralin).

ROSACEA

Rosacea looks like acne, but it starts in middle age. Look for rhinophyma (a bulbous red nose) and coexisting blepharitis. Treat with topical metronidazole or oral tetracycline. The pathogenesis is unknown, but it is not related to diet or caused by alcohol (although alcohol can aggravate it).

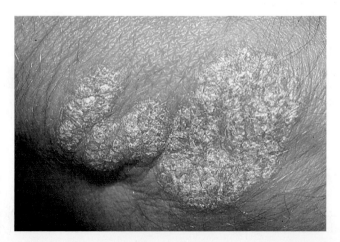

FIGURE 2-8 Psoriasis. Elbow involvement of psoriasis vulgaris demonstrating typical well-demarcated red plaques with silvery scale. *(From Fitzpatrick JE, Aeling JL: Dermatology Secrets. Philadelphia, Hanley & Belfus, 1996.)*

SCABIES

Scabies is caused by the mite *Sarcoptes scabiei*, which tunnel into the skin and leave visible burrows, classically in the finger web spaces and flexor surface of the wrists. Facial involvement sometimes is seen in infants. Patients have severe pruritus, and itching can lead to secondary bacterial infection. Diagnosis is made by scraping the mite out of a burrow and viewing it under a microscope (Fig. 2-9). Treat with permethrin cream applied to the whole body. Remember to treat *all* contacts (e.g., the whole family). Do *not* use lindane to treat unless permethrin is not a choice. Lindane used to be the treatment of choice but can cause neurotoxicity, especially in young children.

SEBORRHEIC DERMATITIS

Seborrheic dermatitis causes the common conditions known as cradle cap and dandruff as well as blepharitis (eyelid inflammation). Look for scaling skin with or without erythema on the hairy areas of the head (scalp, eyebrows, eyelashes, mustache, beard) as well as on the forehead, nasolabial folds, external ear canals, and postauricular creases. Treat with products containing selenium sulfide or zinc. Low-potency topical steroids and ketoconazole cream can also be used.

SQUAMOUS CELL CANCER

Look for preexisting actinic keratoses (hard, sharp, red, often scaly lesions in sun-exposed areas) or burn scars that become nodular, warty, or ulcerated (Fig. 2-10). Do a biopsy if this happens! Squamous cell cancer in situ is known as *Bowen disease*.

STOMATITIS

Stomatitis is an inflammation of the mucous membranes of the mouth. The classic finding is fissuring of the corners of the mouth (angular stomatitis or chelitis). Watch for deficiencies of B-complex vitamins (riboflavin, niacin, pyridoxine) or vitamin C.

TINEA VERSICOLOR

A skin infection with *Malassezia furfur (*formerly known as Pityrosporum*)* that occurs most commonly in young adults. It appears as multiple patches of various size and color (brown, tan, and white) on the torso (Fig. 2-11). It often becomes noticeable in the summer because the affected areas fail to tan and

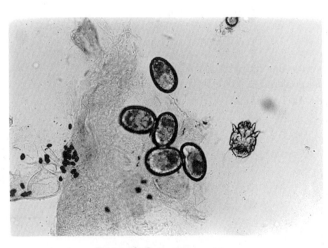

FIGURE 2-9 Scabies scraping.

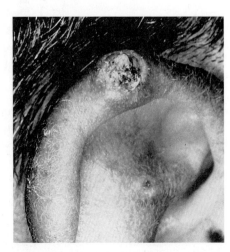

FIGURE 2-10 Squamous cell carcinoma of the ear demonstrating a nodule with central scale and crust. *(From Fitzpatrick JE, Aeling JL: Dermatology Secrets. Philadelphia, Hanley & Belfus, 1996.)*

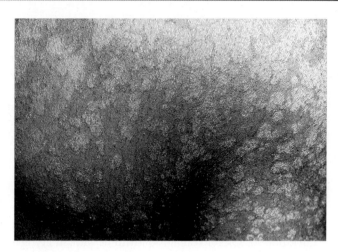

FIGURE 2-11 Tinea versicolor demonstrating hypopigmented, scaly papules. *(From Fitzpatrick JE, Aeling JL: Dermatology Secrets. Philadelphia, Hanley & Belfus, 1996.)*

look white. Diagnose from lesion scrapings (spaghetti and meatball appearance on KOH preparation). Treat with oral or topical imidazoles or selenium sulfide shampoo.

VITILIGO

Vitiligo is depigmentation of unknown etiology, but it can have an autoimmune basis. It is associated with pernicious anemia, hypothyroidism, Addison disease, and diabetes mellitus. Patients often have antibodies to melanin, parietal cells, or thyroid.

WARTS

Warts are caused by human papillomavirus (HPV); infections are most commonly seen in older children, often on the hands. Treatments include salicylic acid, liquid nitrogen, curettage, and others. Genital warts also are caused by HPV (types 16 and 18 [and others] are associated with cervical cancer).

QR CODE

The QR code includes three USMLE-style questions and answers. For more questions, redeem the PIN code on the inside cover for the Crush Step 2 question bank powered by USMLE Consult.

Please see the Introduction for instructions on how to access content using the QR codes.

Question

A 24-year-old white man comes into the office complaining of "white spots" on his skin that he noticed after tanning at the beach. The patient has no other complaints, and the physical examination is unremarkable other than the skin (shown below), which does not itch.

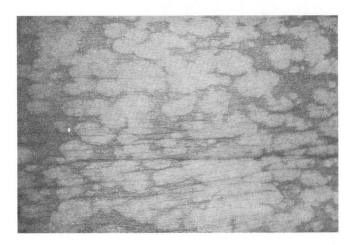

Which of the following is the most likely condition?
(A) Pityriasis rosea
(B) Tinea versicolor
(C) Kaposi's sarcoma
(D) Contact dermatitis
(E) Lichen planus

From Goldman L, Ausiello D: *Cecil Medicine,* 23rd ed. Philadelphia, Saunders, 2008.

3 EAR, NOSE, AND THROAT

EARS

Hearing Loss

The most common cause is aging (**presbycusis**). Treatment options include hearing aids and cochlear implants. The history may suggest other causes:

- Exposure to prolonged or intense loud noise
- **Bacterial meningitis** is the most common cause of acquired hearing loss in children. Follow all children with hearing testing after a bout of meningitis.
- **Congenital TORCH** (**t**oxoplasmosis, **o**ther agents, **r**ubella, **c**ytomegalovirus, **h**erpes simplex virus) **infection**
- **Diabetes mellitus**
- **Drugs** (aminoglycosides, aspirin, quinine, loop diuretics, cisplatin)
- Hypothyroidism
- Labyrinthitis (may be viral or can follow or extend from meningitis or otitis media)
- Ménière disease: accompanied by severe vertigo, tinnitus, nausea and vomiting; treated with anticholinergics, antihistamines (meclizine), or surgery (if refractory)
- Multiple sclerosis
- **Otosclerosis** is the most common cause of progressive **conductive** hearing loss in adults, and **presbycusis** is the most common cause of **sensorineural** hearing loss in adults. Otosclerosis can be differentiated from presbycusis by audiometry. If the patient is found to have conductive hearing loss, the next step is tympanometry. In otosclerosis, the otic bones become fixed together and impede hearing. Otosclerosis can be treated with a hearing aid or a prosthetic stapes implant.
- Pseudotumor cerebri
- Sarcoidosis
- **Tumor** (usually acoustic neuroma; Fig. 3-1)

Sudden Deafness

Sudden deafness develops over a few hours. It is most often caused by a virus (endolymphatic labyrinthitis from mumps, measles, influenza, chickenpox, adenovirus). Hearing usually returns within 2 weeks, but loss may be permanent. No treatment has proved effective; empiric steroids often are used. Trauma with temporal bone fracture is another cause of sudden hearing loss.

Vertigo

Vertigo may be caused by the same eighth cranial nerve lesions that cause hearing loss (Ménière disease, tumor, vestibular neuronitis, multiple sclerosis). Another common cause is benign positional paroxysmal vertigo (BPPV), which is induced by certain head positions and may be accompanied by nystagmus without associated hearing loss. The condition often resolves spontaneously; treatment is not necessary. Whereas BPPV only lasts seconds, the duration of vertigo in Ménière disease is minutes to an hour or so. In addition to vertigo, Ménière disease also includes tinnitus, hearing loss, aural fullness, and occasionally "drop attacks." Whereas vestibular neuronitis classically occurs after an upper respiratory tract infection, a tumor may involve other cranial nerves in addition to the eighth cranial nerve.

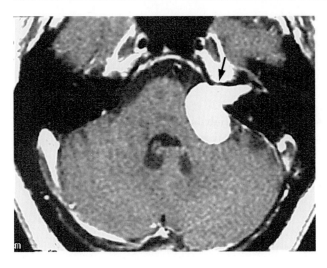

Figure 3-1 Magnetic resonance image revealing an acoustic neuroma *(arrow)*.

Otitis Externa (Swimmer's Ear)

Otitis externa is most commonly caused by infection with *Pseudomonas aeruginosa*. Manipulation of the auricle produces pain; the skin of the auditory canal is erythematous and swollen. Patients might have foul-smelling discharge and conductive hearing loss. Treat with topical antibiotics (e.g., fluoroquinolone drops). Topical steroids can reduce swelling.

Otitis Media

Otitis media is most commonly caused by infection with *Streptococcus pneumoniae*, *Haemophilus influenzae*, and *Moraxella catarrhalis*. Manipulation of the auricle produces no pain. Patients have earache, fever, an erythematous and bulging tympanic membrane (light reflex and landmarks are difficult to see), and nausea and vomiting. Complications include tympanic membrane perforation (bloody or purulent discharge), mastoiditis (fluctuance and inflammation over the mastoid process 2 weeks after otitis), labyrinthitis, palsies of cranial nerves VII and VIII, meningitis, cerebral abscess, lateral sinus thrombosis, and chronic otitis media (permanent perforation of the tympanic membrane). Patients can get cholesteatomas (a destructive, expanding growth consisting of desquamated keratin) with marginal perforations.

Treat cholesteatomas with surgical excision. Treat otitis with antibiotics to avoid complications (e.g., amoxicillin, second-generation cephalosporins such as cefuroxime, or a macrolide).

Recurrent otitis media is a common pediatric clinical problem (as well as prolonged secretory otitis, a result of incompletely resolved otitis) and can cause hearing loss with resultant developmental problems (speech, cognitive functions). Treatment consists of prophylactic antibiotics or tympanostomy tubes. Adenoidectomy is controversial but is thought to help in some cases by preventing blockage of the eustachian tubes.

Infectious myringitis (also known as bullous myringitis) is tympanic membrane inflammation caused by *Mycoplasma* spp., *S. pneumoniae*, or viruses. Otoscopy reveals vesicles on the tympanic membrane. The treatment for infectious myringitis is the same as that for acute otitis media.

NOSE AND SINUSES

Nosebleed

The most common cause of nosebleed in children is nose picking (trauma), but watch out for local tumor, leukemia, and other causes of thrombocytopenia (idiopathic thrombocytopenic purpura, hemolytic uremic syndrome). **Nasopharyngeal angiofibroma** should be suspected in adolescent boys with recurrent nosebleeds or obstruction but no history of trauma or blood dyscrasias. Leukemia can result in pancytopenia; look for associated fever and anemia.

Rhinitis

Rhinitis is edematous, vasodilated nasal mucosa and turbinates with clear nasal discharge. Causes:

Allergic (Hay Fever)

Associated with seasonal flare-ups, boggy and bluish turbinates, early onset (before 20 years old), nasal polyps, sneezing, pruritus, conjunctivitis, wheezing, asthma, eczema, a positive family history, eosinophils in nasal mucus, and elevated immunoglobulin E (IgE). Skin tests might identify an allergen. Treat with avoidance when the antigen (e.g., pollen) is known; treat with antihistamines, nasal steroids or cromolyn. Desensitization is also an option.

Bacterial Infection

These are caused by infection with group A streptococcus *Pneumococcus* spp., or *Staphylococcus* spp. Do a streptococcal throat culture and treat with antibiotics if appropriate (sore throat, fever, tonsillar exudate).

Viral (Common Cold)

These are caused by infection with rhinovirus (most common), influenza, parainfluenza, coxsackie virus, adenovirus, respiratory syncytial virus, coronavirus, or echovirus. Treatment is symptomatic; vasoconstrictors such as phenylephrine are used for short-term treatment but can cause rebound congestion.

Sinusitis

Sinusitis is often caused by *S. pneumoniae*, *H. influenzae*, and other streptococci or staphylococci. Look for tenderness over the affected sinus, headache, and purulent nasal discharge (yellow or green). Radiography or computed tomography (CT) shows opacification of the sinus (Fig. 3-2); CT is preferred to evaluate chronic sinusitis or suspected extension of infection outside the sinus (suggested by high fever and chills).

Treat with antibiotics (amoxicillin, cephalosporin, macrolide, or amoxicillin clavulanate for 2 weeks or up to 6 weeks for chronic cases). Operative intervention may be used for resistant cases (drainage procedure, sinus obliteration) or recurrent sinusitis from a congenital defect (e.g., deviated nasal septum). Remember that the frontal sinuses are not well developed until after the age of 10 years.

 Note *After significant nasal bone fracture (which can be seen on radiography or CT), watch for a septal hematoma, which must be removed to prevent pressure-induced septal necrosis.*

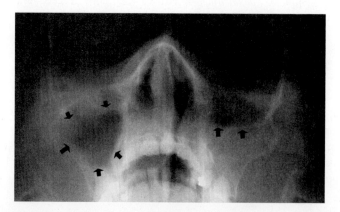

FIGURE 3-2 Radiograph of sinusitis with mucosal thickening of the right maxillary sinus and an air-fluid level in the left maxillary sinus (arrows).

FACE, NECK, AND THROAT

Bell Palsy

Bell palsy is the most common cause of facial paralysis. It has a sudden unilateral onset, usually after an upper respiratory infection. The most common identifiable cause is reactivation of a latent **herpes simplex I** virus infection. Nerve inflammation results in symptoms and signs of a *lower* motor neuron nerve lesion. (Remember how to differentiate stroke from Bell palsy. With an upper motor neuron lesion such as a stroke or tumor, the forehead is spared on the affected side. With a lower motor neuron lesion such as Bell palsy, the forehead is involved on the affected side.) Patients might have hyperacusis; everything sounds loud because the stapedius muscle in the ear is paralyzed. In severe cases, patients may be unable to close the affected eye; use saline drops to protect the eye.

Roughly 75% of patients recover completely without treatment, typically within 3 to 12 weeks. However, some patients have permanent symptoms, so oral steroids and antiviral agents (e.g., valacyclovir, acyclovir) can be given to reduce the risk. Other causes of unilateral facial paralysis:

○ **Fracture** (temporal bone): Patients might have Battle sign or bleeding from the ear.
○ **Herpes zoster** (Ramsay Hunt syndrome): The eighth cranial nerve is also commonly involved. Look for vesicles on the pinna and inside the ear; encephalitis and meningitis may be present.
○ **Lyme disease:** Can cause unilateral or bilateral facial nerve palsy
○ **Meningitis**
○ **Middle ear and mastoid infections**
○ **Tumor:** Especially in the cerebellopontine angle (acoustic neuroma [see Fig. 3-1]; consider neurofibromatosis) or glomus jugulare

Note Get magnetic resonance imaging (MRI) scan (or CT scan as second choice) of the head to evaluate if the cause is not apparent or seems suspicious (especially if additional neurologic signs are present) after history and physical examination.

Neck Mass

In children, 75% of neck masses are benign. In patients older than 40 years of age, 75% are malignant. MRI or CT with contrast helps evaluate. Causes seen typically in children:

○ **Branchial cleft cysts:** Lateral; often become infected
○ **Cystic hygroma:** A type of lymphangioma classically seen in the setting of Turner syndrome; treat with surgical resection
○ **Cervical lymphadenitis:** From streptococcal pharyngitis, Epstein-Barr virus (common in adolescents and adults in their 20s), cat-scratch disease, or infection with *Mycobacterium* spp. (scrofula). Can progress to an abscess (typically caused by a streptococcal infection; Fig. 3-3), which often requires surgical drainage.
○ **Thyroglossal duct cysts:** Midline; elevates with tongue protrusion

In adults, think malignancy first when presented with a neck mass. It can be metastatic adenopathy from a mucosa-based malignancy (e.g., oral cavity, pharynx, or larynx), a lymphoma, or the tumor itself (e.g., thyroid malignancy). In children, if the mass is malignant, the cause is likely leukemia or lymphoma or sometimes a sarcoma.

Workup of an unknown cancer in the neck in adults includes *random* biopsy of the nasopharynx, palatine tonsils, and base of the tongue as well as laryngoscopy, bronchoscopy, and esophagoscopy (with biopsies of any suspicious lesions)—the so-called triple endoscopy with triple biopsy. Positron emission tomography scan can also help identify primary malignancy in some cases.

Peritonsillar Abscess and Retropharyngeal Abscess

Make sure you are able to differentiate between peritonsillar abscess and retropharyngeal abscess and be aware that these are potential airway emergencies.

Peritonsillar abscess typically presents in patients older than the age of 10 years with a "hot potato" voice, drooling, and trismus. Examination reveals a very swollen and fluctuant tonsil with deviation of the uvula to the opposite side. Group A streptococcus is the most common pathogen, although *S. aureus, S. pneumoniae,* and anaerobes are possible. Surgical intervention (needle aspiration, incision

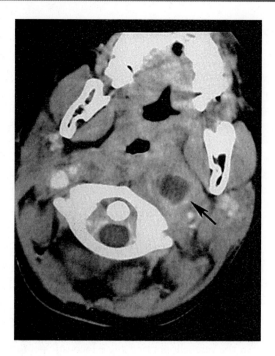

FIGURE 3-3 Computed tomography scan reveals that cervical lymphadenitis has progressed to an abscess *(arrow)*.

and drainage, or tonsillectomy) and broad-spectrum antibiotic therapy (typically ampicillin–sulbactam or clindamycin) are the cornerstones of treatment.

Retropharyngeal abscess typically presents in patients 6 months to 6 years of age who have a fever, odynophagia, a "hot potato" voice, and drooling. Examination typically reveals an ill-appearing child with cervical lymphadenopathy (usually unilateral) and may reveal a mass in the posterior pharyngeal wall (although examination in the operating room may be necessary to permit controlled placement of an airway if needed). Patients with retropharyngeal abscesses demonstrate an unwillingness to move the neck because of pain, and they particularly avoid extension of the neck. Group A streptococcus is the most common pathogen, although *S. aureus* and *Bacteroides* spp. also may cause retropharyngeal abscess. Lateral neck radiographs or contrast-enhanced CT of the neck can be used to help make the diagnosis. Lateral neck radiographs demonstrate a prevertebral space that is increased in depth compared with the anteroposterior measurement of the adjacent vertebral body. Treatment is surgical drainage and broad-spectrum antibiotics.

Parotid Swelling

The classic but now rare cause of parotid swelling is mumps. The best treatment for mumps and the complication of infertility is prevention through immunization. Parotid swelling also may be caused by neoplasm (pleomorphic adenoma is the most common and is benign), alcoholism, Sjögren syndrome, sialolithiasis (a stone in the salivary glands or ducts; more common in the submandibular gland and is associated with significant pain), lymphadenopathy (there are lymph nodes in the parotid gland), and sarcoidosis. The best treatment for pleomorphic adenoma is superficial parotidectomy (not enucleation) to prevent recurrence.

QR CODE

The QR code includes three USMLE-style questions and answers. For more questions, redeem the PIN code on the inside cover for the Crush Step 2 question bank powered by USMLE Consult.

Please see the Introduction for instructions on how to access content using the QR codes.

Question

Which of the following is the most common cause of new-onset sensorineural hearing loss in adults?
(A) Presbycusis
(B) Viral infection
(C) Otosclerosis
(D) Meningitis
(E) Aminoglycosides

4 EMERGENCY MEDICINE

BURNS

Burns may be thermal, chemical, or electrical. Initial management of all burns includes *lots of intravenous (IV) fluids* (use lactated Ringer solution or use normal saline if lactated Ringer solution is not a choice); removal of all clothes and other smoldering items on the body; copious irrigation of chemical burns; and, of course, the ABCs (airway, breathing, and circulation). You should have a very low threshold for intubation; use 100% oxygen until significant carboxyhemoglobin from carbon monoxide inhalation is ruled out. Remember that carbon monoxide poisoning can cause vague constitutional symptoms such as headache, malaise, nausea, and dizziness. It can also cause mental status changes ranging from confusion to coma as well as myocardial ischemia, cardiac arrhythmias, pulmonary edema, and lactic acidosis.

Chemical Burns
Alkali burns are worse than acidic burns because alkali penetrates more deeply. Treat all chemical burns with copious irrigation from the nearest source (e.g., tap water).

Electrical Burns
With electrical burns, most of the destruction is internal and can lead to muscle necrosis, myoglobinuria, acidosis, and renal failure. Use *lots* of IV fluids to prevent such complications. The immediate, life-threatening risk with electricity exposure or burns (including lightning and putting a finger in an electrical outlet) is cardiac arrhythmias. Get an electrocardiogram (EKG).

Thermal Burns
Burn depth terminology no longer includes the use of "first-, second-, and third-degree" burns. Burn severity is now classified as superficial, superficial partial-thickness, deep partial-thickness, and full-thickness burns. The old terminology is included in parentheses below because many physicians have not yet adopted the newer terminology.

Superficial (first-degree) burns are erythematous without blister formation and involve only the epidermis, and pain is localized.

Superficial partial-thickness (second-degree) burns are painful, warm, and moist with blister formation and involve the epidermis and superficial papillary dermis.

Deep partial-thickness (second-degree) burns reveal skin that is mottled, waxy, and white in appearance with ruptured blisters. Pain sensation is absent, but pressure sensation is intact.

Full-thickness (third-degree) burns involve both the epidermis and dermis, have a white to gray leathery appearance, and do not blanch with pressure. Because nerve endings have been burned, these burns are *painless*.

Burns are also graded in severity by the percentage of body surface area (BSA) affected. This can be estimated by the rule of nines: in adults, the head and neck are 9% BSA, each arm is 9% BSA, each leg is 18% BSA, the anterior trunk is 18% BSA, the posterior trunk is 18% BSA, the palm of the hand is 1% BSA, and the perineum is 1% BSA.

Because burn care is very specialized, patients meeting certain criteria must be referred to a burn center for a higher level of care:

○ Partial-thickness and full-thickness burns involving more than 10% BSA in patients ages under 10 or over 50 years
○ Partial-thickness and full-thickness burns more than 20% in any patient
○ Full-thickness burns involving more than 5% BSA
○ Partial-thickness and full-thickness burns of critical areas: face, hands, feet, genitalia, perineum, over major joints
○ Electrical burns
○ Significant chemical injury
○ Inhalational injury

Infection

Burned skin is much more prone to infection, usually by *Staphylococcus aureus* or *Pseudomonas* spp. (with *Pseudomonas* infection, look for a fruity smell or blue-green color). Prophylactic antibiotics are given topically only. Give a tetanus booster to all burn patients unless they received it recently (within the past 5 years).

BODY TEMPERATURE

Hypothermia

Hypothermia is defined as body temperature below 95°F (35°C), usually accompanied by mental status changes and generalized neurologic deficits. It is most important to monitor the EKG for arrhythmias, which are common with hypothermia. You also may see the classic **Osborn J wave**, a small, positive deflection following the QRS complex. Also monitor electrolytes, renal function, and acid–base status.

Patients with hypothermia can be treated with either passive or active rewarming. Passive rewarming can be used for mild cases (32°–35°C) and consists of covering the patient with dry insulating material. Active external rewarming should be done for moderate cases (28°–32°C) and consists of applying heat directly to the skin, such as with a warming blanket. Active core rewarming should be used in the most severe cases (<28°C) and consists of heated IV fluids and irrigation of body cavities (bladder, pleural cavity, and peritoneal cavity) with warmed fluids. Pulmonary bypass is even sometimes used.

○ For **frostnip** (cold, painful areas of skin; mild) and **frostbite** (cold, anesthetic areas of skin; more severe), treat both with warming of affected areas using warm water (not scalding hot) and generalized warming (e.g., blankets). Surgical debridement is necessary for necrotic areas but only after rewarming has been completed.
○ A patient is not considered dead until he or she is *warm and dead*; in other words, **do *not* give up resuscitation efforts until the patient has been warmed above 35°C.**

Hyperthermia

Hyperthermia is the result of heat exposure and may or may not be related to exertion. Patients are at risk for cardiovascular collapse, rhabdomyolysis, and electrolyte abnormalities. Treatment involves first securing the ABCs, IV fluids, and then beginning rapid cooling measures. Patients can be cooled passively with evaporative cooling (spraying water on the patient and placing fans to blow air over the patient), conductive cooling (placing the patient in cold water), or invasive cooling (irrigating body cavities with cooled fluid).

Heat exhaustion is defined as a core body temperature over 40°C with intact thermoregulatory function. Perspiration usually is present.

Heat stroke is defined as a core body temperature over 40.5°C with loss of thermoregulatory function. The classic triad is hyperthermia, central nervous system (CNS) dysfunction, and anhidrosis.

Look for these conditions in addition to infection as other causes of hyperthermia:

○ **Malignant hyperthermia:** Look for succinylcholine or halothane exposure. Treat with **dantrolene.**
○ **Neuroleptic malignant syndrome:** An idiosyncratic, genetically related reaction to an antipsychotic. Look for mental status changes and high levels of creatine phosphokinase in a patient taking

antipsychotics. First, stop the medication. Second, treat with support (especially lots of IV fluids to prevent renal shutdown from rhabdomyolysis), and consider giving dantrolene.

○ **Drug fever:** Idiosyncratic reaction to a medication that usually was started within the past week. Classically caused by medications with anticholinergic activity such as antihistamines, antipsychotics, and antidepressants.

○ **Thyroid storm**

INTRACRANIAL HEMORRHAGE

See Chapter 19 for a discussion of subdural hematoma, epidural hematoma, subarachnoid hemorrhage, intracerebral hemorrhage, and skull fractures.

SHOCK

See Chapter 15 to find out how to identify and treat patients with the different clinical types of shock.

SPINAL CORD TRAUMA

See Chapter 19.

TOXICOLOGY

Toxidromes
Toxidromes are syndromes caused by dangerously high levels of toxic substances in the body.

○ **Cholinergic crisis**: SLUDG (excessive **s**alivation, **l**acrimation, **u**rination, **d**efecation and **g**astrointestinal [GI] activity from the muscarinic stimulation). The patient also will have pinpoint pupils and decreased heart rate.

○ **Anticholinergic crisis:** Blind as a bat (eye muscles unable to focus), hot as a hare (temperature dysregulation), mad as a hatter (CNS disturbance), dry as a bone (decreased secretion of bodily fluids), and red as a beet (flushing). The patients also have dilated pupils and increased heart rate.

○ **Sympathomimetic:** Hypertension, tachycardia, increased activity, anxiety, dilated pupils, diaphoresis, and possibly altered mental status

○ **Opiate:** Coma, pinpoint pupils, and respiratory depression. Use of opiates can lead to bradycardia and hypotension.

Poisonings and Antidotes
Some general principles should be applied to all patients who have overdosed. Start by securing the ABCs and obtaining IV access. Patients with oral ingestions can be given activated charcoal within a few hours of the ingestion. Charcoal works to absorb the toxic substance and decrease the amount absorbed by the GI tract but should not be used if the patient cannot protect the airway. Induced vomiting is no longer used in the case of poisoning because the risk of aspiration is too great. See Table 25-2 in Chapter 25 for antidotes for specific ingestions.

OTHER EMERGENCIES

Near Drowning
Fresh water is classically thought to be worse than sea water (although many dispute this claim), because fresh water, if aspirated, can cause hypervolemia, electrolyte disturbances, and hemolysis. Intubate such patients if they are unconscious and monitor arterial blood gases if they are conscious. Patients who drown in cold water often do better than those who drown in warm water because of decreased metabolic needs. Death usually results from hypoxia or cardiac arrest.

Choking

Leave choking patients alone if they are speaking, coughing, or breathing. If they stop doing all three, perform the Heimlich maneuver.

Tooth Avulsion

Put the tooth back in place with no cleaning (or rinse it only in saline) and stabilize as soon as possible. The sooner this procedure is done, the better the prognosis for salvage of the tooth.

QR CODE

The QR code includes three USMLE-style questions and answers. For more questions, redeem the PIN code on the inside cover for the Crush Step 2 question bank powered by USMLE Consult.

Please see the Introduction for instructions on how to access content using the QR codes.

Question

A 29-year-old man with a history of schizophrenia is brought to the emergency department in an ambulance for high fevers and altered mental status. According to previous records, the patient was recently started on haloperidol. The emergency medical technicians confirm that the patient said he takes haloperidol and is due for another dose. The patient then became unresponsive and could no longer answer questions. The technicians have the patient's haloperidol pill bottle and have not given him the dose that is now overdue. The patient's vital signs are as follows:

Temperature	105.2°F
Blood pressure	182/102 mm Hg
Pulse rate	102 beats/min
Respirations	22 breaths/min

On examination, the patient is difficult to rouse and unable to answer questions. He is markedly diaphoretic and has markedly increased muscle tone in all extremities. The patient is drooling. His chest is clear to auscultation, the heart is tachycardic but with a regular rhythm, and the rest of the examination is unremarkable. Laboratory tests reveal the following:

Hemoglobin	16 g/dL
Mean corpuscular volume	88 μm/cell
Sodium	137 mEq/L
Potassium	5.5 mEq/L
Chloride	104 mEq/L
CO_2	26 mEq/L
Creatine kinase	8460 U/L (reference range, 17–148 U/L)
Creatine kinase MB fraction	<4% of total

What is the appropriate first intervention?
(A) Stop the haloperidol.
(B) Administer a bolus of haloperidol.
(C) Administer diphenhydramine.
(D) Give nitroglycerin.
(E) Perform an MRI of the brain.

5 ENDOCRINOLOGY

It is important to understand the **hypothalamic–pituitary axis** so you can distinguish primary from secondary disorders. In primary endocrine disturbances, the gland itself is malfunctioning (e.g., from tumor, inflammation, enzyme deficiency), but the pituitary and hypothalamus are functioning normally and exhibit the appropriate response to the gland's action. For example, thyroid-stimulating hormone (TSH) is low in Graves disease because the thyroid is overproducing thyroid hormone in response to the presence of thyroid-stimulating antibody. The appropriate response is for the pituitary to secrete less TSH because of feedback inhibition. In a secondary endocrine disturbance, the gland is perfectly normal, but the pituitary or hypothalamus is malfunctioning. For example, if the pituitary secretes low or normal levels of TSH in patients with low thyroid hormone levels, then the pituitary is malfunctioning because it should be secreting *higher* levels of TSH in response to inadequate levels of thyroid hormone.

HYPOTHYROIDISM

Look for classic symptoms such as weakness, lethargy, fatigue, cold intolerance, weight gain with anorexia, constipation, loss of hair, hoarseness, menstrual irregularity (menorrhagia is classic), myalgias and arthralgias, memory impairment, and dementia. Always rule out hypothyroidism as a cause of dementia. Signs of hypothyroidism include bradycardia; dry, coarse, cold, and pale skin; periorbital and peripheral edema; coarse, thin hair; a thick tongue; slow speech; decreased reflexes; hypercholesterolemia; hypertension; carpal tunnel syndrome and paresthesias; vitiligo, pernicious anemia, and diabetes (remember the autoimmune association between these three conditions and Hashimoto disease); and coma (severe disease).

Check thyroid function tests (TSH, thyroxine [T_4], free thyroxine index). Hypothyroidism is usually a primary problem; thus, TSH is high, and T_4 is low. Patients should be treated with thyroid hormone (synthetic T_4). Causes of hypothyroidism:

○ **Hashimoto thyroiditis:** Most common cause; associated with other autoimmune diseases (e.g., pernicious anemia, vitiligo, lupus). Antithyroperoxidase antibodies are present in 90% of cases. Also look for positive **antimicrosomal antibodies.** TSH levels should be increased, and total and free T_4 levels are decreased. Histology shows lymphocyte infiltration of the gland. Women of reproductive age outnumber men eight to one.

○ **Iatrogenic hypothyroidism:** Frequently occurs after treatment for hyperthyroidism (second most common cause in the United States).

○ **Subacute granulomatous thyroiditis:** Acute viral inflammation with fever and an enlarged, *tender* thyroid gland (unlike subacute lymphocytic thyroiditis, which is painless). History of upper respiratory infection is common. Give nonsteroidal antiinflammatory drugs (NSAIDs) for symptom relief. Patients often recover without treatment.

○ **Sick euthyroid syndrome:** Any illness may result in temporary derangements in thyroid function tests that resemble hypothyroidism. TSH ranges from normal to mildly elevated, and serum T_4 ranges from normal to mildly decreased. Clinical circumstances and physical findings are the best guides to whether the patient has true hypothyroidism. In patients with euthyroid sick syndrome, simply treat the underlying illness. If the diagnosis is in doubt, either remeasure thyroid tests after the patient recovers (preferred) or try an empirical dose of levothyroxine (if the patient does not respond to treatment of the underlying illness).

○ **Iodine deficiency:** Rare in the United States. Can cause congenital hypothyroidism in children (stunted growth and mental retardation). For this reason, screening for congenital hypothyroidism is performed at birth. Newborns may not have signs or symptoms of hypothyroidism because of circulating maternal T_3.

○ **Medications:** Amiodarone and lithium are classic examples.

○ **Secondary hypothyroidism:** Caused by pituitary or hypothalamic failure (look for decreased TSH) such as with Sheehan postpartum syndrome.

HYPERTHYROIDISM

Symptoms of hyperthyroidism include nervousness, anxiety, irritability, insomnia, heat intolerance, sweating, palpitations, tremors, weight loss with increased appetite, fatigue, weakness, emotional lability, and diarrhea. Signs include an enlarged thyroid gland, warm skin, thyroid "stare" or "lid lag," exophthalmos, proptosis, ophthalmoplegia (Graves disease), pretibial myxedema (Graves disease), proximal muscle wasting, tremor, tachycardia, and atrial fibrillation. Check thyroid function tests. Hyperthyroidism is usually a primary disturbance; thus, TSH is low, and T_4 is high.

Treatment begins with antithyroid drugs (propylthiouracil or methimazole). Most patients eventually require further therapy. Consider surgery for patients younger than 25 years or pregnant women and radioactive iodine for other patients. Propranolol is used to control symptoms from thyroid storm (the patient decompensates, physically and mentally, from very high thyroid hormone levels) and symptomatic tachycardia, palpitations, and arrhythmias. Causes of hyperthyroidism:

○ **Graves disease:** The most common cause by far. Exophthalmos (Fig. 5-1) and pretibial myxedema (Fig. 5-2) are unique to Graves disease. Exophthalmos is caused by periorbital lymphocytic infiltration and can be worsened by radioactive iodine early in treatment but can be prevented with steroids. Proptosis and ophthalmoplegia also may be present. Patients have positive thyroid-stimulating immunoglobulins, which activate the TSH receptor. Nontender, diffuse goiter also is present. The whole gland takes up excessive radioactive iodine.

○ **Plummer disease (toxic multinodular goiter):** Hyperfunctioning nodules cause a lumpy goiter without positive antibodies or exophthalmos and pretibial myxedema. Radioactive iodine uptake is high in nodules but decreased in the rest of the gland.

○ **Toxic adenoma:** One nodule is palpable and has high radioactive iodine uptake; the rest of the gland shows decreased uptake (thyroid cancer is rarely hyperfunctional).

○ **Thyroiditis:** Hashimoto or subacute thyroiditis can produce a transient hyperthyroidism caused by inflammation before converting to hypothyroidism.

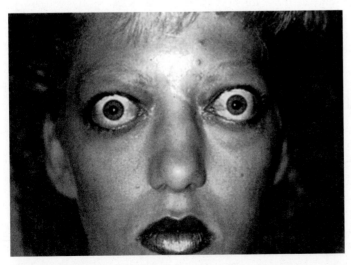

FIGURE 5-1 Thyroid-related ophthalmology with proptosis and eyelid retraction.

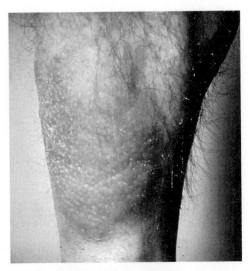

FIGURE 5-2 Example of pretibial myxedema.

- ○ **TSH-producing pituitary tumor**
- ○ **Struma ovarii:** An ovarian teratoma that secretes thyroid hormone.
- ○ **Neonatal thyrotoxicosis:** Presents with goiter, tachypnea, tachycardia, cardiomegaly, diarrhea, and poor weight gain within 1 to 2 days of birth. Can occur even if the mother has a thyroidectomy; caused by maternal immunoglobulin G autoantibodies, which can remain elevated for several months after thyroidectomy.

> *In pregnancy and other states (administration of oral contraceptives or estrogens; infections), thyroid-binding globulin (TBG) may be elevated. Although this causes elevation of total thyroid hormone levels, free thyroid hormone is not elevated, and TSH is normal. Do not treat. The nephrotic syndrome, large protein losses of any kind, and anabolic steroids can decrease TBG and thus decrease total thyroid hormone levels (again, TSH is normal, and you should not treat).*

THYROID NODULES

When presented with a thyroid nodule, your job is to exclude the presence of a malignant thyroid lesion. About 5% of all thyroid nodules are malignant, regardless of size. Be suspicious of cancer in any of the following scenarios: cold nodule on a nuclear scan, male patient, history of childhood irradiation, nodule described as "stony hard," recent or rapid enlargement, and increased calcitonin level (medullary thyroid cancer, usually in patients with multiple endocrine neoplasia type II). Figure 5-3 is an algorithm for the investigation of a thyroid nodule.

HYPOPARATHYROIDISM

The symptoms and signs of primary hypoparathyroidism are the same as those for hypocalcemia (tetany, prolonged QT interval on electrocardiogram). Calcium is low, phosphorus is high, and PTH is low. Treatment generally involves calcium and vitamin D supplementation.

The most common cause is accidental removal or damage after thyroid surgery. Watch for tetany after thyroid surgery. Rare causes are genetic. Watch for DiGeorge syndrome in children with congenital absence of the parathyroid glands, tetany in the first 48 hours of life, an absent thymus gland, immunodeficiency, cardiac anomalies, and midline facial defects.

HYPERPARATHYROIDISM

The symptoms and signs of hyperparathyroidism are the same as those for hypercalcemia ("bones, stones, groans, and psychiatric overtones"). In primary cases, serum calcium is high, phosphorus is normal to low, and parathyroid hormone (PTH) is increased. In secondary cases, calcium is low. Hyperparathyroidism is associated with multiple endocrine neoplasia (MEN) types 1 and 2.

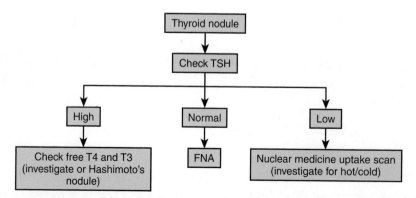

FIGURE 5-3 Steps in investigating a thyroid nodule.

Ninety percent of primary cases are caused by a parathyroid adenoma, which can usually be confirmed with a nuclear medicine scan. Other causes include parathyroid hyperplasia and parathyroid carcinoma. Secondary cases include low calcium levels (e.g., from renal failure), to which an increase in PTH is a normal physiologic response. Tertiary hyperparathyroidism occurs when PTH has been elevated for too long (secondary to long-standing hypocalcemia) and continues to be oversecreted even when calcium is normalized with treatment. Translation: Put all patients with renal failure on calcium supplements to prevent this complication.

HYPOADRENALISM

The symptoms of hypoadrenalism are anorexia, weight loss, weakness, apathy. Signs include hypotension, hyperkalemia, hyponatremia, hyperpigmentation (only if the pituitary is functioning because of proopiomelanocortin, a common pimp on the wards), nausea and vomiting, diarrhea, abdominal pain, mild fever, hypoglycemia, acidosis, eosinophilia, and shock.

Addison disease (*primary* adrenal insufficiency) is most commonly idiopathic (probably autoimmune). Patients may have other autoimmune diseases, such as hypothyroidism, pernicious anemia, vitiligo, diabetes, or hypoparathyroidism. Look for increased skin pigmentation, weight loss, dehydration, anorexia, nausea and vomiting, dizziness and syncope, hyponatremia, and hyperkalemia. Under metabolic stress (infection, surgery), patients might have an adrenal crisis: abdominal pain, hypotension or cardiovascular collapse, renal shutdown, and death. Adrenocorticotropic hormone (ACTH) is increased in Addison disease (in contrast to a decreased ACTH in secondary adrenal insufficiency). Treat with hydrocortisone and IV fluids to avoid adrenal crisis.

The diagnosis of hypoadrenalism, when not obvious, is done by administering ACTH and seeing whether levels of plasma cortisol increase over baseline. If the patient is in adrenal crisis, do not delay giving IV steroids and fluids while you do this test; the patient may die while you wait for the results.

Secondary adrenal insufficiency is a commonly tested disorder and is most often caused by previous use of corticosteroids. After patients take steroids for more than 1 month, they might not be able to mount an appropriate increase in ACTH when needed for *up to 1 year!* The classic setting is the patient on steroids who stops taking all medications before surgery and then develops refractory hypotension and electrolyte disturbances (hyperkalemia is classic) after surgery. Give corticosteroids! Patients who take steroids chronically should be given stress doses of corticosteroids in the setting of an illness, operation, or other stressor to prevent adrenal crisis.

Other secondary causes of adrenal insufficiency are Sheehan syndrome (pituitary apoplexy; history of postpartum hypotension, inability to breastfeed, amenorrhea, fatigue, loss of pubic and axillary hair), neoplasms (pituitary adenomas and craniopharyngiomas), metastatic cancer, infection (tuberculosis, fungal infections, opportunistic infections in AIDS and other immunosuppressed states), and ketoconazole. In secondary hypoadrenalism, mineralocorticoid (aldosterone) secretion is not affected because it is not directly under pituitary control; thus, the electrolyte disturbance is not as severe, and there is *no* skin hyperpigmentation. ACTH is decreased, as is melanocyte-stimulating hormone, which is thought to cause the skin hyperpigmentation in *primary* adrenal insufficiency.

HYPERADRENALISM (CUSHING SYNDROME)

In the United States, Cushing syndrome is usually caused by prescribed steroids. Look for moon facies, truncal obesity, buffalo hump, striae, poor wound healing, hypertension, osteoporosis, secondary diabetes or glucose intolerance, menstrual abnormalities, and psychiatric disturbances (depression, psychosis).

Cushing *disease* is Cushing syndrome caused by pituitary overproduction of ACTH, which usually is caused by a pituitary adenoma. Women of reproductive age outnumber men five to one. Other causes include ectopic ACTH production (classically by small cell lung cancer) and adrenal adenomas or carcinomas (more common in children).

The first test is either a 24-hour measurement of free cortisol in urine (free cortisol levels are abnormally elevated) or a dexamethasone suppression test. A high-dose dexamethasone suppression test can be used to differentiate pituitary from other causes of excess ACTH production. In Cushing disease, cortisol levels are suppressed several hours after administration of high doses of dexamethasone. Other causes of excess ACTH production such as adrenal neoplasms and small cell cancer of the lung do not respond to high-dose dexamethasone suppression.

A random cortisol level is an inappropriate test because of wide inter- and intrapatient variations. **Remember that ACTH is elevated in Cushing disease but decreased with an adrenal adenoma.** If ACTH is increased, a magnetic resonance imaging (MRI) scan of the brain should be obtained to look for a pituitary adenoma. If ACTH is decreased and the patient has no history of taking steroids, an abdominal computed tomography (CT) or MRI should be obtained to look for an adrenal tumor. Primary cancer is usually obvious when ectopic ACTH is the cause (e.g., weight loss, hemoptysis with lung mass on chest radiograph in patients with small cell lung cancer). Treatment is based on the cause and usually involves surgery.

HYPERALDOSTERONISM

Primary hyperaldosteronism is known as *Conn syndrome* and is caused by an adrenal adenoma. Look for hypertension, hypernatremia, hypokalemia (can lead to muscle weakness), metabolic alkalosis, increased aldosterone, and *low* renin (caused by a negative feedback loop). An early morning plasma aldosterone to plasma renin ratio (value >30 is suggestive of Conn syndrome) can be used as a screening test. Get a CT scan of the abdomen to find the adrenal tumor.

Secondary hyperaldosteronism is much more common than primary hyperaldosteronism. It is caused by low perfusion of the kidney, as in congestive heart failure, renal artery stenosis (bruit), dehydration, nephrotic syndrome, and cirrhosis. Look for hypertension, edema, renal bruit, variable sodium and potassium, and *high* renin. The key mechanism is that the kidney senses hypoperfusion and secretes renin; therefore, the renin level is high. Treatment of the underlying disorder (if possible) resolves the hyperaldosteronism. Potassium levels may be normal or even high. Of note, hyperkalemia may be the cause of increased aldosterone release just as hypocalcemia causes increased release of PTH. Both are normal physiologic responses.

PHEOCHROMOCYTOMA

Pheochromocytoma is popular on the boards and wards despite rarity in real life. Look for intermittent hypertension that is very high, wild swings in blood pressure, tachycardia, postural hypotension, headaches, sweating, dizziness, mental status changes, or a feeling of impending doom. Patients also may have glucose intolerance caused by high catecholamines. Pheochromocytoma may also be associated with other syndromes such as neurofibromatosis and von Hippel-Lindau disease and as a component of MEN syndromes 2A and 2B.

If you are suspicious, first screen with a 24-hour urine test to look for catecholamines and their breakdown products (vanillylmandelic acid, homovanillic acid, or metanephrines). If the screen result is positive, do an abdominal CT to look for an adrenal mass and remove the tumor after stabilizing the patient with α-sympathetic blockers followed by β-sympathetic blockers.

DIABETES INSIPIDUS

Diabetes insipidus (DI) is a lack of antidiuretic hormone (ADH or vasopressin) effect in the body. Patients with DI secrete inappropriately dilute urine because of a lack of ADH effect and may urinate up to 25 L of urine per day, resulting in dehydration and hypernatremia. Such patients die rapidly if they are unable to drink water. In the presence of central nervous system dysfunction or significant dehydration, treat with IV normal saline. Hypertonic fluids can be given after the intravascular volume improves. Do not do a water deprivation test on someone who is hypovolemic.

Normally, when the body is dehydrated, ADH causes the urine to become highly concentrated through retention of free water. Giving ADH and measuring urine osmolarity determine whether the cause is central or nephrogenic. Whereas central disease responds to ADH (urine osmolarity increases with ADH challenge), nephrogenic disease does not (urine remains inappropriately dilute).

○ **Nephrogenic DI:** Nephrogenic DI is caused by kidney unresponsiveness to ADH. Look for medications (lithium, methoxyflurane, demeclocycline) as the cause. Treat by stopping the offending drug and giving thiazide diuretics (paradoxical effect; ADH does not help).

○ **Central DI:** Central DI is caused by a lack of ADH production by the posterior pituitary. Central DI may be idiopathic or result from trauma, neoplasm, sarcoidosis, or granulomatous disease. Treat with ADH or vasopressin and treat any possible underlying cause.

SYNDROME OF INAPPROPRIATE SECRETION OF ANTIDIURETIC HORMONE

The syndrome of inappropriate secretion of ADH (SIADH) is a consideration in patients with hyponatremia and normal volume status (euvolemic). In SIADH, serum osmolarity is low, but urine osmolarity is high (inappropriate urine concentration). Look for the values of all electrolytes and laboratory tests to be low (the classic example is uric acid) because of dilution of the serum with free water secondary to inappropriate ADH. Look for medications (narcotics, chlorpropamide, antiepileptic agents, and oxytocin—be careful in pregnant patients), trauma (pain is a powerful stimulus for ADH), small cell lung cancer, lung infections (pneumonia), and postoperative status (watch for the postoperative patient who is receiving fluids or narcotics and has pain to develop SIADH).

Treat with **water restriction.** Demeclocycline can be used to inhibit ADH action. For board purposes, *do not* give hypertonic saline and *do not* try to correct hyponatremia aggressively or quickly unless the patient is having active seizures. Rapid correction can cause brainstem damage (osmotic myelinolysis, also known as central pontine myelinolysis). Demeclocycline is sometimes used to treat SIADH if water restriction fails because it induces nephrogenic DI, which allows the patient to get rid of free water.

OBESITY

IMPORTANT POINTS

Obesity increases the risk of:
1. Overall mortality (at any age)
2. Cancer, especially endometrial cancer
3. Gallstones (cholesterol stones)
4. Gastroesophageal reflux disease, Barrett esophagus, and esophageal adenocarcinoma
5. Heart disease and coronary artery disease
6. Hypertension
7. Hypertriglyceridemia (also weakly associated with hypercholesterolemia)
8. Hypoventilation, pickwickian syndrome, sleep apnea
9. Insulin resistance and diabetes mellitus
10. Osteoarthritis
11. Thromboembolism
12. Varicose veins

HIRSUTISM

Hirsutism is a male hair growth pattern in women or prepubescent children. The most common causes are familial, genetic, or idiopathic hirsutism, but on the boards, watch for polycystic ovary syndrome (Stein-Levinthal syndrome), Cushing syndrome, and drugs (minoxidil, phenytoin, cyclosporine). These disorders do not produce virilization. If virilization (clitoral enlargement, deepening of the voice, temporal balding) accompanies the hirsutism, an androgen-secreting ovarian tumor (e.g., Sertoli-Leydig cell tumor or arrhenoblastoma) or adrenal source (congenital adrenal hyperplasia, Cushing syndrome, or adrenal tumor) is likely.

QR CODE

The QR code includes three USMLE-style questions and answers. For more questions, redeem the PIN code on the inside cover for the Crush Step 2 question bank powered by USMLE Consult.

Please see the Introduction for instructions on how to access content using the QR codes.

Question

A 32-year-old woman complains of excessive perspiration, palpitations, and fatigue. On questioning, she admits to anxiety, difficulty sleeping, and diarrhea. She was diagnosed with generalized anxiety disorder by her previous physician and given buspirone, which she is still taking. On examination, you note tachycardia with an irregular rate and shiny, red, indurated skin over both shins. Which of the following is true concerning the most likely diagnosis?

(A) It is mediated by a viral infection.
(B) Alprazolam is most effective for treatment.
(C) Thymectomy usually is indicated.
(D) Radioactive ablation is used commonly in treatment.
(E) Markedly elevated urinary catecholamine breakdown products are likely.

6 ETHICS AND PATIENT ENCOUNTERS

CONSENT

- Do not force adult Jehovah's Witness patients to accept blood products (or force any competent adults to accept any treatment they don't want!), and do not give a treatment behind a competent patient's back without consent because it's "in his or her best interest."
- If a child has a life-threatening condition and the parents refuse a simple, curative treatment (e.g., antibiotics for meningitis), first try to persuade the parents to change their minds. If they will not, your second option is to get a court order to give the treatment and get hospital support services involved. Do not give the treatment until you talk to the courts if you can avoid it.
- Let competent people die if they want to do so. Never force treatments on adults of sound mind. Respect wishes for passive euthanasia but avoid active euthanasia.
- Informed consent involves giving the patient information about the diagnosis (his or her condition and what it means), the prognosis (the natural course of the condition without treatment), the proposed treatment (description of the procedure and what the patient will experience), the risks and benefits of the treatment, and the alternative treatments. The patient then can choose what he or she wants to do. The documents seen on hospital wards that patients are made to sign are neither required nor sufficient for informed consent; they are used for documentation and medicolegal purposes (i.e., lawsuit paranoia).
- Living wills and do-not-resuscitate (DNR) orders should be respected and followed if done correctly. For example, if in a living will the patient says that a ventilator should not be used if he or she is unable to breathe independently, do not put the patient on a ventilator even if the spouse, son, or daughter makes the request.

CONFIDENTIALITY

- Do not tell anyone how your patient is doing unless he or she is directly involved with care and needs to know or is an authorized family member. If a colleague asks about a friend who happens to be your patient, refuse to answer.
- Break confidentiality only in the following situations:
  - The patient asks you to do so.
  - Child abuse is suspected.
  - The courts mandate you to tell.
  - You have a duty to protect life. (If the patient says that he or she is going to kill someone or him- or herself, tell the intended victim and the authorities.)
  - The patient has a reportable disease. You must report it to the authorities. They will deal with it.
  - The patient is a danger to others. If the patient is blind or has seizures, let the proper authorities know so they can take away the patient's license to drive. If the patient is an airplane pilot and a paranoid, hallucinating schizophrenic, authorities need to know.

COMPETENCE

○ When the patient is incompetent, a guardian (surrogate decision maker or health care power of attorney) should be appointed by the court.

○ Depression always should be evaluated as a reason for the patient's "incompetence." Patients who are suicidal might refuse all treatment; this decision should not be respected until the depression is treated.

○ Patients can be hospitalized against their will in psychiatry (if they are a danger to themselves or others or gravely disabled) for a limited time. After 1 to 3 days, patients usually get a hearing to determine whether they have to remain in custody. This practice is based on the principle of beneficence (a principle of doing good for the patient and avoiding harm).

○ Restraints can be used on an incompetent or violent patient (delirious, psychotic) if needed, but their use should be brief and reevaluated often. Restraints have caused injuries and even death in some cases and can do more harm than good.

○ Patients younger than 18 years do not require parental consent in the following situations:
  ○ If they are emancipated (married, living on their own and financially independent, parents of children, serving in the armed forces)
  ○ If they have a sexually transmitted disease, want contraception, or are pregnant
  ○ If they want drug treatment or counseling

○ Some states have exceptions to these rules, but for the boards, let such minors make their own decisions.

○ If a patient is comatose and no surrogate decision maker has been appointed, the wishes of the family generally should be respected. If there is a family disagreement or ulterior motives are evident, talk to your hospital ethics committee. Use courts as a last resort.

○ In a pediatric emergency when parents and other family members are not available, treat the patient as you see fit. In incompetent or comatose adults, the same principle is followed if no responsible parties, caregivers, or relatives can be located.

COMMUNICATION

○ Do not hide a diagnosis from patients (including pediatric patients) if they want to know the diagnosis even if the family asks you do so. Do not lie to any patient because the family asks you to do so. The flip side also applies: Do not force patients to receive information against their will. If they don't want to know the diagnosis, don't tell them.

○ If a patient cannot communicate, give any required emergency care unless you know that the patient does not want it.

○ Ask patients open-ended questions (cannot be answered "yes" or "no") and always ask "why" if a patient's actions, words, or requests puzzle you.

○ Don't get mad at patients and yell at them even if they deserve it.

○ Parents might ask you to test their child for drugs or sexually transmitted diseases without telling the child. Don't do it.

○ Be a patient advocate, always.

○ When confronting patients, don't be harsh or judgmental.

○ Always try to get more history and information from the patient when given the option unless the patient is unstable and needs immediate intervention.

CARE

○ Patients might refuse your treatment and instead choose to use a wild Tanzanian root they read about on the Internet for their condition. Support their decision and agree to help however you can.

○ "Withdrawing" and "withholding" care are no different in a legal sense. Just because the patient is on a respirator does not mean that you cannot stop the use of the respirator.

○ In terminally ill patients, give enough medication to relieve pain. Don't be afraid to give narcotics if needed and don't worry about addiction in this setting.

○ Consultation of a subspecialist is appropriate in many settings. For example, if a patient has a thoracic aortic dissection, a vascular or cardiothoracic surgical consult is not only reasonable but expected. The boards want you to know the treatment options, but they might ask a question or two to make sure you are not too cocky in your abilities.

QR CODE

The QR code includes three USMLE-style questions and answers. For more questions, redeem the PIN code on the inside cover for the Crush Step 2 question bank powered by USMLE Consult.

Please see the Introduction for instructions on how to access content using the QR codes.

Question

A 68-year-old male patient you have been caring for has been diagnosed with terminal pancreatic cancer. After a discussion between the two of you about his condition, the patient decided to draft a living will. The will states that he is not to be intubated or given CPR under any circumstances. Three weeks later, the patient's wife, who is upset, calls you to the emergency department (ED). When you arrive in the ED, the patient has extremely labored respirations, tachycardia, and delirium. The ED physician refused to perform aggressive intervention because of the diagnosis and living will. The wife demands that you save the patient's life, including putting him on a respirator. She does not care about the living will. She threatens to sue if prompt intervention is not performed. What should you do?
(A) Intubate the patient temporarily until you can contact an attorney.
(B) Tell the woman her behavior is inappropriate and leave the ED.
(C) Tell the woman you understand why she is upset but refuse to intubate the patient.
(D) Respect the wife's wishes and intubate the patient. Later schedule elective extubation after the wife has come to accept the patient's terminal condition.
(E) Schedule an emergency family meeting and have them vote on the issue.

7 GASTROENTEROLOGY

GASTROESOPHAGEAL REFLUX DISEASE

Gastroesophageal reflux disease (GERD) is caused by inappropriate, intermittent lower esophageal sphincter (LES) relaxation. It classically presents as heartburn, often related to eating and lying supine. However, GERD can also manifest as chest pain, regurgitation, cough or asthma, sore throat, dysphagia, laryngitis or hoarseness, or recurrent pneumonia.

IMPORTANT POINTS

1. The incidence of GERD is increased in those with a sliding-type hiatal hernia and obesity.
2. Symptoms include heartburn, chest pain, painful swallowing, and asthma-type symptoms. Initial treatment is to lose weight; elevate the head of the bed; and avoid coffee, alcohol, tobacco, chocolate, spicy and fatty foods, and medications with anticholinergic properties. If this fails, antacids, H2-blockers, or proton pump inhibitors may be tried; often these are started empirically at initial presentation.
3. Surgery (e.g., Nissen fundoplication) is reserved for severe or resistant cases.
4. Sequelae include esophagitis, esophageal stricture (can mimic esophageal cancer), esophageal ulcer, hemorrhage, Barrett metaplasia, and esophageal adenocarcinoma. Adenocarcinoma has become the leading type of esophageal cancer, and its incidence has rapidly increased, paralleling the rapid increase in obesity. In contrast, esophageal squamous cell carcinoma is associated with alcohol and tobacco use.
5. In cases that are atypical or do not respond to medical therapy, consider endoscopy. Endoscopic evaluation is particularly important when alarm symptoms are present, including nausea or vomiting, dysphagia, odynophagia, weight loss, melena, or anemia. The gold standard for diagnosis of GERD is 24-hour esophageal pH monitoring (i.e., a probe inserted into the esophagus).

HIATAL HERNIA

This term, when used without a qualifier, implies a sliding hiatal hernia; that is, the entire gastroesophageal junction moves above the diaphragm, pulling the stomach with it—a common and benign finding that is associated with GERD. A *paraesophageal hiatal hernia* means that the gastroesophageal junction stays below the diaphragm but the stomach herniates through the diaphragm into the thorax. This is an uncommon, more serious type of hernia that can become strangulated and should be repaired surgically when found. Hiatal hernias are illustrated in Figure 7-1.

PEPTIC ULCER DISEASE

Peptic ulcer disease manifests with chronic, intermittent, epigastric pain—burning, gnawing, or aching—that is localized and often relieved by antacids or milk. Look for epigastric tenderness. Patients may have occult blood in the stool and nausea or vomiting. Peptic ulcer disease is more common in male patients. There are two types of peptic ulcer disease: gastric and duodenal (Table 7-1).

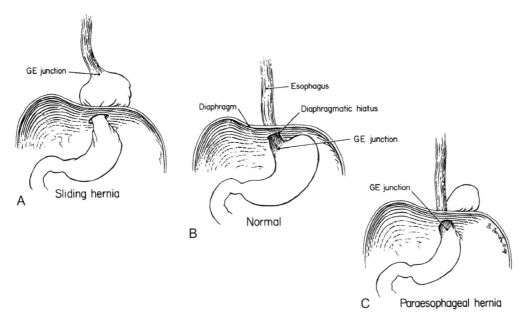

Figure 7-1 Hiatal hernias. **A,** In the sliding hiatal hernia, the gastroesophageal (GE) junction slides freely above and below the diaphragmatic hiatus. **B,** Normal GE junction. C, In a paraesophageal hernia, the GE junction is fixed below the diaphragm, allowing part of the stomach to herniate into the chest. *(From Crapo JD, Hamilton MA, Edgman S: Medicine and Pediatrics. Philadelphia, Hanley & Belfus, 1988.)*

TABLE 7-1 Characteristics of Duodenal and Gastric Ulcers

CHARACTERISTIC	DUODENAL	GASTRIC
Percentage of cases	75	25
Acid secretion	Normal to high	Normal to low
Main etiology	*Helicobacter pylori*	NSAIDs
Peak age	40s	50s
Eating food	Pain improves and then worsens 2–3 h later	Pain not relieved or made worse

NSAID, nonsteroidal antiinflammatory drug.

IMPORTANT POINTS

1. Endoscopy is becoming the first-line diagnostic study (upper gastrointestinal [GI] barium radiography study was classically done first) and is more sensitive (but more expensive) than radiography.
2. Always biopsy any gastric ulcer to exclude malignancy (duodenal ulcers do not have to be biopsied initially because malignancy is rare). If a gastric ulcer is present, a repeat endoscopy should be performed after treatment to confirm resolution of the ulcer.
3. The feared complication of peptic ulcer disease is perforation. Look for peritoneal signs, a history of peptic ulcer disease, or free air on abdominal radiography. Treat with antibiotics and laparotomy with repair of perforation. Another complication of peptic ulcer disease is obstruction caused by inflammation or stricture.
4. If ulcers are severe, atypical, or nonhealing, think about Zollinger-Ellison syndrome (gastrin levels are >1000 pg/ml; endoscopy reveals prominent gastric folds and ulcers beyond the duodenal bulb) or stomach cancer.
5. Diet changes are not thought to help heal ulcers (but reduced alcohol and tobacco probably help).
6. Start treatment with H2 blockers or proton pump inhibitors (latter favored). If *Helicobacter pylori* is present, treat with antibiotics. Triple or quadruple drug therapy (e.g., amoxicillin, clarithromycin, and a proton pump inhibitor such as lansoprazole) for 2 weeks is generally given, and many regimens are in use.

(Continued)

IMPORTANT POINTS—Cont'd

7. Surgical options are considered only after failure of medical treatment or in patients with complications (perforation, bleeding). Common procedures include antrectomy, vagotomy, and Billroth I and II procedures. After surgery (especially Billroth procedures) watch for dumping syndrome (weakness, dizziness, sweating, nausea or vomiting after eating). The following also may develop: hypoglycemia 2 to 3 hours after the meal (causes recurrence of dumping symptoms), afferent loop syndrome (bilious vomiting after a meal relieves abdominal pain), bacterial overgrowth, and vitamin deficiencies (vitamin B_{12} or iron, causing anemia).

8. Gastric acid seems to be necessary, but not sufficient, to cause ulcers. Patients with achlorhydria (most commonly caused by pernicious anemia, in which acid-secreting parietal cells are destroyed by antiparietal cell antibodies) generally do not get ulcers, but patients with ulcers may have normal or even low gastric acid secretion.

UPPER VERSUS LOWER GASTROINTESTINAL BLEEDING

Table 7-2 compares upper and lower GI bleeding.

TABLE 7-2 Upper versus Lower Gastrointestinal Bleeding

CHARACTERISTIC	UPPER	LOWER
Location	Proximal to ligament of Treitz	Distal to ligament of Treitz
Common causes	Gastritis, peptic ulcer disease, varices	Vascular ectasia, diverticulosis, colon cancer, colitis or inflammatory bowel disease, hemorrhoids
Stool	Tarry, black stool (melena)	Red blood seen in stool (hematochezia)
Nasogastric tube aspirate	Positive for blood	Negative for blood

IMPORTANT POINTS

1. The first step is to make sure that the patient is stable (airway, breathing, and circulation [ABCs], IV fluids, and blood if needed); then get a diagnosis. Next place a nasogastric tube and test the aspirate for blood to help determine whether the patient has an upper or lower GI bleed.

2. Endoscopy is usually the first test performed (upper or lower, depending on symptoms and nasogastric tube aspirate).
   ○ Endoscopically treatable lesions include polyps, vascular ectasias, and varices.
   ○ A radionuclide or nuclear medicine scan can detect slow or intermittent bleeding if the source cannot be found with endoscopy. Angiography can detect more rapid bleeding, and embolization of bleeding vessels can be done with this procedure.

3. Surgery is reserved for severe or resistant bleeding and usually involves resection of affected bowel (often the colon).

4. The most common cause of a lower GI bleed in elderly adults is diverticulosis. The second most common cause is vascular ectasia.

DIVERTICULOSIS

Diverticulosis (Figs. 7-2 and 7-3) is extremely common (roughly half of 50-year-old adults in the United States have it), and the incidence increases with age. Diverticulosis is characterized by saclike mucosal projections through the muscular layer of the colon, rectum, or both. It is thought to be partially caused

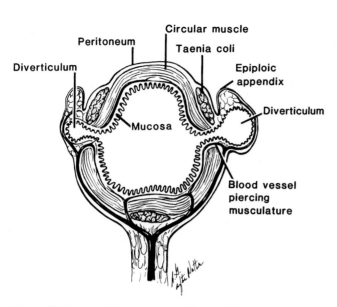

FIGURE 7-2 Diverticulosis. Herniation of mucosa between two taeniae. Note the point of weakness where the main blood vessel passes into the mucosa. *(From James EC, Corry RJ, Perry JF: Principles of Basic Surgical Practice. Philadelphia, Hanley & Belfus, 1987.)*

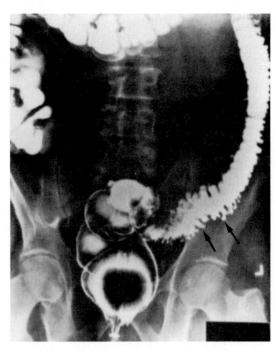

FIGURE 7-3 Simple diverticulosis *(arrows)* without muscle thickening.

by a low-fiber, high-fat diet. Complications are lower GI bleeding (a common cause of painless lower GI bleeds) and diverticulitis (inflammation of a diverticulum).

Diverticulitis causes left lower quadrant pain or tenderness, fever, diarrhea or constipation, and an increased white blood cell count. The pathophysiology is thought to be similar to that of appendicitis. Stool or other debris impacts within the diverticulum and causes obstruction, leading to bacterial overgrowth and inflammation. The diagnosis can be confirmed with a computed tomography (CT) scan, if needed, which can also help to rule out complications such as perforation or abscess. In the absence of complications, the treatment is antibiotics that cover bowel flora (e.g., a fluoroquinolone plus metronidazole) and bowel rest (i.e., no oral intake). Surgery is needed for perforation or abscess.

After a treated episode of diverticulitis, all patients need colon cancer screening with endoscopy or barium enema (colon carcinoma with perforation can mimic diverticulitis clinically and on CT). These studies should be avoided during active diverticulitis, however, because of an increased risk for perforation.

DIARRHEA

Diarrhea has multiple etiologies and is best broken down into categories:
○ **Systemic causes:** Any illness can cause diarrhea as a systemic symptom, particularly in children (e.g., hyperthyroidism, infection).
○ **Osmotic diarrhea:** Nonabsorbable solutes remain in the bowel, where they retain water (e.g., lactose or other sugar intolerances). When the patient stops ingesting the substance (e.g., no more milk or a trial of not eating), the diarrhea stops—an easy diagnosis.
○ **Secretory diarrhea:** Results when the bowel secretes too much fluid. Causes include bacterial toxins (cholera, some strains of *Escherichia coli*), vasoactive intestinal peptide-secreting tumor (pancreatic islet cell tumor), or bile acids (after ileal resection). Secretory diarrhea continues even when the patient stops eating.
○ **Malabsorption:** Causes include celiac sprue (look for dermatitis herpetiformis, and stop gluten in the diet), Crohn disease, gastroenteritis (caused by depletion of brush border enzymes), Whipple disease

(chronic malabsorptive diarrhea caused by *Tropheryma whippelii* leading to weight loss, migratory arthritis, lymphadenopathy, and fever), and exocrine pancreatic insufficiency. Malabsorptive diarrhea improves when the patient stops eating.

○ **Infectious causes:** Look for fever, white blood cells in the stool (not with toxigenic bacteria; only with invasive bacteria such as *Shigella*, *Salmonella*, *Yersinia*, and *Campylobacter* spp.), and travel (Montezuma revenge caused by *E. coli*). *Campylobacter* infection may cause bloody diarrhea, abdominal cramping, and fever. *Campylobacter* infection may be associated with Guillain-Barré syndrome, hemolytic uremic syndrome (HUS), or thrombotic thrombocytopenic purpura. Hikers and stream drinkers can get infected with *Giardia* spp., which manifests with steatorrhea (fatty, greasy, malodorous stools that float) from small bowel involvement and unique protozoal cysts in the stool. Treat with metronidazole. Tropical sprue should be considered in persons with chronic diarrhea, megaloblastic anemia, flatulence, and a history of living in an endemic area. The cause is not known, but it is thought to be infectious. Small intestine biopsy reveals abnormal flattening of the villi. Treatment consists of folic acid and vitamin B$_{12}$ plus antibiotics (tetracycline or sulfa drugs) for 3 to 6 months.

○ **Exudative diarrhea:** Results from inflammation in bowel mucosa that causes seepage of fluid. Mucosal inflammation usually is caused by inflammatory bowel disease (Crohn disease or ulcerative colitis) or cancer. Patients commonly have fever and white blood cells in the stool, as in infectious diarrhea, but lack pathogenic organisms.

○ **Altered intestinal transit:** This type of diarrhea is seen after bowel resections, in patients taking medications that interfere with bowel function, and in patients with hyperthyroidism or neuropathy (e.g., diabetic diarrhea). Watch for factitious diarrhea, which is caused by secret laxative abuse.

IMPORTANT POINTS

1. With all diarrhea, watch for dehydration and electrolyte disturbances (e.g., metabolic acidosis, hypokalemia), a common and preventable cause of death in underdeveloped areas.
2. Do a rectal examination; look for occult blood in stool; and examine stool for ova or parasites, fat content (steatorrhea), and white blood cells.
3. If the patient has a history of antibiotic use, think of *Clostridium difficile* and test the stool for *C. difficile* toxin. If the test result is positive, treat with oral metronidazole (if it fails or is not a choice, use oral vancomycin).
4. Do not forget about factitious diarrhea (surreptitious laxative abuse, usually by medical personnel), hyperthyroidism, colorectal cancer, and diabetes as causes of diarrhea.
5. Irritable bowel syndrome (IBS) is a common cause of GI complaints. Patients may be anxious or neurotic and have a history of diarrhea aggravated by stress, bloating, abdominal pain relieved by defecation, or mucus in the stool. Look for psychosocial stressors in the history and normal physical findings and diagnostic test results. This diagnosis of exclusion requires basic laboratory tests, rectal and stool examination, and sigmoidoscopy, but because it is very common, it is the most likely diagnosis in the absence of positive findings, especially in young adults. IBS is three times more common in women than men. Treat with reassurance and try increased dietary fiber. Avoid treating with medications on the boards.
6. After bacterial diarrhea (especially *E. coli* or *Shigella* spp.) in children, watch for HUS: thrombocytopenia, hemolytic anemia (schistocytes, helmet cells, fragmented red blood cells on peripheral smear), and acute renal failure. Treat supportively. Patients might need dialysis, transfusions, or both.
7. The most common cause of acute infectious diarrhea in children is rotavirus. The second most common cause is Norwalk virus.

INFLAMMATORY BOWEL DISEASE

Crohn disease and ulcerative colitis are compared in Table 7-3.

Both Crohn disease (Fig. 7-4) and ulcerative colitis can cause uveitis, arthritis, ankylosing spondylitis, erythema nodosum, erythema multiforme, primary sclerosing cholangitis, failure to thrive in children, toxic megacolon, anemia of chronic disease, and fever. Both are treated with 5-aminosalicylic acid with or without a sulfa drug (e.g., sulfasalazine). Corticosteroids and other immunosuppressants (e.g., infliximab, azathioprine) are used for more severe disease and flare-ups. Avoid antidiarrheal medications, which can precipitate toxic megacolon.

Toxic megacolon (Fig. 7-5) is classically seen with inflammatory bowel disease (more common in ulcerative colitis) and infectious colitis (especially *C. difficile*). It may be precipitated by antidiarrhea medications. Symptoms include a high fever, leukocytosis, abdominal pain, rebound tenderness, and a markedly dilated colon on abdominal radiography. Toxic megacolon is an emergency. Start treatment by discontinuing all antidiarrhea medications; then place the patient on NPO (nothing by mouth) status, insert a nasogastric tube, and administer IV fluids. Give antibiotics to cover bowel flora (coverage equivalent to ampicillin, gentamicin, and metronidazole) and steroids if the cause is inflammatory bowel disease. Surgery is required if perforation occurs (free air on abdominal radiography).

TABLE 7-3 Comparison of Crohn Disease and Ulcerative Colitis		
CHARACTERISTIC	**CROHN DISEASE**	**ULCERATIVE COLITIS**
Site of origin	Distal ileum, proximal colon	Rectum
Thickness of pathology	Transmural	Mucosa and submucosa only
Progression	Irregular (skip lesions)	Proximal, continuous from rectum; no skipped areas
Location	From mouth to anus	Involves colon and rectum; rarely extends to ileum
Change in bowel habits	Obstruction, abdominal pain	Bloody diarrhea
Classic lesions	Fistulas or abscesses, cobblestoning, string sign on barium radiographs	Pseudopolyps, lead-pipe colon on barium radiographs, toxic megacolon
Colon cancer risk	Slightly increased	Markedly increased
Surgery cures bowel disease?	No (can worsen it)	Yes (proctocolectomy with ileoanal anastomosis)

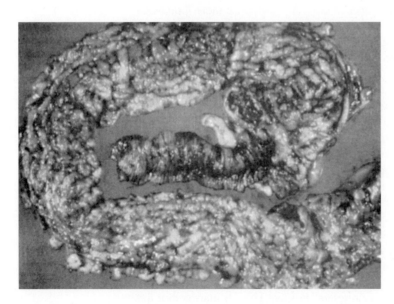

FIGURE 7-4 Cobblestone appearance of Crohn disease colitis.

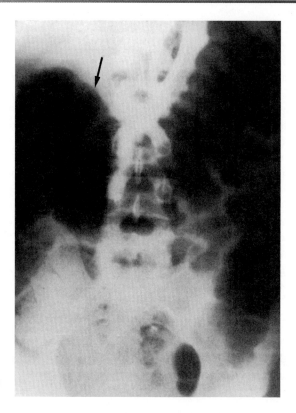

FIGURE 7-5 Dilated transverse colon with air (*arrow*) in toxic megacolon.

LIVER DISEASE

Acute Liver Disease

Signs of acute liver disease include elevated liver function tests (aspartate aminotransferase [AST], alanine aminotransferase [ALT], bilirubin, alkaline phosphatase, or prothrombin time [PT] and international normalized ratio [INR]), jaundice, nausea and vomiting, right upper quadrant pain or tenderness, or hepatomegaly.

IMPORTANT POINTS

1. **Acute alcoholic hepatitis:** Elevated liver function tests; AST levels are more than twice as high as ALT levels in many cases (fairly specific). AST and ALT levels usually are not more than 500IU/L. Histology shows balloon degeneration with a polymorphic cellular infiltrate.
2. **Hepatitis A:** An RNA virus transmitted by the fecal–oral route. Look for outbreaks from foodborne sources; no long-term sequelae, although acute liver failure is a remote possibility. Serology is positive immunoglobulin M (IgM) antibody to hepatitis A virus during jaundice or shortly thereafter. The incubation period for hepatitis A is about 4 weeks, although IgM may be detected by the time symptoms begin.
3. **Hepatitis B:** Prevention is the best treatment (vaccination). Hepatitis B is acquired through needles, sex, or perinatally. Transfused blood is now screened for hepatitis B, but a history of transfusion years ago (before 1972 in the United States) is still a risk factor. Hepatitis B immunoglobulin and hepatitis B vaccination or hepatitis B vaccination alone have been demonstrated to be effective in preventing transmission after exposure to hepatitis B virus. Serology (Table 7-4) is hepatitis B surface antigen (HBsAg) positive with unresolved infection (acute or chronic). Hepatitis B e antigen (HBeAg) is a marker for infectivity (hepatitis B e antibody [HBeAb]-positive patients have low likelihood of spreading disease). The first antibody to appear is IgM hepatitis B core antibody (HBcAb), during the window phase, when both HBsAg and hepatitis B surface antibody (HBsAb) results are negative. Positive HBsAb means that the patient is immune (either because of recovery from infection or vaccination). HBsAb

IMPORTANT POINTS—Cont'd

never appears if the patient develops chronic hepatitis. Sequelae of chronic hepatitis B infection are cirrhosis and hepatocellular cancer (only with chronic infection). Hepatitis B infection is associated with membranous glomerulonephritis. Interferon alfa-2b, peginterferon alfa-2a, adefovir, dipivoxil, entecavir, telbivudine, or tenofovir can be tried in patients with chronic hepatitis and elevated liver enzymes.

4. **Hepatitis C:** The new king of chronic hepatitis (causes two thirds of cases); usually transmitted through shared IV needles (rarely transmitted sexually; donated blood is now screened). Similar to hepatitis B, it can also progress to chronic hepatitis (≈75% of cases), cirrhosis, and cancer. Serology shows antibody to hepatitis C virus indicating evidence of prior exposure but not immunity because most have chronic, active infection. A test for hepatitis C virus RNA detects virus directly and allows better determination of infection status and prognosis. Treatment is not curative but can help slow progression to cirrhosis (e.g., pegylated interferon-α and ribavarin). If a patient has persistently normal levels of liver enzymes, then initiation of antiviral treatment can be delayed. Genotype 1 is the most common in the United States, but treatment success rates are higher with genotypes 2 and 3. Hepatitis C infection is associated with membranoproliferative glomerulonephritis.

5. **Hepatitis D:** Seen only in patients with hepatitis B. Acquired in same ways as hepatitis B. Coinfection of hepatitis B virus (HBV) and hepatitis D virus (HDV) results in acute hepatitis and is usually transient and self-limited. Elimination of HBV leads to elimination of HDV. Superinfection with HDV in a chronic HBsAg carrier may present as severe acute hepatitis and leads to chronic HDV infection. IgM antibodies to hepatitis D antigen show recent resolution of infection. The presence of hepatitis D antigen, hepatitis D virus RNA, and high levels of IgM antibodies to hepatitis D indicates chronicity.

6. **Hepatitis E:** Similar to hepatitis A (food- and waterborne; no chronic state). Often fatal in pregnant women as a result of fulminant hepatitis.

7. **Drug induced:** Look for acetaminophen, isoniazid and other tuberculosis drugs (rifampin and gyrazinamide), halothane, carbon tetrachloride, tetracycline, and HMG Co-A reductase inhibitors. Stop the drug!

8. **Reye syndrome:** Develops in a child given aspirin for fever; caused by mitochondrial injury. Look for the triad of encephalopathy, fatty liver degeneration, and transaminase elevation.

9. **Acute fatty liver of pregnancy:** Develops in the third trimester. Treat with immediate delivery.

10. **Ischemia or shock:** History of shock

11. **Idiopathic autoimmune hepatitis:** 20- to 40-year-old women with anti–smooth muscle or antinuclear antibodies and no risk factors or laboratory markers of other causes for hepatitis. Liver enzyme levels typically are >1000 IU/L. Histology reveals infiltration with lymphocytes and plasma cells. Treat with steroids.

12. **Biliary tract disease:** See later section; look for markedly elevated alkaline phosphatase.

Make sure you know and understand Table 7-4. It is high yield.

TABLE 7-4 Serologic Markers at Different Stages of Disease

	HBsAg	HBeAg	HBeAb	HBsAb	HBcAb
Incubation	+	+	−	−	−
Acute stage	+	+	−	−	+
Persistent carrier	+	+/−	−/+	−	+
Recovery (immune)	−	−	+	+	+
Immunization	−	−	−	+	−

The presence of HBeAg and anti-HBe depends on degree of infectivity.
HBcAb, hepatitis C surface antibody; HBeAb, hepatitis B e antibody; HBeAg, hepatitis B e antigen;
HBsAb, hepatitis B surface antibody; HBsAg, hepatitis B surface antigen.
Adapted from Cohen J, Powderly WG, Berkley SF, et al. *Infectious Diseases*, 2nd edition. Edinburgh, Mosby, 2004, p. 2015.

Chronic Liver Disease

Often caused by alcohol, hepatitis, or metabolic diseases (hemochromatosis, Wilson disease, α-1 antitrypsin deficiency). Stigmata of chronic liver disease include gynecomastia, testicular atrophy, palmar erythema, spider angiomas on the skin, and ascites.

IMPORTANT POINTS

1. **Alcoholism:** The most common cause of cirrhosis in the United States. Positive history, Mallory bodies on histology (not specific). The three stages of alcoholic liver disease are (1) alcoholic fatty liver, (2) alcoholic hepatitis (Mallory bodies and neutrophil inflammation; a reversible state), and (3) alcoholic cirrhosis (an irreversible state).

2. **Hepatitis B or C:** Positive history and serology. Hepatitis D also can cause chronic infection but only in the setting of coexisting hepatitis B infection. Use liver biopsy to evaluate the extent of damage to the liver (fibrosis) in chronic disease.

3. **Hemochromatosis:** Primary form is autosomal recessive disease (look for family history) characterized by excessive iron absorption that is deposited in liver (potentially causing cirrhosis, hepatocellular carcinoma), pancreas (potentially causing diabetes), heart (resulting in dilated cardiomyopathy), skin (causing pigmentation classically called "bronze diabetes"), and joints (arthritis). Impotence, amenorrhea, loss of libido, hair loss, and koilonychia ("spooning" of the fingernails) also occur. Most common inherited disorder in whites. Men are symptomatic earlier and three times more often in part because women lose iron with menstruation. Suspect diagnosis based on elevated serum iron, transferrin saturation, and ferritin levels. Confirm with DNA testing. Treat with phlebotomy, deferoxamine, and genetic counseling. Secondary iron overload can cause a hemochromatosis-like picture, which is classically seen in the setting of anemia that results from ineffective erythropoiesis (e.g., thalassemia) and excessive iron intake.

4. **Wilson disease:** Autosomal recessive disease that results in excessive copper accumulation. Serum ceruloplasmin (a copper transport protein) is low, and urinary copper is high. Serum copper usually is low but can be normal; liver biopsy shows excessive copper and confirms diagnosis. Patients classically have liver disease with central nervous system or psychiatric manifestations (copper deposits in basal ganglia and lentiform nucleus; another name for this disease is hepatolenticular degeneration) and Kayser–Fleischer rings in the eye (nearly pathognomonic). Treat with penicillamine (copper chelator); zinc and trientine are other agents used. Use zinc in pregnancy because of its efficacy and safety for the fetus.

5. **α-1 Antitrypsin deficiency:** The classic description is a younger adult who develops cirrhosis or emphysema without risk factors for either; autosomal recessive inheritance. Confirm diagnosis with low blood levels of α-1 antitrypsin or DNA testing. Replacement therapy can be given to slow progression and delay complications. For severe cases, liver transplantation is the only cure.

Metabolic derangements that accompany liver failure:

○ **Coagulopathy:** Prolonged PT; in severe cases, partial thromboplastin time may be prolonged. Because the damaged liver cannot use vitamin K, patients must be treated with fresh-frozen plasma.

○ **Jaundice and hyperbilirubinemia:** Elevated conjugated and unconjugated bilirubin with hepatic damage (vs. biliary tract disease, which is associated with a conjugated bilirubin that is more elevated than unconjugated bilirubin; see next section on biliary tract disease for more details).

○ **Hypoalbuminemia:** Liver synthesizes albumin.

○ **Ascites:** Caused by portal hypertension or hypoalbuminemia. Ascites can be detected on physical examination by shifting dullness or a positive fluid wave. Possible complication is spontaneous bacterial peritonitis (infected ascitic fluid that can lead to sepsis). Look for fever or a change in mental status in a patient with known ascites. Do a paracentesis and examine the ascitic fluid for white blood cells (especially an elevated neutrophil count), Gram stain, culture and sensitivity, glucose (low with infection), and protein (high with infection). Usually caused by *E. coli*, *S. pneumoniae*, or other enteric bugs. Treat with broad-spectrum antibiotics.

- ○ **Portal hypertension:** Seen with cirrhosis (chronic liver disease); causes hemorrhoids, esophageal varices, and caput medusae (engorged veins in the abdominal wall).
- ○ **Hyperammonemia:** The liver clears ammonia. Treat with decreased protein intake (source of ammonia) and lactulose (prevents absorption of ammonia). The last choice is neomycin (kills bowel flora that produce ammonia).
- ○ **Hepatic encephalopathy:** At least partly caused by hyperammonemia; often precipitated by protein intake, GI bleed, or infection. Look for asterixis and mental status changes.
- ○ **Hepatorenal syndrome:** Liver failure causes kidney failure (idiopathic).
- ○ **Hypoglycemia:** The liver stores glycogen.
- ○ **Disseminated intravascular coagulation:** Activated clotting factors are usually cleared by the liver.

BILIARY TRACT DISEASE

Jaundice may be caused by bile duct obstruction. Look for markedly elevated alkaline phosphatase and conjugated bilirubin that is more elevated than unconjugated bilirubin. Conjugated bilirubin is more elevated than unconjugated bilirubin because the liver still functions and can conjugate bilirubin, but conjugated bilirubin cannot be excreted because of biliary tract disease. Symptoms include pruritus, clay-colored stools, and dark urine that is strongly bilirubin positive. Unconjugated bilirubin is not excreted in the urine because it is tightly bound to albumin.

Causes include:

- ○ **Cholestasis:** Often from medications (oral contraceptives, phenothiazines, androgens) or pregnancy.
- ○ **Common bile duct obstruction with gallstone:** Look for history of gallstones or the four Fs (female, 40, fertile, fat). Ultrasonography can sometimes image the stone; if not, use endoscopic retrograde cholangiopancreatography (ERCP) or magnetic resonance cholangiopancreatography (MRCP). Cholangitis usually is precipitated by a gallstone that blocks the common bile duct with subsequent infection of the bile duct system. The tip-off is the presence of Charcot triad: fever, right upper quadrant pain, and jaundice. Treat with antibiotics and remove gallstones surgically or endoscopically.
- ○ **Common bile duct obstruction from cancer:** Look for weight loss. Pancreatic cancer is the most common cause; look for Courvoisier sign (jaundice with a palpably enlarged gallbladder). Sometimes cholangiocarcinoma or bowel cancer blocks the common bile duct. Always be suspicious of cancer in a patient presenting with painless jaundice!
- ○ **Primary biliary cirrhosis:** Usually seen in middle-aged women with no risk factors for liver or biliary disease. It causes marked pruritus, jaundice, and positive antimitochondrial antibodies. The rest of the work-up is negative. Patients with primary biliary cirrhosis have an increased risk of hepatocellular carcinoma. It is also associated with xanthomas, Sjögren syndrome, Raynaud syndrome, scleroderma, and hypothyroidism. Cholestyramine helps with pruritus. Ursodeoxycholic acid can help to slow progression of the disease, however, not all patients respond.
- ○ **Primary sclerosing cholangitis:** Classically seen in young adults with inflammatory bowel disease (usually ulcerative colitis); manifests like cholangitis. Highly irregular biliary tree on cholangiography. There is an increased risk for cholangiocarcinoma and colon cancer. Patients with newly diagnosed primary sclerosing cholangitis should undergo colonoscopy to evaluate for ulcerative colitis. Patients with ulcerative colitis and primary sclerosing cholangitis should undergo colonoscopy every 1 to 2 years because of their high risk of colonic dysplasia.
- ○ **Acalculous cholecystitis:** Often seen in hospitalized, critically ill patients. Imaging shows gallbladder distension, gallbladder wall thickening, and pericholecystic fluid. Treat with broad-spectrum antibiotics and cholecystectomy with abscess drainage.
- ○ **Emphysematous cholecystitis:** Caused by secondary infection of the gallbladder wall with gas-forming organisms such as *Clostridium welchii*, *E. coli*, staphylococci, streptococci, and *Pseudomonas* spp.

ESOPHAGEAL DISORDERS

Dysphagia (difficulty swallowing) and odynophagia (painful swallowing) are the classic symptoms of esophageal disease. Patients can also present with atypical chest pain.

Causes include:

○ **Achalasia:** Caused by a hypertensive lower esophageal sphincter (LES), incomplete relaxation of the LES, and loss or derangement of peristalsis. Achalasia is usually idiopathic but may be secondary to Chagas' disease (South America). Patients have intermittent dysphagia for solids and liquids classically without heartburn because the LES stays tightly closed and does not allow acid reflux. Barium swallow reveals a dilated esophagus with distal "bird-beak" narrowing. Diagnosis can be made with esophageal manometry. Treat with pneumatic balloon dilation, local botulinum toxin injection, calcium channel blockers, or, as a last resort, surgery (myotomy).

○ **Barrett esophagus:** A columnar metaplasia of the normally squamous cell esophageal mucosa due to long-standing acid reflux. Must be followed with periodic endoscopy and biopsies to rule out progression to esophageal adenocarcinoma.

○ **Boerhaave tears:** Full-thickness esophageal ruptures, which can cause a GI bleed. If not iatrogenic (from endoscopy), they are usually caused by vomiting or retching (people with alcoholism or bulimia). Diagnosis is usually made endoscopically or with imaging such as chest radiography (pleural effusion with or without pneumothorax, both usually and classically on the left, and/or pneumomediastinum), water-soluble contrast esophagram, or CT scan. Treat with immediate surgical repair and drainage.

○ **Diffuse esophageal spasm or nutcracker esophagus:** Both have irregular, forceful, painful esophageal contractions that cause intermittent chest pain. Diagnose with esophageal manometry. Treat with calcium channel blockers, nitroglycerin as needed, and surgery (myotomy) if needed.

○ **Mallory-Weiss tears:** Superficial esophageal erosions that can cause a GI bleed. They usually are seen with vomiting and retching (people with alcoholism or bulimia) or are iatrogenic (from endoscopy). Diagnosis and treatment are done endoscopically (sclerose any bleeding vessels).

○ **Scleroderma:** Can cause aperistalsis in the lower esophagus caused by fibrosis and atrophy of smooth muscle. The lower esophageal sphincter becomes incompetent, and patients often develop GERD symptoms. Look for positive antinuclear antibody results (anticentromere antibody specific for CREST and antitopoisomerase antibody specific for scleroderma), masklike facies, and other autoimmune symptoms. Remember the CREST syndrome includes calcinosis, Raynaud phenomenon, esophageal dysmotility, sclerodactyly, and telangiectasias.

 With suspected GI perforation, use water-soluble contrast (e.g., Gastrografin) first instead of barium (which can cause chemical peritonitis or mediastinitis when a perforation or leak is present). If aspiration is a concern, remember that the lungs tolerate barium well, but they can develop chemical pneumonitis from water-soluble contrast.

 The epidemiology of esophageal cancer has recently changed because adenocarcinoma is now more common than squamous cell carcinoma. Squamous cell carcinoma is usually caused by alcohol and tobacco (synergistic effect) and classically is seen in black men over the age of 40 years who smoke and drink alcohol. Patients complain of weight loss and food "sticking" in the chest (solids more than liquids). The tumor is usually in the proximal esophagus. Adenocarcinoma is caused by the long-standing effects of gastric acid reflux and thus occurs in the distal esophagus.

PANCREATITIS

Acute Pancreatitis

More than 80% of cases of acute pancreatitis are caused by alcohol or gallstones. Other causes include hypertriglyceridemia, viral infections (mumps, coxsackie virus), trauma, hypercalcemia, peptic ulcer disease, medications (steroids, azathioprine), and the dreaded scorpion bite. Patients have abdominal pain radiating to the back; nausea and vomiting that does not relieve the pain; leukocytosis; and elevated amylase and lipase. Perforated peptic ulcer disease also may have elevated amylase and manifests similarly, but patients have free air on abdominal radiography and history of peptic ulcer disease.

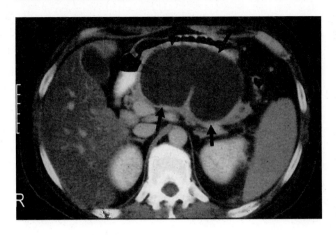

FIGURE **7-6** Large pancreatic pseudocyst (*arrows*) demonstrated on computed tomography.

Treatment includes NPO status, nasogastric tube, IV fluids, and pain control. For pain control, use meperidine (which has a risk of seizures) or morphine (which causes sphincter of Oddi spasm, although clinical evidence of this is lacking).

Chronic pancreatitis in the United States is almost always caused by alcoholism and usually results from repeated bouts of acute pancreatitis. Gallstones do not cause chronic pancreatitis. Chronic pancreatitis may lead to diabetes, steatorrhea (excessive fat in stool caused by lack of pancreatic enzymes), calcification of the pancreas (which may be seen on a plain abdominal radiograph), and fat-soluble vitamin deficiencies (caused by malabsorption). The incidence of pancreatic cancer is slightly increased in patients with pancreatitis, although smoking is a greater risk factor than alcohol for pancreatic cancer. Treat chronic pancreatitis with alcohol abstinence, oral pancreatic enzyme replacement, and fat-soluble vitamin supplements.

Severe Pancreatitis

Grey Turner sign is blue-black flanks, and Cullen sign is a blue-black umbilicus. Both are caused by hemorrhagic exudate.

Complications include pseudocyst (Fig. 7-6) (drain surgically if chronic and symptomatic), abscess or infection (antibiotics and surgical abscess drainage), and diabetes (with chronic pancreatitis). Chronic pancreatitis is a risk factor for pancreatic cancer. Other risk factors include family history, tobacco use, diabetes, obesity, and a high-fat diet.

QR CODE

The QR code includes three USMLE-style questions and answers. For more questions, redeem the PIN code on the inside cover for the Crush Step 2 question bank powered by USMLE Consult.

Please see the Introduction for instructions on how to access content using the QR codes.

Question

A 32-year-old woman is brought to see you by her husband for bizarre behavior. The woman has been accusing neighbors of stealing water from her garden hose and using the water to grow plants with the ability to take over the world. The woman has a resting tremor, which has been present for the past 4 years. She has not seen a physician since childhood. On examination, the woman is uncooperative, paranoid, and refuses to answer questions. You notice a coarse resting tremor of the upper extremities and note the woman's clumsiness when she undoes the buttons of her jacket. She has marked ataxia on testing. The liver is enlarged and nodular with a firm liver edge. Laboratory tests reveal the following:

Ceruloplasmin	Undetectable (reference range, 23–43 mg/dL)
AST	60 U/L (reference range, 7-27 U/L)
ALT	84 U/L (reference range, 1–21 U/L)
Hepatitis B surface antigen	Negative
Hepatitis B surface antibody	Positive

Which of the following is true regarding diagnosis and treatment of the most likely disorder?
(A) Progression of cirrhosis can be slowed by antiviral treatment.
(B) Iron supplements commonly are used to slow progression of the disorder.
(C) An abnormal serum copper level is the gold standard test to confirm the diagnosis.
(D) Penicillamine often is the treatment of choice.
(E) The patient could not have received the hepatitis B vaccine.

8 GENERAL SURGERY

COMMON DISORDERS REQUIRING SURGERY

Abdominal Pain

Abdominal pain is an extraordinarily common reason for a general surgeon to see a patient. When reading a question about abdominal pain, it is important to approach the pain by the region of the abdomen affected (Fig. 8-1):

○ **Right upper quadrant:** Think of the gallbladder (cholecystitis, cholangitis, choledocholithiasis), liver disease (abscess), or Fitz-Hugh-Curtis syndrome. Don't forget hepatic adenoma in the classic scenario of a young woman taking oral contraceptive pills.
○ **Left upper quadrant:** Think of the spleen (rupture with blunt trauma) or peptic ulcer disease.
○ **Right lower quadrant:** Think of the appendix (appendicitis), ileocecal disease (Crohn disease), or adnexal pathology in a reproductive-age female patient.
○ **Left lower quadrant:** Think of the sigmoid colon (diverticulitis) or adnexal pathology in a reproductive-age female patient.
○ **Epigastric:** Think of the stomach (penetrating ulcer, gastric carcinoma) or pancreas (pancreatitis).
○ **Diffuse:** Consider bowel obstruction, peritonitis, and mesenteric ischemia.

Nonsurgical causes of abdominal pain that should be in your differential diagnosis include spontaneous bacterial peritonitis, pneumonia and pleural effusion (upper quadrants), myocardial ischemia (upper quadrants), herpes zoster, diabetic ketoacidosis, Addison disease, porphyrias, multiple myeloma (think of an elderly patient with hypercalcemia leading to constipation and abdominal pain), abdominal wall hematoma, cystitis, hernias, renal or ureteral stones, abdominal aortic aneurysm, ectopic pregnancy, and testicular or ovarian torsion.

Acute Abdomen

An inflamed peritoneum often leads to a laparotomy because it signifies a potentially life-threatening condition (important exceptions to laparotomy are pancreatitis, many cases of diverticulitis, and spontaneous bacterial peritonitis). The best physical confirmations of peritonitis are rebound tenderness and involuntary guarding. Voluntary guarding and tenderness to palpation are softer signs because both are often present in more benign diseases. When you are in doubt about the diagnosis and the patient is stable, get a computed tomography (CT) scan of the abdomen and pelvis and do serial abdominal exams. The traditional teaching was to withhold pain medications so as to not mask symptoms before a diagnosis is made. However, multiple studies have shown that the administration of pain medication *does not* mask symptoms in a way that makes a diagnosis more difficult to make. In fact, because patients are more relaxed when pain is relieved, it may even be easier to perform an abdominal examination and make a diagnosis. If the patient is unstable or worsening, proceed to laparoscopy or laparotomy.

Adrenal Masses

Adrenal masses may be found incidentally on CT scans of the abdomen. Look for signs and symptoms in the question stem that might lead you toward any of the adrenal disease syndromes.

○ **Pheochromocytoma:** Flushing, hypertension, sweating
○ **Cushing syndrome:** Moon facies, elevated serum sodium, hypertension, truncal obesity, abdominal striae
○ **Conn syndrome** (an aldosterone-secreting tumor): Hypertension, elevated serum sodium, decreased serum potassium, metabolic alkalosis

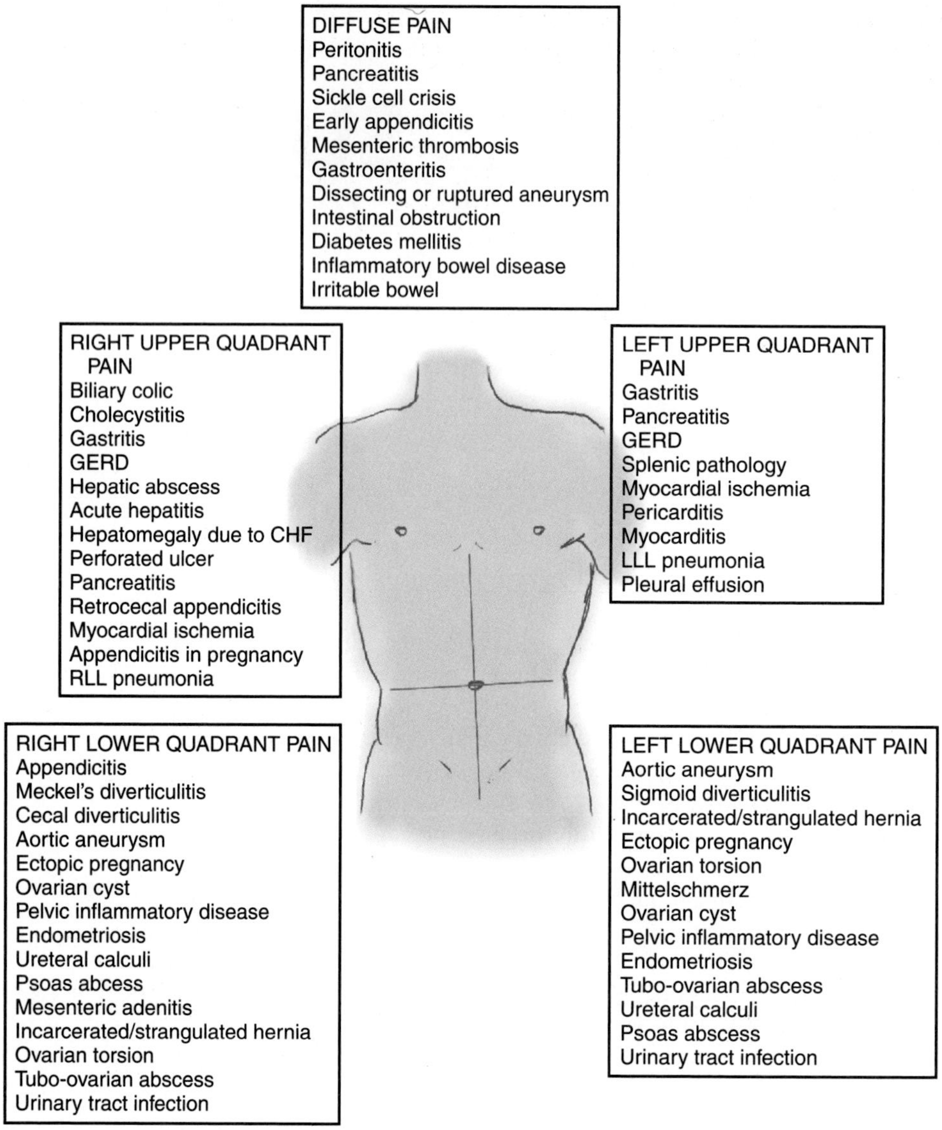

DIFFUSE PAIN
Peritonitis
Pancreatitis
Sickle cell crisis
Early appendicitis
Mesenteric thrombosis
Gastroenteritis
Dissecting or ruptured aneurysm
Intestinal obstruction
Diabetes mellitus
Inflammatory bowel disease
Irritable bowel

RIGHT UPPER QUADRANT PAIN
Biliary colic
Cholecystitis
Gastritis
GERD
Hepatic abscess
Acute hepatitis
Hepatomegaly due to CHF
Perforated ulcer
Pancreatitis
Retrocecal appendicitis
Myocardial ischemia
Appendicitis in pregnancy
RLL pneumonia

LEFT UPPER QUADRANT PAIN
Gastritis
Pancreatitis
GERD
Splenic pathology
Myocardial ischemia
Pericarditis
Myocarditis
LLL pneumonia
Pleural effusion

RIGHT LOWER QUADRANT PAIN
Appendicitis
Meckel's diverticulitis
Cecal diverticulitis
Aortic aneurysm
Ectopic pregnancy
Ovarian cyst
Pelvic inflammatory disease
Endometriosis
Ureteral calculi
Psoas abcess
Mesenteric adenitis
Incarcerated/strangulated hernia
Ovarian torsion
Tubo-ovarian abscess
Urinary tract infection

LEFT LOWER QUADRANT PAIN
Aortic aneurysm
Sigmoid diverticulitis
Incarcerated/strangulated hernia
Ectopic pregnancy
Ovarian torsion
Mittelschmerz
Ovarian cyst
Pelvic inflammatory disease
Endometriosis
Tubo-ovarian abscess
Ureteral calculi
Psoas abscess
Urinary tract infection

FIGURE 8-1 Differential diagnosis of acute abdominal pain. CHF, Congestive heart failure; GERD, gastroesophageal reflux disease; LLL, left lower lobe; RLL, right lower lobe. *(From Marx J, Hockberger R, Walls R: Rosen's Emergency Medicine, 7th edition. Philadelphia, Mosby, 2010.)*

You then want to think about ordering labs (cortisol, electrolytes, urinary catecholamine metabolites such as metanephrines) to rule out any of these syndromes. If these test results are suggestive of one of the syndromes, you can make a diagnosis and proceed to surgery. Adrenal masses also may be caused by metastases (especially lung cancer), adrenal carcinoma, cysts, and lipomas. Surgical removal of masses larger than 4 cm should be considered because of the risk of adrenal carcinoma.

Anorectal Disease

Anal fissure: These are most commonly the result of passing hard stool. Patients complain of sharp, cutting pain when passing a bowel movement and may also report bright red blood on toilet paper or in the stool. You can usually see the fissure on physical exam; it appears as a superficial linear defect in the anal skin. Treatment includes topical anesthetics, Sitz baths (sitting in warm water), a high-fiber diet, stool softeners, and topical nitroglycerin to relax the musculature. Other treatment options include botulinum toxin injections or lateral sphincterotomy.

Anal abscess and **anal fistula** are the acute and chronic manifestations of the same process, an infected anal gland. A patient with an abscess will complain of severe anal pain that is not necessarily associated with bowel movements, and fever may be present. Drainage is required. An anal fistula presents with chronic drainage after an abscess, and there may be pain with defecation. Surgical treatment may be required. Think of Crohn disease in the patient with recurrent anal fistulae. Surgery should be avoided in patients with Crohn disease.

External hemorrhoids: Patients complain of anal pain and itching, particularly in the case of a thrombosed hemorrhoid. External hemorrhoids are also associated with passing hard stool and may be the result of straining. External hemorrhoids can be diagnosed by physical exam; they usually appear as a small swelling around the anus. Thrombosed external hemorrhoids appear as a larger, bluish purple, tender swelling around the anus. Treatment includes a high-fiber diet, Sitz baths, and stool softeners. In the case of thrombosed external hemorrhoids, the clot can be excised to help the patient's pain improve faster.

Internal hemorrhoids: These are painless because they originate above the dentate line. Patients complain of bright red blood from the rectum. In the case of prolapsed internal hemorrhoids, the patient may complain of a mass protruding from the rectum. For nonprolapsed hemorrhoids, treatment is the same as that for external hemorrhoids. Prolapsed internal hemorrhoids can be ligated with a rubber band, treated with a sclerosing agent, or cauterized. In rare cases, surgical excision is required.

Don't get fooled by hemorrhoids on the USMLE. An older patient with known hemorrhoids who presents with rectal bleeding still needs a digital rectal examination and colonoscopy to evaluate for colon cancer even though a "known source" of bleeding is present.

Appendicitis

Appendicitis peaks in 10- to 30-year-old children and adults. The classic history is crampy, poorly localized periumbilical pain followed by nausea and vomiting. Pain then localizes to the right lower quadrant, and patients develop peritoneal signs with worsening of nausea and vomiting. If the appendix ruptures, the pain may initially improve, but peritoneal signs will quickly develop, and the patient's condition will worsen. Leukocytosis is variable but classically is present. Patients who are hungry and ask for food classically do *not* have appendicitis. Remember the positive Rovsing sign (pushing on the left lower quadrant produces pain at McBurney point) and McBurney point tenderness (Fig. 8-2). The psoas sign (extension of the hip causes pain in the case of an inflamed retrocecal appendix) and the turator sign (flexion of the hip with internal rotation causes pain) are two other signs on physical exam that can suggest appendicitis. CT scan of the abdomen and pelvis with oral and intravenous (IV) contrast (or ultrasonography in pediatric and pregnant patients to spare radiation) can be used to confirm the diagnosis, assess for complications such as perforation and abscess, and exclude other causes. Treatment is appendectomy.

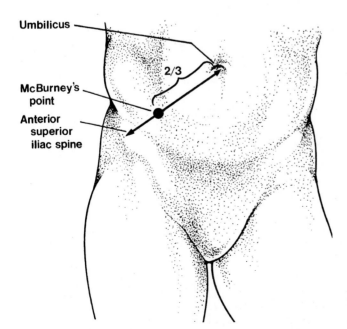

FIGURE 8-2 McBurney point. This is the usual point of maximal tenderness in the right lower quadrant in appendicitis. *(From James EC, Corry RJ, Perry JF: Principles of Basic Surgical Practice. Philadelphia, Hanley & Belfus, 1987.)*

Bowel Obstruction

In **small bowel obstruction** (SBO), symptoms include bilious vomiting (seen early), abdominal distension, constipation, hyperactive bowel sounds (high-pitched, rushing sounds), and pain that usually is diffuse and poorly localized. Patients often have a history of previous surgery; the most common cause of SBOs in adults is adhesions, which usually develop from prior surgery. The second most common cause of SBO is a hernia, so be wary of bowel obstruction in patients with hernias. In children, think of intussusception, Meckel diverticulum, or incarcerated hernia. Start treatment with nothing by mouth (NPO), nasogastric tube put to suction, and IV fluids. The diagnosis can easily be made by seeing the characteristic bowel gas pattern of an SBO on abdominal plain radiography (Fig. 8-3). CT scan with IV contrast can help confirm the diagnosis, exclude complications, and assess the cause. If symptoms do not resolve or peritoneal signs occur, laparotomy is needed to relieve the obstruction.

Symptoms in **large bowel obstruction** include gradually increasing abdominal pain, abdominal distension, constipation, and feculent vomiting (seen late). In older patients, the most common causes are diverticulitis, colon cancer, and volvulus. Treat early with the patient NPO and a nasogastric tube. The diagnosis can be made by seeing the characteristic bowel gas pattern of a large bowel obstruction on abdominal plain radiography (Fig. 8-4). CT scan with IV contrast is used to confirm the diagnosis and assess the cause. A sigmoid volvulus (Fig. 8-5) often can be decompressed with an endoscope. Other causes or refractory cases require surgery to relieve the obstruction. In children, watch for Hirschsprung disease. In adults, perform colon cancer screening after the bout has resolved.

An **ileus** is a disruption of bowel motility from nonmechanical causes. Signs and symptoms include diffuse abdominal discomfort, abdominal distension, nausea and vomiting, and lack of bowel movements or flatulence. There are very little (if any) bowel sounds on auscultation. Ileus is common postoperatively, which is why patients are maintained NPO after surgery until bowel function returns. Certain medications, such as opiates, as well as abnormal electrolytes, spinal cord injury, and peritonitis can also cause an ileus. An ileus can be diagnosed by seeing the characteristic bowel gas pattern of an ileus on abdominal plain radiography (Fig. 8-6). Treatment usually consists of keeping patients NPO, nasogastric suction, discontinuing any medications that may be making it worse (e.g., narcotics), reversing any underlying conditions that may be causing it, and using medications to stimulate bowel movements.

Diverticulitis

Left lower quadrant pain in a patient older than 50 years is diverticulitis unless you have a good reason to think otherwise and is generally accompanied by a change in bowel habits, fever, and leukocytosis. The diagnosis is generally confirmed with a CT scan of the abdomen and pelvis using oral and IV contrast, which can also rule out a complicating abscess. Treat medically with broad-spectrum antibiotics and

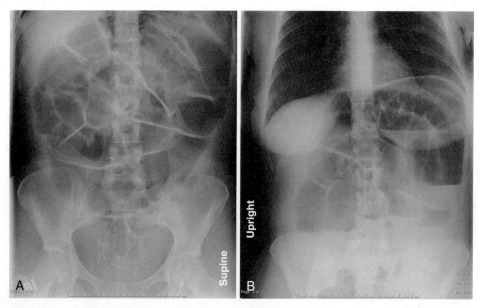

FIGURE 8-3 A, Supine plain abdominal radiograph showing dilated loops of small bowel in a patient with small bowel obstruction. **B,** Upright abdominal radiograph revealing multiple air-fluid levels and small bowel dilation consistent with a diagnosis of small bowel obstruction. *(From Marx J, Hockberger R, Walls R: Rosen's Emergency Medicine, 7th edition. Philadelphia, Mosby, 2010.)*

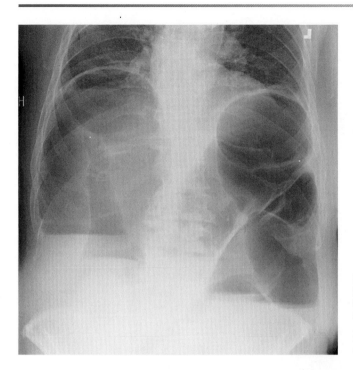

FIGURE 8-4 Large bowel obstruction. Note the dilated colon and air-fluid levels. The haustra can be seen, distinguishing large bowel obstruction from small bowel obstruction. *(From Cameron JL, Cameron AM: Current Surgical Therapy, 10th edition. Philadelphia, Churchill Livingstone, 2011, p. 155.)*

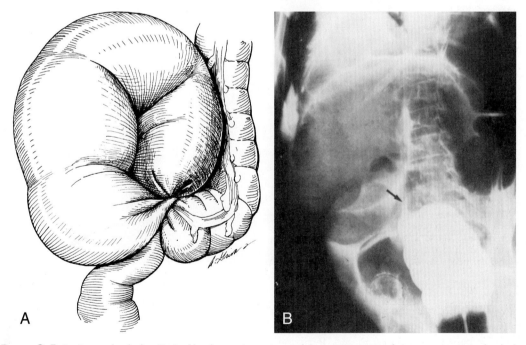

FIGURE 8-5 A, Sigmoid volvulus. **B,** Bird-beak sign *(arrow)* on meglumine (Gastrografin) enema in sigmoid volvulus.

avoidance of oral ingestion (NPO). If the disease is recurrent or refractory to medical therapy, consider sigmoid resection. Perform colon cancer screening (e.g., colonoscopy or barium enema) after the bout has resolved (not during active symptoms!) to exclude underlying colorectal carcinoma. Additionally, endoscopy is usually avoided during active diverticulitis secondary to the increased risk of perforation.

Gallbladder Disease

Ultrasonography is the best first imaging study for suspected gallstones or gallbladder disease (Fig. 8-7). For cholecystitis, a nuclear hepatobiliary or scintigraphy study (e.g., a hepatoiminodiacetic acid [HIDA] scan) can be used to clinch a difficult diagnosis (nonvisualization of the gallbladder) if ultrasonography is nondiagnostic. For disease involving the common bile duct, endoscopic retrograde

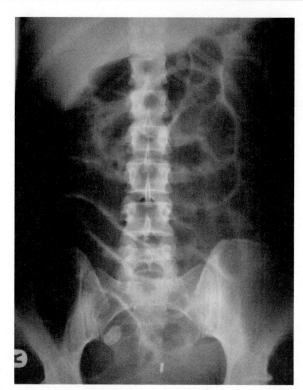

FIGURE 8-6 Generalized ileus in a patient with a perforated appendicitis. Also note the appendicolith in the right ileac fossa. *(From Adam A, Dixon A: Grainger & Allison's Diagnostic Radiology, 5th edition. London, Churchill Livingstone, 2008.)*

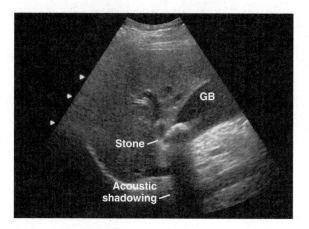

FIGURE 8-7 Typical ultrasonographic appearance of cholelithiasis. There is a gallstone present within the lumen of the gallbladder (GB), casting an acoustic shadow. *(From Feldman M, Friedman LS, Brandt LJ: Sleisenger and Fordtran's Gastrointestinal and Liver Disease, 9th edition. Philadelphia, Saunders, 2010.)*

cholangiopancreatography (ERCP) or magnetic resonance cholangiopancreatography (MRCP) can be helpful to visualize the common bile duct.

○ **Cholelithiasis:** The classic patient is fat, 40 years old, fertile, and female (the 4 Fs of cholelithiasis). Pain is usually crampy, localized to the right upper quadrant, and intermittent. The pain comes after meals, particularly meals high in fat. Ultrasonography is the best modality for diagnosing gallstones, and there should be no laboratory abnormalities. Patients initially can be treated with pain medication and avoidance of fatty foods, but for symptomatic gallstones, the definitive treatment is cholecystectomy. It is very important to note, though, that not every patient with gallstones needs surgery. If you find gallstones incidentally on an ultrasonography and the patient is not symptomatic, he or she does not need surgery. Only patients with *symptomatic* gallstones go to the operating room.

○ **Cholecystitis:** The classic patient with cholecystitis is the same as that for cholelithiasis because cholecystitis most commonly results from a gallstone obstructing the cystic duct. Patients complain of constant right upper quadrant pain as well as nausea, vomiting, and bloating. It is important to note that the pattern of pain is very different in cholecystitis than in cholelithiasis. Patients may be febrile, and on examination, they should have a positive Murphy sign (cessation of inspiratory effort during palpation of the right upper quadrant). The diagnosis is made by ultrasonography with findings of gallstones, gallbladder wall thickening greater than 4 to 5 mm, and pericholecystic fluid. A HIDA scan can be used if ultrasonography is equivocal. Laboratory analysis may show an elevated white blood cell (WBC) count with neutrophilic predominance. Treatment includes IV antibiotics followed by cholecystectomy when the inflammation or infection has resolved.

○ **Choledocholithiasis:** The classic patient with choledocholithiasis is the same as that for cholelithiasis. Choledocholithiasis results from a gallstone obstructing the common bile duct. Patients will be jaundiced and will also complain of colicky right upper quadrant abdominal pain. Diagnosis is often made by ultrasonography because gallstones may be seen in the common bile duct or the common bile duct may be dilated over 6 mm. However, because ultrasonography may not visualize common bile duct stones, MRCP may be required for making the diagnosis of retained stones. Because bile is blocked, laboratory studies should show an elevated bilirubin and alkaline phosphatase (ALP). Depending on the severity of the disease, aspartate aminotransferase (AST) and alanine aminotransferase (ALT) may be elevated as well (although usually not a marked elevation). Treatment is ERCP with sphincterotomy to release the retained stone and relieve the obstruction. It is important to note that choledocholithiasis can cause pancreatitis if the obstructing stone is close to the ampulla of Vater (because the common bile duct and pancreatic ducts meet here).

○ **Cholangitis:** Patients with cholangitis present with right upper quadrant abdominal pain, fever, and jaundice. In severe disease, patients can have altered mental status and hypotension. Patients often have a history of gallstones. Diagnosis can be made with ultrasonography, which shows a dilated common bile duct. Patient will have elevated AST, ALT, bilirubin, alkaline phosphatase, gamma-glutamyl transpeptidase (GGT), and WBC count (the WBC count is often much higher than in cholecystitis). This is a very severe infection, so antibiotics must be started. For patients who do not respond to conservative management and antibiotic therapy, biliary drainage is required and can be performed by ERCP, percutaneously, or open surgical decompression.

Hernia

There are four common types (Fig. 8-8), and all can be treated with surgical repair:

○ **Indirect:** *Most common type* in both sexes and all age groups. The hernia sac travels through the inner and outer inguinal rings (protrusion begins lateral to the inferior epigastric vessels) and *into the scrotum* or labial region because of a patent processus vaginalis (congenital defect).

○ **Direct:** The hernia *(no sac)* protrudes medial to the inferior epigastric vessels because of weakness in the abdominal musculature of Hesselbach triangle.

○ **Femoral:** More common in women. Hernia (no sac) goes through the femoral ring onto the anterior thigh (located *below the inguinal ring*). This type is most susceptible to incarceration and strangulation.

○ **Incisional:** After any wound (especially surgical), a hernia can occur through the site of the incision.

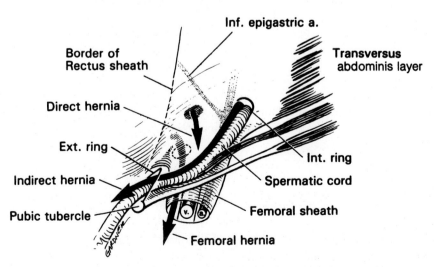

FIGURE 8-8 The transversus abdominis layer in the groin, with *arrows* indicating the areas where the common groin hernias may occur. Ext., external; Inf. epigastric a., inferior epigastric artery; Int., internal.

Complications of hernias:

○ **Incarceration:** Herniated organs become trapped and swollen or edematous. Incarcerated hernias are the *most common* cause of SBO in patients who have never had abdominal surgery and the *second most common* cause in patients who have had abdominal surgery. Treatment is prompt surgery.

○ **Strangulation:** The entrapment becomes so severe that the blood supply is cut off; necrosis can occur. Strangulation is a surgical emergency; the patient might present with symptoms of SBO and shock.

Meckel Diverticulum

This is the most common congenital anomaly of the small intestine. Most patients are asymptomatic, but some patients can develop bleeding. A Meckel diverticulum can act as a lead point in the bowel for processes such as volvulus or intussusception. Diagnosis is made by a Meckel can (Tc-99 scan), and treatment is surgical resection.

Mesenteric Ischemia

Acute mesenteric ischemia: An acute occlusion of a mesenteric vessel, most commonly from arterial embolism or intestinal vasoconstriction. The classic presentation is pain out of proportion to the exam, which means patients have a relatively normal abdominal exam results but complain of excruciating pain. The decrease in blood flow leads to bowel infarction, which can be diagnosed with a CT scan. Treatment may consist of surgical embolectomy if possible, but in most cases, treatment includes resection of the already infarcted bowel. Broad-spectrum antibiotics are needed for necrotic bowel.

Chronic mesenteric ischemia: The result of long-standing atherosclerosis of the mesenteric vessels. Symptoms are caused by poor blood flow to the intestine after meals, leading to the hallmark symptoms of postprandial pain (so-called "intestinal angina"). Treatment is similar to treatment for peripheral vascular disease—reversing predisposing or precipitating causes such as quitting smoking.

Pancreatic Disease

Pancreatitis: Look for epigastric pain in an alcohol abuser or patient with history of gallstones. Pain might radiate to the back. Serum amylase or lipase, if given, is elevated; if they have not been given, order them (generally ordered in all cases of abdominal pain of unknown etiology)! Common signs and symptoms include decreased bowel sounds, local ileus (sentinel loop of bowel on radiography), and nausea and vomiting with anorexia. Treat with narcotics (meperidine, which has a risk of seizures, has traditionally been favored over morphine because of the concern about sphincter of Oddi spasm, although clinical evidence of this is lacking; fentanyl is another option), NPO, nasogastric tube, IV fluids, and supportive care. In the case of necrotic pancreatitis, antibiotics are required. Watch for acute respiratory distress syndrome (ARDS) and pleural effusion, both of which are well-documented sequelae of severe pancreatitis.

Pancreatic pseudocyst: Most often a complication of pancreatitis. A pancreatic pseudocyst consists of a circumscribed peripancreatic fluid collection consisting of pancreatic enzymes, blood, and necrotic tissue. When small, pseudocysts can be managed with observation. If large or symptomatic, drainage of the collection is performed endoscopically, percutaneously, or laparoscopically.

Pancreatic abscess: Also a complication of pancreatitis. This is a collection of pus resulting from tissue necrosis and infection that usually presents with abdominal pain, fever, and leukocytosis 1 to 2 weeks after an episode of pancreatitis. A pancreatic abscess can be drained percutaneously, although surgical debridement may be necessary.

Perforated Ulcer

Patients often have no history of alcohol consumption or gallstones. *Helicobacter pylori* infection and nonsteroidal antiinflammatory drug use are the most common causes of peptic ulcers. Radiography classically shows free air under the diaphragm, and patients have a history of peptic ulcer disease. Amylase may be mildly elevated (Step 2 question might provide amylase value to trick you), but lipase is often normal, and free air doesn't occur in pancreatitis. Treat with emergent surgery.

Pilonidal Disease

Pilonidal disease affects people most commonly between 15 and 30 years of age. Pilonidal sinuses and abscesses are open wounds in the sacral region of the back resulting from a small area of folliculitis that grows into a deep subcutaneous cavity. Pilonidal disease is diagnosed by physical exam—look for open wounds in the sacral area of the back. Pilonidal abscesses are managed by incision, drainage, and curettage. Chronic pilonidal sinuses are managed by surgical excision of the sinus tract.

Splenic Rupture

History of blunt abdominal trauma, hypotension, tachycardia, shock, and the Kerr sign (referred pain in the left shoulder). CT confirms the severity of injury, with observation and monitoring done for all but the most severe injuries. With active bleeding or complete rupture, endovascular embolization of the spleen or splenectomy is advised. Patients with Epstein-Barr virus infection (i.e., infectious mononucleosis) and splenomegaly should *not* play contact sports because they have an increased risk of splenic rupture. Immunize all patients after splenectomy against encapsulated bacterial pathogens, if not already done (i.e., *Haemophilus influenzae*, pneumococcal and meningococcal vaccines).

Volvulus

A volvulus is a portion of bowel that rotates on the axis of its mesentery, leading to compromised blood flow. Volvulus is more common in elderly patients. Look for an acute onset of crampy abdominal pain and distension. Plain abdominal radiographs show very dilated loops of bowel with a "bird beak" sign at the site of obstruction. There are two types:
- **Cecal volvulus:** Less common; treated with surgery.
- **Sigmoid volvulus:** More common; may be reduced initially by rectal tube, endoscopy, or enema. Usually needs surgery for definitive treatment because there is a high risk of recurrence.

PULMONARY FUNCTION, CARDIAC HISTORY, AND SURGERY

The role for preoperative pulmonary function testing remains controversial. Spirometry is generally recommended in patients with a history of dyspnea and tobacco use who are undergoing upper abdominal or coronary artery bypass surgery. A baseline chest radiograph is commonly ordered for patients older than 60 years and patients with known pulmonary or cardiovascular disease. The best indicator of possible **postoperative pulmonary complications** is preoperative pulmonary function. Overall, the best way to reduce pulmonary postoperative complications is to *stop smoking* preoperatively (preferably at least 8 weeks before surgery). Aggressive pulmonary toilet, incentive spirometry, minimal narcotics, and early ambulation help to prevent or minimize postoperative pulmonary complications. Spirometry and a good history are the best preoperative tests for assessment of pulmonary function. Spirometry evaluates forced vital capacity (FVC), forced expiratory volume in one second (FEV_1), FEV_1/FVC (%), and maximal voluntary ventilation.

Surgery carries a risk of morbidity and death from cardiovascular disease, including myocardial infarction, so patients also should be evaluated for cardiac disease. Minor surgeries (e.g., breast biopsy, cataracts) usually place only a small stress on the body and thus do not need much in the way of cardiac workup. Algorithms exist for the evaluation of patients with known coronary artery disease or coronary risk factors who are undergoing surgery. Recommendations do not call for preoperative testing in all patients. The need for cardiac evaluation is determined by the clinical risk factors identified from the patient's history, physical examination, functional status, electrocardiography, and risks inherent to the procedure being considered. Noninvasive testing (e.g., exercise stress test, adenosine thallium stress test, dobutamine echocardiography) or invasive testing (coronary angiography) may be needed for higher risk patients.

IMPORTANT POINTS ABOUT SURGERY

1. Before surgery, the patient should avoid oral ingestion for at least 8 hours to reduce the risk of aspiration. For this reason, general anesthesia is higher risk (usually avoided) in obstetrics, because patients have not been NPO when they go into labor.
2. Use compressive or elastic stockings, early ambulation, or low-molecular-weight heparin (or a combination of these) to help prevent deep vein thrombosis and pulmonary embolism.
3. The most common cause of postoperative fever in the first 24 hours is atelectasis. Treat or prevent this with early ambulation, chest physiotherapy and percussion, incentive spirometry, and proper pain control. Both too much pain and too many narcotics increase risk of atelectasis.
4. "**W**ater, **w**ind, **w**alk, **w**ound, and **w**onder drugs" helps to recall causes of postoperative fever. Water = urinary tract infection, wind = atelectasis or pneumonia, walk = deep vein thrombosis, wound = surgical wound infection, and wonder drugs = drug fever. If daily fever spikes occur, think about an intraabdominal abscess and order a CT scan to locate it. Drainage is required.
5. Perioperative β-blockers can reduce the risk of myocardial infarction in those with coronary artery disease and possibly those with coronary disease risk factors, but it is usually reserved for those already taking β-blockers.
6. Fascial or wound dehiscence classically occurs *5 to 10 days postoperatively*. Look for leakage of serosanguineous fluid from the wound, particularly after the patient coughs or strains, which is often associated with infection. Treat with antibiotics (if secondary to infection) and reclosure of the incision.

TRAUMA

If you spent your free time during your surgery rotation trying to catch up on lost sleep, go back and read a chapter about trauma from a general surgery text. Trauma and its management are high yield for Step 2.

The mnemonic **ABCDE** is to help you remember the steps to the primary survey in trauma. These five steps are the key to the initial management of patients with trauma. Always do them in order. For example, if the patient is bleeding to death and has a blocked airway, you must choose which problem to address first. The answer is airway management.

○ **A = Airway:** Provide, protect, and maintain an adequate airway at all times. If the patient can answer questions, the airway is fine. You can use an oropharyngeal airway in uncomplicated cases and give supplemental oxygen. If the patient is unstable, if the patient is unable to protect his or her airway (unconscious, altered mental status), if the patient is having difficulty breathing, or if the patient is not breathing, you need to intubate. If intubation fails, do a cricothyroidotomy.
○ **B = Breathing:** Similar to airway, but even when the airway is patent, the patient might not be breathing spontaneously. The end result is the same: If the patient is unable to breathe adequately on his or her own, the patient should be intubated and given respiratory support with a ventilator. It is extremely important on this portion of the primary survey to assess for equal and bilateral breath sounds, or you may be missing a pneumothorax or hemothorax. In case the patient does have one of these two processes, you must treat it ASAP.
○ **C = Circulation:** If a trauma patient does not have any pulses, you need to realize that this is different from a patient who has purely cardiac arrest. You need to start resuscitating the patient with fluid and, if indicated, do an emergency thoracotomy. Indications for emergency thoracotomy include traumatic arrest resulting from penetrating chest trauma with previously witnessed cardiac activity (e.g., an EMS call that gives you the vital signs but now the patient has no pulses). If the patient does have pulses but seems hypovolemic (tachycardia, bleeding, weak pulse, paleness, diaphoresis, capillary refill >2 sec), give IV fluids, blood products, or both. The initial procedure is to start two large-bore IV catheters and give a bolus of lactated Ringer solution (IV fluid of choice in trauma). Reassess the patient after the bolus for improvement. Give another bolus if needed. If the patient does not respond to 2 L of IV fluids, you should start resuscitation with blood (Table 8-1).

○ **D = Disability:** Check neurologic function. Know the Glasgow Coma Scale (Table 8-2) because you may be asked to calculate (roughly) a patient's Glasgow Coma Scale score.

○ **E = Exposure:** Strip the patient and "put a finger in every orifice" so you do not miss any occult injuries. Also remove any garments that the patient is wearing that may be wet, cold, or contaminated and make sure that the patient is warm.

○ Care of the trauma patient after the primary survey has been completed is very simple. If the patient is bleeding, find the bleeding and stop the bleeding. It is important to know that any patient who is bleeding into the abdomen should go to the operating room for a laparotomy, and any patient who is bleeding into the pelvis should go to the angiography suite for embolization.

○ If the patient is otherwise stable, do a complete secondary survey of the patient, looking for all possible injuries that may have been sustained. If the patient becomes unstable at any point, return to "A" and start the primary survey over again.

IMPORTANT POINTS

1. All trauma patients generally get cervical spine, chest, and pelvic radiographs. CT scans of any affected areas are used liberally with significant injuries or symptoms.

2. Evaluate any head trauma with a noncontrast CT (better than magnetic resonance imaging [MRI] for acute trauma).

3. Injuries below the fourth intercostal space count as abdominal trauma and should be evaluated as such.

4. In **blunt abdominal trauma**, initial findings determine the course of action: If the patient is awake and stable and your exam is benign, observe and repeat the abdominal exam later. You can also do a FAST (focused assessment by sonography in trauma) scan to check for free fluid in the abdomen and pelvis. Meanwhile, perform CT scan of the abdomen and pelvis with oral and IV contrast.

○ If the patient is hemodynamically unstable (hypotension or shock that does not respond to a fluid challenge), proceed directly to laparotomy.

○ If the patient has a positive FAST scan (i.e., there is free fluid, presumably blood, in the abdomen), proceed to laparotomy.

○ If the patient has altered mental status, the abdomen cannot be examined, or an obvious source of blood loss explains the hemodynamic instability, order a CT scan of the abdomen and pelvis with oral and IV contrast (also get CT of the head and cervical spine with altered mental status). Diagnostic peritoneal lavage is no longer used because it is nonspecific and less sensitive than CT; it can also alter CT scan results.

5. In **penetrating abdominal trauma**, the type of injury and initial findings determine the course of action:

○ With any gunshot wound that penetrates the abdominal cavity, proceed directly to laparotomy.

○ With a wound from a sharp instrument or weapon, management is more controversial. Either proceed directly to laparotomy (the better choice if the patient is unstable) or do CT scan of the abdomen and pelvis with oral and IV contrast. If the CT scan results are positive, do a laparotomy; if they are negative, observe and repeat the abdominal exam later. If the wound appears superficial, you can explore the wound. If you see that the wound has entered the peritoneal cavity, then proceed to laparotomy.

6. Always make sure to maintain cervical spine precautions during a trauma evaluation, even when intubating. Spinal cord injury, especially at a high level of the cord, can be devastating.

Thoracic Trauma

Six thoracic injuries that can be rapidly fatal and that you should be able to recognize:

○ **Airway obstruction:** No audible breath sounds. Patients cannot answer questions even though they may be awake and gurgling. Treat with intubation. If intubation fails, do a cricothyroidotomy (or a tracheostomy in the operating room if time allows).

TABLE 8-1 Blood and Fluid Loss

	CLASS I	CLASS II	CLASS III	CLASS IV
Blood loss (mL)	<750	750–1500	1500–2000	>2000
Blood loss (% blood volume)	<15	15–30	30–40	>40%
Heart rate (beats/min)	<100	>100	>120	>140
Blood pressure	Normal	Decreased	Decreased	Decreased
Respiratory rate (breaths/min)	14–20	20–30	30–40	>35
Urine output (mL/h)	>30	20–30	5–15	Negligible
Mental status	Slightly anxious	Mildly anxious	Anxious, confused	Confused, lethargic
Replacement fluid	Crystalloid	Crystalloid	Crystalloid and blood	Crystalloid and blood

TABLE 8-2 Glasgow Coma Scale

Eye opening
4 = Spontaneous
3 = Open to verbal stimuli
2 = Open to pain
1 = Do not open

Motor function
6 = Follows commands
5 = Localizes pain (moves to remove painful stimulus)
4 = Withdraws from pain
3 = Flexor posturing (decorticate posturing)
2 = Extensor posturing (decerebrate posturing)
1 = No movement to pain

Verbal response
5 = Alert and oriented
4 = Confused
3 = Patient utters recognizable words
2 = Grunts or incomprehensible noises
1 = No speech

Total the number of points from each of the three sections:
14 to 15: Mild head injury
9 to 13: Moderate head injury
3 to 8: Severe head injury

○ **Open pneumothorax:** Open defect in the chest wall that causes poor ventilation and oxygenation. Treat with intubation, positive-pressure ventilation, and closure of the defect in the chest wall. You can use gauze and tape it *on three sides only* to allow excessive pressure to escape. Otherwise you could convert an open pneumothorax into a tension pneumothorax.
○ **Tension pneumothorax:** Usually occurs after blunt or penetrating trauma to the chest. Air forced into pleural space cannot escape and collapses the affected lung and then shifts the mediastinum and trachea to the opposite side of the chest. You should be able to recognize this condition on a chest radiograph (Fig. 8-9). There are no breath sounds on the affected side, and chest percussion produces a hypertympanic sound. Hypotension and distended neck veins can result from impaired cardiac filling. Treat with needle thoracentesis in the second intercostal space at the midclavicular line followed by insertion of a chest tube.
○ **Cardiac tamponade:** The classic history is penetrating trauma to the left chest (where the heart is located). Patients have hypotension (caused by impaired cardiac filling), distended neck veins, muffled heart sounds, **pulsus paradoxus** (exaggerated decrease in blood pressure on inspiration), and normal breath sounds. Treat with pericardiocentesis if the patient is unstable (put a needle in the pericardial sac and aspirate the blood or fluid). If the patient is stable, you can do an echocardiogram or CT scan to confirm the diagnosis first.
○ **Massive hemothorax:** Loss of more than 1 L of blood into the thoracic cavity. Patients have decreased (not absent) breath sounds in the affected area, dull note on percussion, hypotension or

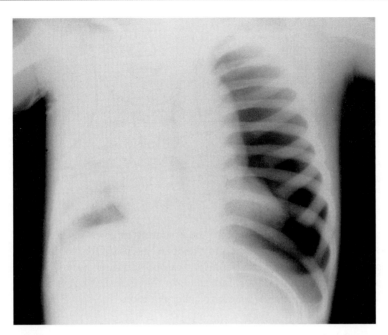

FIGURE 8-9 Left tension pneumothorax. *(From James EC, Corry RJ, Perry JF: Principles of Basic Surgical Practice. Philadelphia, Hanley & Belfus, 1987.)*

collapsed neck veins (from blood leaving the vascular tree), and tachycardia. Placement of a chest tube causes the blood to come out. Give IV fluids, blood, or both before you place the chest tube. If bleeding stops after the initial outflow, get a radiograph and CT of chest to check for remaining blood or pathology and treat supportively. If more than 20 mL/kg of blood (≈1500 mL for the average person) comes out of the chest tube right after you place it, the patient needs a thoracotomy. Additionally, if the patient bleeds from the chest tube at a rate of more than 3 mL/kg/h (≈200 mL/h for the average person), perform a thoracotomy.

○ **Flail chest:** When several adjacent ribs are broken in multiple places, the affected part of the chest wall can move paradoxically during respiration (in during inspiration; out during expiration). There is almost always an associated pulmonary contusion, which, combined with pain, can make respiration inadequate. When you are in doubt or the patient is not doing well, intubate and give positive-pressure ventilation.

Other Thoracic Injuries

○ **Aortic rupture:** The most common cause of immediate death after an automobile accident or fall from a great height. Look for widened mediastinum on radiography and appropriate trauma history. Get a CT scan of the chest with IV contrast if you are suspicious (the second—less desirable—choice is conventional angiography). Treat with surgical repair.

○ **Liver lacerations and contusions:** Detected and graded by CT scan. Usually treated conservatively unless there is active bleeding or a shattered liver (endovascular embolization or surgical repair is needed in this setting).

○ **Pulmonary contusion:** Lung "bruise" that causes immediate consolidation that can be detected on initial chest radiography or CT. Main problem is difficulty in ventilation and oxygenation. Treat supportively with oxygen (use intubation if needed).

○ **Diaphragm rupture:** Usually results after blunt trauma and occurs on the left because the liver "protects" the right side. Look for bowel herniated into the chest on chest radiography. Can often be detected by CT scan if the diagnosis is in doubt. Fix surgically.

Neck Trauma

The neck is divided into three zones for trauma (Fig. 8-10):

○ **Zone I:** Base of the neck (from the clavicles to the cricoid cartilage)

○ **Zone II:** Midcervical region (from the cricoid cartilage to the angle of the mandible)

○ **Zone III:** From the angle of the mandible to the base of the skull

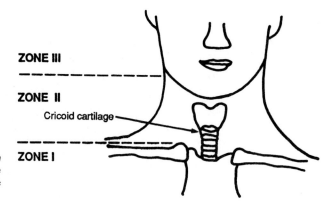

FIGURE 8-10 Neck zones for trauma. *(From Markovchick V, Pons P: Emergency Medicine Secrets, 2nd edition. Philadelphia, Hanley & Belfus, 1999.)*

With zone I and III injuries, do a CT angiogram before going to the operating room. With zone II injuries, the traditional and now outdated wisdom is to proceed to the operating room for surgical exploration without doing an arteriogram first, but CT angiography (or carotid ultrasonography) is now more commonly done before surgery to see if exploration is indicated. In the presence of obvious bleeding or a rapidly expanding hematoma, proceed to immediate surgical exploration.

QR CODE

The QR code includes three USMLE-style questions and answers. For more questions, redeem the PIN code on the inside cover for the Crush Step 2 question bank powered by USMLE Consult.

Please see the Introduction for instructions on how to access content using the QR codes.

Question

A patient comes into the emergency department after an automobile accident in which he was unrestrained. He says his chest hurts, but he does not remember the accident. He is breathing rapid, shallow breaths because of pain and shortness of breath. His vital signs are as follows:

Temperature	98.9 °F
Blood pressure	110/60 mm Hg
Pulse rate	108 beats/min
Respirations	24 breaths/min

On examination, the neck veins are not distended; the anterior chest wall has a bruise in the right midclavicular area; and the underlying fourth, fifth, and sixth ribs are markedly tender to palpation. On auscultation of the chest, there is fairly poor air movement because the patient refuses to take a deep breath, with absent breath sounds on the right. The left side is clear to auscultation. On the right side of the chest, there is marked hyperresonance with percussion compared with the left. During the examination, the patient begins to get restless, his breathing becomes more labored, and his neck veins start to become distended. What is the appropriate intervention at this time?

(A) CT scan of the chest with contrast enhancement
(B) Pericardiocentesis
(C) Lateral and posteroanterior chest radiographs done in the radiology department to ensure adequate film quality
(D) Intubation with positive-pressure ventilation
(E) Needle thoracentesis

9 GENETICS

Step 2 questions often ask you to give genetic counseling to a parent or to predict the likelihood of having a second affected child after the first is born with a given disease. Because it is assumed that you know the inheritance pattern of the disease, the following information should come in handy. Many of the diseases discussed in this chapter are also presented in other chapters, but hey, a little extra review never hurt anyone.

AUTOSOMAL DOMINANT

Look for an affected mother or father who passes the disease to 50% of offspring:
- **von Willebrand disease:** The most common hereditary coagulation disorder. Results from dysfunctional platelets. Three types exist; types 1 and 2 are autosomal dominant, and type 3 (the most severe) is autosomal recessive. Look for easy bruising, nosebleeds, heavy menses, and bleeding gums.
- **Neurofibromatosis type 1:** Café-au-lait spots (Fig. 9-1), profuse peripheral nerve tumors (neurofibromas), and Lisch nodules (hamartomas of the iris). Neurofibromatosis type 2: bilateral acoustic neuromas.
- **Multiple endocrine neoplasia (MEN) syndromes**
  - Type 1: three Ps—Parathyroid adenomas, pancreatic endocrine tumors, pituitary adenomas
  - Type 2A: two Ps—Parathyroid adenomas, pheochromocytoma, medullary thyroid carcinoma
  - Type 2B: one P—Pheochromocytoma, medullary thyroid carcinoma, mucosal neuromas, marfanoid habitus
- **Achondroplasia:** common cause of dwarfism. You may be asked to make the diagnosis by looking at a picture of a patient.
- **Marfan syndrome:** Tall patient with arachnodactyly, hyperextensible joints, mitral valve prolapse, aortic dissection, and lens dislocation.
- **Huntington disease:** Triplet repeat disorder characterized by chorea (involuntary writhing movements). The late course of the disease includes behavioral and psychiatric disturbances, eventually leading to dementia. This is a commonly tested topic. Understand the concept of **anticipation**, which is described at the end of this chapter.
- **Familial hypercholesterolemia:** Look for xanthomas, early coronary artery disease, and markedly elevated cholesterol.
- **Familial polyposis coli** (aka **familial adenomatous polyposis**): Affected patients develop hundreds to thousands of polyps in the colon. Extremely high risk of malignancy; often managed with prophylactic total colectomy before age 25 years.
- **Adult polycystic kidney disease** (aka **autosomal dominant polycystic kidney disease**): Kidneys (and sometimes liver and pancreas) are filled with numerous fluid-filled cysts. Causes secondary hypertension and eventually leads to renal failure.
- **Hereditary spherocytosis:** Inherited hemolytic anemia; diagnosed by osmotic fragility test.
- **Tuberous sclerosis:** Hypopigmented skin macules, facial angiofibromas (i.e., adenoma sebaceum; Fig. 9-2), seizures, mental retardation, central nervous system hamartomas, rhabdomyomas, renal tumors.
- **Myotonic dystrophy:** Muscle weakness with an inability to release grip, balding, cataracts, mental retardation, cardiac arrhythmias. Triplet repeat disorder.

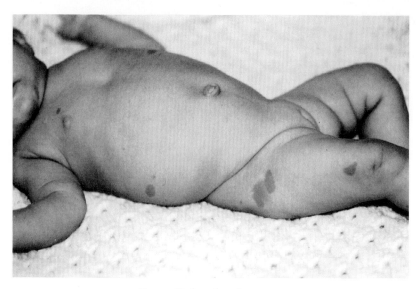

FIGURE 9-1 Café-au-lait spots.

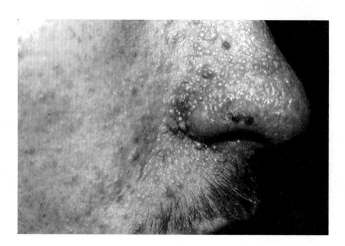

FIGURE 9-2 Facial aniofibromas.

AUTOSOMAL RECESSIVE

Look for family history and unaffected parents who pass the disease to 25% of children:
- **Sphingolipidoses** (e.g., Tay-Sachs disease and Gaucher disease; the exception is Fabry disease, which is X-linked)
- **Mucopolysaccharidoses** (e.g., Hurler disease; the exception is Hunter disease, which is X-linked)
- **Glycogen storage diseases** (e.g., Pompe and McArdle disease)
- **Cystic fibrosis:** Diagnosed by a sweat chloride test; leads to progressive lung disease and pancreatic insufficiency. Look for meconium ileus as an infant.
- **Galactosemia:** Look for congenital cataracts, neonatal sepsis; avoid galactose- and lactose-containing foods
- **Amino acid disorders** (e.g., phenylketonuria, alkaptonuria)
- **Sickle cell disease:** More common in African Americans; commonly presents with acute painful vaso-occlusive crisis. Hemoglobin S is the abnormal hemoglobin that leads to sickling.
- **Children's polycystic kidney disease** (aka **autosomal recessive polycystic kidney disease**): Cystic dilation of the renal collecting ducts and hepatic abnormalities. Babies may present with large palpable flank masses.
- **Wilson disease** (hepatolenticular degeneration): Disease of copper metabolism leading to cirrhosis and neuropsychiatric disturbances. Look for Kayser-Fleischer rings around the iris.

○ **Hemochromatosis:** There are four types of hemochromatosis, and all but type 4 are autosomal recessive. Characterized by excessive absorption of dietary iron, leading to cirrhosis, diabetes, skin pigment changes, and congestive heart failure. Often referred to as "bronze diabetes."
○ **Adrenogenital syndrome** (aka **congenital adrenal hyperplasia**): A group of diseases characterized by dysfunctional or lacking adrenal enzymes that alter primary or secondary sex characteristics. 95% are caused by 21-hydroxylase deficiency, which causes salt wasting (vomiting and dehydration) in addition to virilization.
○ **Werdnig-Hoffman disease:** Degeneration of the anterior horn cells in the spinal cord and brainstem (lower motor neurons). Most infants are hypotonic at birth, and all are affected by age 6 months. Look for a positive family history and a long and slowly progressive course of disease.

X-LINKED RECESSIVE

Only males are affected. Females are carriers.
○ **Hemophilia:** Hemophilia A (factor VIII deficiency) is more common than hemophilia B (factor IX deficiency). Look for hemarthroses and bleeding into the soft tissues.
○ **Glucose-6-phosphatase dehydrogenase deficiency:** A hemolytic anemia that can be triggered by infection or medication. Look for hemolysis that occurs when antimalarial or sulfa drugs are given.
○ **Fabry disease:** Sphingolipidosis, as above
○ **Hunter disease:** Mucopolysaccharidosis, as above
○ **Lesch–Nyhan syndrome:** Hypoxanthine-guanine phosphoribosyltransferase enzyme deficiency. Look for mental retardation, uric acid crystals in urine (found in the diaper), and self-mutilation (patients may bite off their own fingers).
○ **Duchenne (and Becker) muscular dystrophy:** Progressive loss of muscular strength. Look for pseudohypertrophy and Gower sign (child gets up by using the upper extremities to push self up). Becker muscular dystrophy is less severe.
○ **Wiscott–Aldrich syndrome:** Look for eczema, thrombocytopenia, and immunodeficiency.
○ **Bruton agammaglobulinemia** (aka X-linked agammaglobulinemia): Look for recurrent respiratory tract infections.
○ **Fragile X syndrome**: Second most common cause of mental retardation in males (after Down syndrome). Patients have large testes, long faces, and large ears. Triplet repeat disorder.

POLYGENIC DISORDERS

Relatives are more likely to have disease, but there is no obvious heritable pattern (yet …):
○ Pyloric stenosis
○ Cleft lip or palate
○ Type 2 diabetes
○ Obesity
○ Neural tube defects
○ Schizophrenia
○ Bipolar disorder
○ Ischemic heart disease
○ Alcoholism

CHROMOSOMAL DISORDERS

Down syndrome (trisomy 21; Figs. 9-3 and 9-4) is the most common known cause of mental retardation. The major risk factor is age of the mother (one in 1500 offspring of 16-year-old mothers; one in 25 for 45-year-old mothers). At birth, look for hypotonia, a transverse palmar crease, and characteristic facies. Congenital cardiac defects (especially ventricular septal defect) are common, and patients are at increased risk for leukemia, duodenal atresia (and other bowel atresias), Hirschsprung disease, celiac disease, hypothyroidism, obstructive sleep apnea, gastroesophageal reflux, upper respiratory tract infections, infertility, visual problems, and early Alzheimer disease.

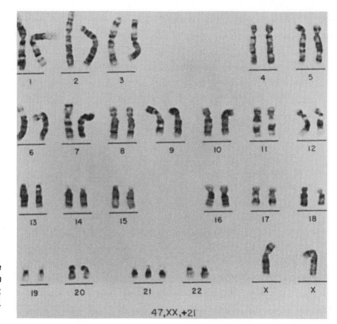

FIGURE 9-3 This karyotype in Down syndrome reveals three copies of chromosome 21. *(From Gabbe SG, Niebyl JR, Simpson JL: Obstetrics: Normal and Problem Pregnancies, 5th ed. Philadelphia, Churchill Livingstone, 2007.)*

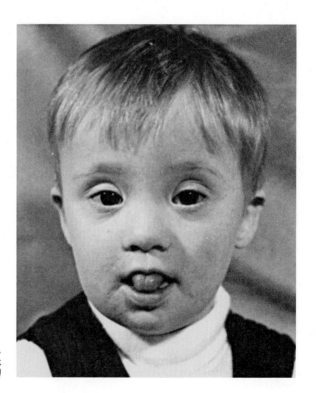

FIGURE 9-4 Down syndrome. *(From Kliegman RM, Behrman RE, Jenson HB, Stanton BF: Nelson Textbook of Pediatrics, 18th edition. Copyright 2007, Elsevier.)*

Edward syndrome (trisomy 18) is more common in females than males. Patients are small for their age and have mental retardation, a small head, a hypoplastic mandible, low-set ears, and clenched fists with the index fingers overlapping the third and fourth fingers (almost pathognomonic). Early pediatric death is typical.

Patau syndrome (trisomy 13) includes mental retardation, apnea, deafness, holoprosencephaly (fusion of cerebral hemispheres), myelomeningocele, cardiovascular abnormalities, rocker-bottom feet. Early pediatric death is typical.

Patients with **Turner syndrome** (XO instead of XX) have lymphedema of the neck at birth, short stature, a webbed neck, widely spaced nipples (a so-called shield chest), amenorrhea, and lack of breast development (caused by primary ovarian failure). Coarctation of the aorta is common (may cause secondary hypertension), and patients may have horseshoe kidneys or cystic hygroma (benign neck mass or lymphangioma). A buccal smear classically reveals absent Barr bodies.

In **Klinefelter syndrome** (XXY), the patient is tall and has microtestes (<2 cm in length), gynecomastia, sterility (the classic presentation is for infertility), and a mildly decreased IQ.

Cri-du-chat syndrome is caused by a deletion on the short arm of chromosome 5; look for a high-pitched cry like a cat along with severe mental retardation.

OTHER KEY CONCEPTS IN GENETICS

Penetrance is the proportion of individuals with a particular genotype that express the associated phenotype. It is important to know that not all genes are 100% penetrant. Expressivity is used to describe variations in the phenotype of individuals carrying a particular genotype. This basically means that patients with a particular genotype may not all have the same severity of disease.

Triplet repeat disorders (trinucleotide repeat disorders) are a group of genetic diseases caused by varying numbers of repeats of a specific three nucleotide combination. Examples include Huntington disease (CAG) and fragile X (CGG). These diseases have a critical number of repeats, above which the patient gets the disease (e.g., for Huntington disease, patients with under 35 CAG repeats do not get the disease, but patients with more than 40 repeats do get the disease). Triplet repeat disorders also demonstrate anticipation in which the severity of disease increases with each successive generation. Anticipation also often involves the manifestations of disease starting earlier in life with each successive generation.

QR CODE

The QR code includes three USMLE-style questions and answers. For more questions, redeem the PIN code on the inside cover for the Crush Step 2 question bank powered by USMLE Consult.

Please see the Introduction for instructions on how to access content using the QR codes.

Question

What is the most likely method of inheritance for schizophrenia?
(A) Autosomal dominant
(B) Autosomal recessive
(C) X-linked recessive
(D) Polygenic disorder

10 GERIATRICS

IMPORTANT POINTS

1. The most rapid increase in population in the United States (percentage-wise) is in people older than 65 years (now roughly 15% of the population). Within this group, the over-85 subgroup is increasing most rapidly.

2. At age 80 years, patients have half the lean body mass of a 30-year-old adult. Because basal metabolic rate depends on lean body mass, elderly patients need fewer calories.

3. Normal changes in elderly people include slightly impaired immune response, visual (presbyopia) and hearing (presbycusis) impairment, decreased muscle mass, increased fat deposits, osteoporosis, brain changes (decreased weight, enlarged ventricles and sulci), and a slightly decreased ability to learn new material.

4. Normal sexual function changes in men: Elderly men take longer to get an erection and have an increased refractory period (after ejaculation, it takes longer before the patient can have another erection). Delayed ejaculation is common, and the patient might ejaculate only one of every three times that he has sex. Impotence and lack of sexual desire are *not* normal and should be investigated. Look for psychological (depression) as well as physical causes such as vascular disease and neurologic disease. Medications, especially antihypertensives, are notorious culprits.

5. Normal sexual function changes in women: For decreased lubrication, advise water-soluble lubricants. Atrophy of the clitoris, labia, and vaginal tissues can cause dyspareunia; treat with estrogen cream (or hormone replacement therapy if desired by the patient). Delayed orgasm is common, but lack of sexual desire is *not* normal and should be investigated (psychological or physical causes).

6. The best prophylaxis for pressure ulcers in an immobilized patient is frequent turning at least every 2 hours. The most common sites for pressure ulcers are the sacral and coccygeal areas, ischial tuberosities, and greater trochanteric areas.

7. Sleep changes: Elderly people sleep less deeply, wake up more frequently during the night, and awaken earlier in the morning. They take longer to fall asleep (longer sleep latency) and have less stage 3 and 4 and rapid eye movement (REM) sleep.

8. Depression in elderly people can manifest as dementia (i.e., pseudodementia). Look for a history that would trigger depression (e.g., loss of a spouse, terminal or debilitating disease).

9. After age 65 years, 15% of people have dementia. The most common causes of dementia, in decreasing order, are Alzheimer disease (gradually progressive, with neurofibrillary tangles) and multi-infarct (stepwise, with risk factors for cerebrovascular accident). Other causes include hypothyroidism, HIV, and Pick disease. Test for reversible causes of dementia such as hypothyroidism, depression, and vitamin B_{12} deficiency. Be sure to be able to differentiate dementia from delirium (see the psychiatry chapter for a thorough discussion).

IMPORTANT POINTS—Cont'd

10. Only 5% of people older than 65 years live in nursing homes. The most common cause of pneumonia in nursing homes is *Streptococcus pneumoniae* infection. If the patient is at risk for aspiration, then a pneumonia is most likely caused by anaerobes.

11. More than 90% of hip fractures are associated with falls. Most occur in patients older than 70 years of age. Decrease the risk of falls in elderly individuals with mobility problems by fall-proofing the home (e.g., repair broken handrails or steps and slippery floors, remove items that can be tripped over), watching for medications that decrease the patient's sense of balance (the classic offenders are sedatives and anticholinergic drugs), and treating gait abnormalities (use of physical therapy and appropriate walking devices and shoes).

QR CODE

The QR code includes two USMLE-style questions and answers. For more questions, redeem the PIN code on the inside cover for the Crush Step 2 question bank powered by USMLE Consult.

Please see the Introduction for instructions on how to access content using the QR codes.

Question

Which of the following is true concerning persons older than age 65 years?
(A) About 40% have dementia.
(B) Only about 5% live in nursing homes.
(C) Approximately 2% to 3% of the population is older than age 65 years.
(D) *Sundowning* is a normal phenomenon in elderly adults.
(E) Elderly people are less likely to commit suicide than younger people are.

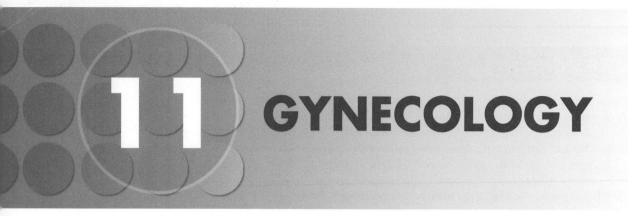

11 GYNECOLOGY

ADENOMYOSIS

In adenomyosis, the endometrial glands are found within the uterine musculature (i.e., part of the spectrum of endometriosis but confined to the uterus). Patients usually are older than 40 years and have dysmenorrhea and menorrhagia. Physical exam reveals a large, boggy uterus. Ultrasonography might suggest and magnetic resonance image (MRI) can confirm this diagnosis, which is usually clinical.

Do dilation and curettage (D&C) to rule out endometrial cancer and consider a total abdominal hysterectomy to relieve severe symptoms. Gonadotropin-releasing hormone agonists also can relieve symptoms.

AMENORRHEA

Primary Amenorrhea

Any girl who has not menstruated by age 16 years has primary amenorrhea. In the absence of secondary sexual characteristics by age 14 years or absence of menstruation within 2 years of developing secondary sex characteristics, patients also should be evaluated.

IMPORTANT POINTS

1. The first step is to rule out pregnancy! (Yes, pregnancy can manifest as primary amenorrhea.)
2. If the patient is older than 14 years and has no secondary sexual characteristics, she most likely has a congenital problem (i.e., Kallman syndrome).
3. In a phenotypically normal female patient (normal breast development) with an absence of both axillary and pubic hair, think of androgen insensitivity syndrome. The uterus is absent.
4. In the presence of normal breast development and a uterus, the first step is to get a prolactin level to rule out pituitary adenoma. If prolactin is high, get an MRI of the brain. If it is normal, administer progesterone and follow the same procedures as for evaluation of secondary amenorrhea.

Although it is not necessary to memorize the algorithm in Figure 11-1, it may be helpful in understanding the evaluation of primary amenorrhea. Don't forget to first rule out pregnancy.

Secondary Amenorrhea

Secondary amenorrhea is defined as the absence of menses for 3 months in a woman who has previously menstruated. The diagnosis is pregnancy until proven otherwise. Amenorrhea is not uncommon in hard-training athletes (caused by exercise-induced depression of gonadotropin-releasing hormone [GRH]). Watch for amenorrhea as a presenting symptom for anorexia (amenorrhea is required for a diagnosis of anorexia), especially in a ballet dancer or model. Another common cause is polycystic ovarian syndrome (PCOS; see later discussion). Secondary amenorrhea also may be caused by endocrine disorders (headaches, galactorrhea, and visual field defects can indicate a pituitary tumor), antipsychotics (caused by increased prolactin), or previous chemotherapy (which causes premature ovarian failure and menopause).

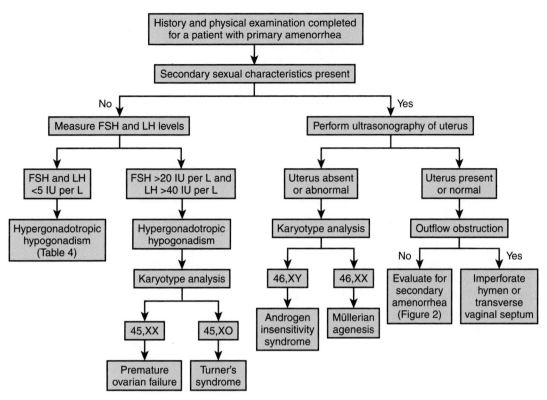

FIGURE 11-1 Evaluation of primary amenorrhea. Algorithm for the evaluation of primary amenorrhea. FSH, follicle-stimulating hormone; LH, = luteinizing hormone. *(From Master-Hunter T, Heiman DL. Amenorrhea: evaluation and treatment. Am Fam Physician. 2006;73(8):1374–1382.)*

The first step after a negative pregnancy test result and no obvious abnormality in the history or physical exam is to administer progesterone, which tells you the patient's estrogen status:

○ If the patient has vaginal bleeding within 2 weeks, she has sufficient estrogen. Next, check luteinizing hormone (LH). If the level is high, think of PCOS. If it is low or normal, check the prolactin level to rule out pituitary adenoma and the thyroid-stimulating hormone (TSH) level to rule out hypothyroidism (a high TSH level causes high prolactin level). If prolactin is high with normal TSH, get an MRI of the brain. If prolactin is normal, look for drug-, stress-, or exercise-induced depression of GRH. Any of these patients may try clomiphene to become pregnant.

○ If the patient does not have vaginal bleeding after the administration of progesterone, she has insufficient estrogen. Check follicle-stimulating hormone (FSH) next. If the level is elevated, the patient has premature ovarian failure (i.e., menopause); check for autoimmune disorders, karyotype abnormalities, and history of chemotherapy. If FSH is low or normal, the patient might have a craniopharyngioma or other central nervous system tumor; get an MRI of the brain. When in doubt, follow these steps *in order* to evaluate any amenorrhea:

1. Do a pregnancy test.
2. Administer progesterone.
3. Further testing depends on results of progesterone challenge (bleeding or no bleeding).

Any sexually active woman of reproductive age who has amenorrhea should have a pregnancy test as the first step in evaluation.

BIRTH CONTROL

○ There are four major types of birth control: behavioral (rhythm and withdrawal methods), barrier (condoms, diaphragm, cervical cap, copper IUD), hormonal (oral contraceptive pills [OCPs], injectable hormone depot preparations, implantable hormone devices, intravaginal hormone devices, and hormone-impregnated intrauterine devices), and sterilization.

○ The most effective forms of birth control are sterilization (e.g., tubal ligation or vasectomy), implants (etonogestrel implant) or an intrauterine device followed by injectable hormone depot preparations, then birth control pills or birth control patch or a hormonal vaginal ring.

○ OCPs are a good choice if the patient is a candidate and does not desire sterilization. OCPs do *not* reduce transmission of sexually transmitted infections (STIs).

○ An intrauterine device is most appropriate for older women, preferably those who are monogamous, because it increases the risk of ectopic pregnancy and pelvic inflammatory disease (PID) (look for *Actinomyces* spp.).

○ Condoms are good because they prevent transmission of STIs.

Oral Contraceptives

Absolute contraindications: Past or current venous thromboembolism (deep venous thrombosis or pulmonary embolism), cerebrovascular disease (stroke), coronary artery disease, complicated valvular heart disease, diabetes with complications, breast cancer, pregnancy, lactation (<6 weeks postpartum), liver disease, headaches with focal neurologic symptoms, major surgery with prolonged immobilization, age older than 35 years and smoking 15 or more cigarettes per day, and hypertension (blood pressure >160/100 mm Hg or with concomitant vascular disease).

Relative contraindications: Postpartum less than 21 days, lactation (6 weeks to 6 months), undiagnosed vaginal or uterine bleeding, age older than 35 years and smoking less than 15 cigarettes per day, history of breast cancer but no recurrence in the past 5 years, interacting drugs (e.g., certain anticonvulsants, rifampin), gallbladder disease, headaches without aura in patient age 35 years or older, and hypertension (well-controlled or blood pressure 140–159/90–99 mm Hg).

Side effects: Glucose intolerance (check for diabetes mellitus annually in women at high risk), depression, edema (bloating), weight gain, cholelithiasis, benign liver adenomas (Fig. 11-2), melasma ("the mask of pregnancy"), nausea, vomiting, headache, and hypertension.

Benefits: A 50% reduction in ovarian cancer; decrease in the incidence of endometrial cancer, menorrhagia, dysmenorrhea, benign breast disease, functional ovarian cysts (often prescribed for the previous four effects), premenstrual tension, iron-deficiency anemia, ectopic pregnancy, and salpingitis.

IMPORTANT POINTS

1. OCPs are one of the most common causes of secondary hypertension. All patients taking birth control pills who are noted to have increased blood pressure should discontinue the pills and then have their blood pressure rechecked at a later date.

2. Because of the risks of thromboembolism, OCPs should be stopped 1 month before elective surgery and not restarted until 1 month after surgery.

3. OCPs have little, if any, effect on the risk of developing breast cancer.

4. Cervical neoplasia may be increased in users of birth control pills, but this effect also may be caused by the confounding factor of increased sexual relations or number of partners. Nonetheless, users of birth control pills should have regular Pap smears.

5. The effectiveness of OCPs may be reduced by medications that induce the P450 system. It is important to warn your female patients taking OCPs that they may want to use a second form of birth control when starting a new medication, particularly antibiotics.

BREAST DISORDERS

Breast Discharge

First get the patient's history of OCPs, hormone therapies, antipsychotic medications, or hypothyroidism symptoms, all of which can cause discharge. When bilateral and nonbloody, the discharge is *not* caused by breast cancer; rather, the cause may be a prolactinoma (check prolactin) or endocrine disorder (check the TSH level). A discharge that is unilateral, bloody, or associated with a mass should raise concern about breast cancer. Biopsy all masses.

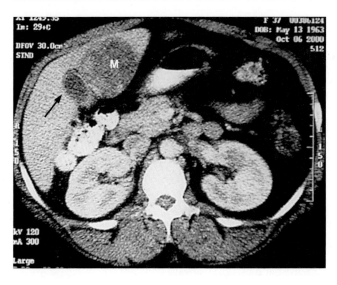

FIGURE 11-2 Liver adenoma. Contrasted computed tomography (CT) image demonstrating a nonspecific solid mass (M) in the left hepatic lobe adjacent to the gallbladder (*arrow*). The gallbladder is darker than the mass because of lower density of normal fluid in the gallbladder. Given a history of birth control pill use, this would be a slam dunk diagnosis for a hepatic adenoma on the boards (even without the CT image), but in the real world, it would likely have to be biopsied to exclude other tumor histology.

Breast Mass in a Woman Younger than 35 Years

○ **Fibrocystic disease:** *Bilateral*, multiple, tender (especially premenstrually) *cystic lesions*. Most common of all breast diseases. Generally, no further workup is needed—just routine follow-up. OCPs, progesterone for 1 week at the end of each month, or danazol might help to relieve symptoms.

○ **Fibroadenoma:** Painless, discrete, sharply circumscribed, unilateral, rubbery, mobile mass. Most common benign tumor of the female breast. Observe the patient for one or more menstrual cycles in the absence of symptoms. Pregnancy or OCPs can stimulate growth; menopause causes regression (estrogen-dependent growths). Excision is curative but not required (unless the patient desires it or there is clinical concern for cancer). Recurrence is common.

○ **Mastitis or abscess:** Lactating women typically in the first few months postpartum may develop painful, swollen erythematous breast(s). The nipple may be cracked or fissured. The patient should be treated with analgesics (e.g., acetaminophen, ibuprofen) and instructed to continue breastfeeding with the affected breast(s) even though it is painful (use a breast pump to empty the breast if needed) to prevent further milk duct blockage and abscess formation. An antistaphylococcal antibiotic (e.g., cephalexin, dicloxacillin) is given for more than mild symptoms. Methicillin-resistant *Staphylococcus aureus* (MRSA) is becoming an increasingly important pathogen in mastitis. Use trimethoprim–sulfamethoxazole or clindamycin if MRSA is a concern or is cultured. If a fluctuant mass develops or there is no response to antibiotics within a few days, an abscess is likely present and must be drained.

○ **Fat necrosis:** History of trauma in the area of the mass.

IMPORTANT POINTS

1. If a breast mass is found in a young woman (i.e., younger than age 35 years), you still must confirm that it is benign.

2. When presented with a young woman with a new dominant breast mass that persists through a few menstrual cycles, proceed to ultrasonography and possibly biopsy. Although it is most likely to be a fibroadenoma, this cannot be assumed.

Avoid mammography in women younger than 30 years (breast tissue is too dense to give interpretable films). If suspicious of cancer (exceedingly rare in this age group), use ultrasonography for evaluation.

Breast Mass in a Woman 35 Years or Older

○ **Fibrocystic disease:** As above, but aspiration of cyst fluid and baseline mammography are recommended. If the cyst fluid is nonbloody and the mass resolves after aspiration, the patient needs only reassurance, follow-up, and a baseline mammogram. If the fluid is bloody or the cyst recurs quickly, do a biopsy to rule out cancer.

○ **Fibroadenoma:** Get baseline mammogram. Observe briefly if the mass is small *and* seems benign clinically *and* the woman is premenopausal *and* she has no risk factors for breast cancer. Otherwise, do a biopsy. Watch for phyllodes tumor (previously called cystosarcoma phyllodes) that masquerades as fibroadenoma. Phyllodes tumors are typically large and fast growing.

○ **Fat necrosis:** As for younger women

○ **Mastitis or abscess:** As for younger women

○ **Breast cancer:** You might not get a classic presentation of nipple retraction or peau d'orange in a nulliparous woman with a strong family history. In a woman 35 years or older, you will rarely be faulted for doing a biopsy of any new mass. In the absence of a classic benign presentation (e.g., trauma to the breast with fat necrosis or bilaterality with premenstrual mastalgia), always consider biopsy. Also get a diagnostic mammogram (first imaging study) and potentially ultrasonography or breast MRI. (See Chapter 21, Oncology.)

IMPORTANT POINTS

1. If the patient is postmenopausal (or older than 50 years) and develops a new breast mass, you should be highly suspicious of malignancy on the boards.

2. In patients with a clinically evident breast mass, the decision to perform a biopsy is a clinical one. Mammography (and ultrasonography and increasingly MRI) is often done to help evaluate the mass and in a woman older than 35 years can serve as a baseline for future comparison. If a mass is detected on imaging and not clearly or probably benign, biopsy is generally recommended.

3. Conversely, any suspicious lesion found on mammography (or other imaging) should be biopsied even if it is inapparent or seems benign on physical exam.

ABNORMAL UTERINE BLEEDING

In women of childbearing age, abnormal uterine bleeding includes any change in menstrual period frequency, duration, or amount of flow, as well as bleeding between cycles. When abnormal uterine bleeding is evaluated, it is important to make certain that the bleeding is not from a gastrointestinal or urinary source. After it is clear that the bleeding is vaginal, pregnancy should be the first consideration in women of childbearing age. Common causes of abnormal bleeding include medications (e.g., anticoagulants, hormonal contraception), systemic conditions (e.g., thyroid, hematologic, pituitary, and hypothalamic disorders), and genital tract disease (e.g., cervical cancer, STD, trauma, uterine fibroids, endometrial polyps, endometrial hyperplasia, endometrial cancer).

Dysfunctional uterine bleeding (DUB) is defined as abnormal uterine bleeding not associated with tumor, inflammation, or pregnancy. DUB is the most common cause of abnormal uterine bleeding and is a diagnosis of exclusion. More than 70% of cases are associated with anovulatory cycles (unopposed estrogen, as occurs in PCOS). The age of the patient is important. After menarche and just before menopause, DUB is extremely common and, in fact, physiologic. Most other patients have polycystic ovaries, the most common nonphysiologic cause of DUB.

Postmenopausal bleeding is defined as vaginal bleeding starting 12 months or more after the cessation of menses or unscheduled bleeding in a postmenopausal woman who has been taking hormone replacement therapy (HRT) for 12 months or more.

Always do a D&C to rule out endometrial cancer in women older than 35 years. Also get hemoglobin and hematocrit to make sure that the patient is not anemic from excessive blood loss.

Uncommon causes of DUB are infections, endocrine disorders (thyroid, adrenal, pituitary or prolactin), coagulation defects, and estrogen-producing neoplasm.

> ## IMPORTANT POINTS
>
> **1.** In the absence of pathology, treat with nonsteroidal antiinflammatory drugs (NSAIDs) if the patient desires pregnancy or levonorgestrel intrauterine device if pregnancy is not desired.
> **2.** OCPs are also a first-line agent for menorrhagia and DUB if the patient does not desire pregnancy and cycles are irregular.
> **3.** Progesterone can be used to help stop severe bleeding.

ENDOMETRIOSIS

Endometriosis is endometrial glands outside the uterus (ectopic). Patients usually are nulliparous and older than 30 years with the following symptoms: **dysmenorrhea, dyspareunia** (painful intercourse), **dyschezia** (painful defecation), or perimenstrual spotting. The most common site is the ovaries (look for tender adnexae in an afebrile patient) followed by the broad or uterosacral ligament (classic signs are nodularities on physical exam and sequela of a retroverted uterus) and peritoneal surface. The gold standard of diagnosis is laparoscopy with visualization of endometriosis. Ultrasonography or MRI can sometimes make the diagnosis noninvasively.

> ## IMPORTANT POINTS
>
> **1.** Endometriosis is the most likely cause of infertility in a menstruating woman older than 30 years (in the absence of a PID history).
> **2.** Treat first with OCPs (danazol, gonadotropin-releasing hormone agonists, and progestins are second-line agents).
> **3.** Surgery and cautery may be used to destroy the endometriomas in an attempt to restore fertility. In an older patient, consider total abdominal hysterectomy and bilateral salpingo-oophorectomy for severe symptoms.

HORMONE REPLACEMENT THERAPY

HRT (i.e., estrogen with or without progesterone) is now controversial and probably best used only as a means of symptom relief. Observation during therapy is necessary because estrogen and progesterone are not harmless. Every woman should make the decision on her own after weighing the risks and benefits.

The known benefits of estrogen therapy include a decreased risk of osteoporosis and decreased fractures, reduced hot flashes and genitourinary symptoms of menopause (e.g., dryness, urgency, atrophy-induced incontinence, frequency), and decreased risk of colorectal cancer (according to the Women's Health Initiative, with combined estrogen and progesterone therapy).

The known risks of estrogen therapy include an increased risk of endometrial cancer (decreased by co-administration of progesterone), a small increase in the risk of coronary heart disease with combined estrogen and progesterone therapy (although the risk is not increased in women who are less than 10 years postmenopausal or 50–59 years of age), an increased risk of venous thromboembolism, an increased risk of breast cancer (according to the Women's Health Initiative, when combined estrogen and progesterone therapy is used there was a slightly decreased risk of breast cancer with estrogen only, although this decrease was not statistically significant), an increased risk of stroke (according to the Women's Health Initiative, with either estrogen only or combined estrogen and progesterone therapy), and an increased risk of gallbladder disease.

INFERTILITY

Infertility is defined as the inability to achieve pregnancy after 12 months of unprotected sexual activity. In two-thirds of couples, infertility is a female problem; in one-third, it is a male problem. If nothing is apparent after history and physical exam, the first step is **semen analysis** (cheap, easy, noninvasive). Normal semen has the following properties:

○ Ejaculate volume >1 mL
○ Sperm concentration >20 million/mL
○ Initial forward motility >50% of sperm
○ Normal morphology >60% of sperm

The next step is documentation of ovulation. History might suggest an ovulatory problem (irregular cycle length, duration, or amount of flow; lack of premenstrual symptoms). Basal body temperature, luteal phase progesterone levels, or an endometrial biopsy can be done to check for ovulation.

Tubal and uterine evaluation is done by a hysterosalpingogram (Figs. 11-3 and 11-4). History might suggest a tubal problem (PID, previous ectopic pregnancy) or a uterine problem (previous D&C [can cause intrauterine synechiae], adhesions, scarring [Asherman syndrome], fibroids or endometriosis).

Cervical factor may be a cause of infertility and is suggested by a history of cervicitis, birth trauma, or previous cone biopsy. Evaluate cervical mucus and do a postcoital test.

Laparoscopy is a last resort or is done in patients with a history suggestive of endometriosis. Lysis of adhesions and destruction of endometriosis lesions can restore fertility.

Medical therapy for infertility is usually clomiphene citrate to induce ovulation, but this approach requires that the woman is producing adequate estrogen. If the woman is hypoestrogenic, use human menopausal gonadotropin (hMG), which is a combination of FSH and LH. If these methods fail, use in vitro fertilization.

LEIOMYOMA

Leiomyomas are also called fibroids and are benign tumors (Fig. 11-5). However, they are the most common indication for hysterectomy (when they grow too large or cause symptoms). Look for rapid growth during pregnancy or use of OCPs with regression after menopause (tumors are estrogen dependent). Fibroids can cause infertility; myomectomy might restore fertility. Other symptoms include pain and menorrhagia or metrorrhagia. Anemia caused by leiomyoma is an indication for hysterectomy. D&C rules out endometrial cancer and malignant transformation

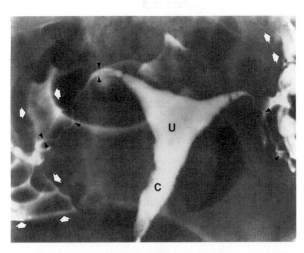

FIGURE 11-3 Normal hysterosalpingogram. Contrast is seen filling the endocervical canal (C) and the uterine cavity (U). The fallopian tubes (*black arrowheads*) and bilateral free spillage of contrast (*white arrows*) are demonstrated.

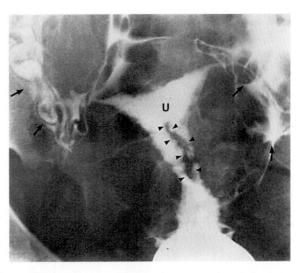

FIGURE 11-4 Uterine synechiae (Asherman syndrome) shown as an irregular filling defect (*arrowheads*) in the lower uterine cavity (U) on this abnormal hysterosalpingogram. Bilateral free spillage of contrast (*arrows*) confirms patency of the fallopian tubes.

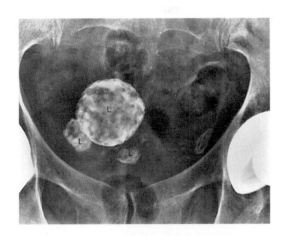

FIGURE 11-5 Plain radiograph of the pelvis shows typical calcifications within three separate uterine leiomyomas (L).

in women older than 35 years. Patients might present with a polyp protruding through the cervix. Malignant transformation is rare (<1%). Treatments include medroxyprogesterone acetate or danazol to slow or stop bleeding. GnRH analogs are also used because they decrease the size of leiomyomas, suppress further growth, and decrease surrounding vascularity. Uterine artery embolization also may be tried.

 Any sexually active woman of reproductive age with abnormal uterine bleeding should have a pregnancy test as the first diagnostic step.

If a uterine mass continues to grow after menopause, make sure to rule out malignancy.

MENOPAUSE

Menopause is defined as the cessation of menses for a minimum of 12 months because of the cessation of follicular development. The average age at menopause is 51 years. Cessation of menses and ovarian failure before age 40 years is considered premature menopause or premature ovarian failure.

Perimenopausal and menopausal patients have irregular cycles or amenorrhea, hot flushes, mood swings, and elevated FSH levels. Patients also might complain of dysuria; dyspareunia; incontinence; or vaginal itching, burning, or soreness—symptoms that often are caused by atrophic vaginitis in this age group. Look for vaginal mucosa to be thin, dry, and atrophic, with increased parabasal cells on cytology. Topical estrogens can be used to relieve vaginal symptoms. Long-term systemic estrogens (HRT with or without progestin) are seldom used these days because of the increased risk of cardiovascular disease, cerebrovascular accident, venous thromboembolism, invasive breast cancer, and gallbladder disease (see the previous discussion on HRT).

PELVIC INFLAMMATORY DISEASE

PID is typically caused by an ascending sexually transmitted infection of the upper female genital tract that may involve the endometrial cavity (endometritis), fallopian tubes (salpingitis), ovaries (oophoritis), parametrial tissues or ligaments (parametritis), or peritoneal cavity (peritonitis). Look for a female patient ages 13 to 35 years with abdominal pain, adnexal tenderness, and cervical motion tenderness (all three must be present). PID also requires one or more of the following: elevated erythrocyte sedimentation rate (or C-reactive protein), leukocytosis, fever, purulent cervical discharge, or purulent fluid from culdocentesis. Treat with more than one antibiotic (e.g., cefoxitin or ceftriaxone and doxycycline on an outpatient basis; clindamycin and gentamicin on an inpatient basis) to cover multiple organisms (e.g., *Neisseria gonorrhoeae*, *Chlamydia* spp., *Escherichia coli*). With a history of intrauterine device use, think *Actinomyces israelii*.

IMPORTANT POINTS

1. PID is the most common cause of preventable infertility (causes scarring of the fallopian tubes) and the most likely cause of infertility in a normally menstruating woman younger than age 30 years.
2. Watch for progression to tuboovarian abscess (palpable on exam) and its rupture. Treat with antibiotics on an inpatient basis initially; perform laparotomy with excision of the affected tube (unilateral disease) or total abdominal hysterectomy and bilateral salpingo-oophorectomy (bilateral disease) if there is no response or worsening symptoms over the first 24 to 48 hours.

PELVIC RELAXATION AND VAGINAL PROLAPSE

Pelvic relaxation and vaginal prolapse are caused by weakening of pelvic supporting structures. Look for history of several vaginal deliveries, a feeling of heaviness or fullness in the pelvis, backache, worsening of symptoms with standing, and resolution with lying down.

○ **Cystocele:** Bladder bulges into the upper anterior vaginal wall. Symptoms: urinary urgency, frequency, incontinence.
○ **Rectocele:** Rectum bulges into the lower posterior vaginal wall. Major symptom: difficulty with defecating.
○ **Enterocele:** Loops of bowel bulge into the upper posterior vaginal wall.
○ **Urethrocele:** Urethra bulges into the lower anterior vaginal wall. Symptoms: urinary urgency, frequency, incontinence.

 Conservative treatment involves pelvic strengthening exercises, a pessary (an artificial device inserted into the vagina to provide support), or both. Surgery is used for refractory or severe cases.

POLYCYSTIC OVARIAN SYNDROME

The classic presentation is an overweight woman with hirsutism, amenorrhea, and infertility. PCOS is the most likely cause of infertility in women younger than 30 years with abnormal menstruation. Multiple ovarian cysts may be seen on ultrasonography (although not needed for diagnosis). A high LH level and androgen excess (e.g., testosterone, androstenedione) are present and the ratio of LH to FSH is greater than 2 to 1. Unopposed estrogen increases the risk for endometrial hyperplasia and cancer. Spironolactone can be used to treat hirsutism associated with PCOS.

Treat with OCPs or cyclic progesterone. If the patient desires pregnancy, use clomiphene. Patients have an increased risk of insulin resistance and diabetes; metformin is often used in the treatment of PCOS.

VAGINAL INFECTIONS

Vaginal infections are described in Table 11-1. Figure 11-6 shows gram-negative diplococci that probably indicate gonorrhea.

IMPORTANT POINTS

1. Chlamydia is treated with erythromycin or amoxicillin if the patient is pregnant. If compliance is an issue (alcoholic, drug-abusing, homeless, or unreliable patient), you can give azithromycin, 1 g orally all at once, and watch the patient take it.
2. Any patient with gonorrhea is generally treated for presumed chlamydial coinfection (e.g., give ceftriaxone *and* doxycycline). The reverse, however, is not true.
3. With all infections except *Candida* and *Gardnerella* spp., treat the patient's sexual partners and give counseling (e.g., condoms).
4. All of the above information is similar for men (except candidal infection), but all lesions and discharges are on or come from the penis.

TABLE 11-1 Vaginal Infections 101

BUG	FINDINGS	TREATMENT
Candida albicans	"Cottage cheese" discharge, pseudohyphae on KOH preparation; history of diabetes mellitus, antibiotic treatment, pregnancy	Topical or oral antifungal
Chlamydia trachomatis	Most common sexually transmitted disease; dysuria, positive culture or antibody test result	Doxycycline, azithromycin
Gardnerella vaginalis	Malodorous discharge; fishy smell on KOH preparation; clue cells	Metronidazole
Herpes	Multiple shallow, painful ulcers; recurrence and resolution	Acyclovir, valacyclovir
Human papillomavirus	Venereal warts, koilocytosis on Pap smear	Many (acid, cryotherapy, laser, podophyllin)
Molluscum contagiosum	Characteristic appearance of lesions, intracellular inclusions	Many (curettage, cryotherapy, coagulation)
Neisseria gonorrhoeae	Mucopurulent cervicitis; gram-negative bugs on Gram stain	Ceftriaxone or cefixime
Pediculosis	"Crabs"; itching, lice on pubic hairs	Permethrin cream
Primary syphilis	Painless chancre, spirochete on dark-field microscopy	Penicillin
Secondary syphilis	Condyloma lata, maculopapular rash on palms, serology	Penicillin
Trichomonas vaginalis	Bugs can be seen swimming under microscope; pale green, frothy, watery discharge; "strawberry" cervix	Metronidazole

KOH, potassium hydroxide.

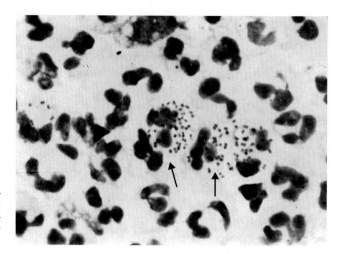

FIGURE **11-6** Gram stain of an endocervical or urethral exudate or discharge revealing leukocytes containing gram-negative diplococci (*arrows*). This is virtually diagnostic for gonorrhea.

QR CODE

The QR code includes three USMLE-style questions and answers. For more questions, redeem the PIN code on the inside cover for the Crush Step 2 question bank powered by USMLE Consult.

Please see the Introduction for instructions on how to access content using the QR codes.]

Question

A 29-year-old woman comes to you concerned about the risks versus the benefits of oral contraceptive pills for birth control. Which of the following is true regarding oral contraceptive pills?
(A) They usually worsen dysmenorrhea.
(B) They commonly cause weight loss.
(C) They reduce the incidence of ovarian cancer.
(D) They reduce the incidence of hypertension.
(E) They are often given to women with active liver disease because they tend to lessen liver inflammation.

12 HEMATOLOGY

ANEMIA

Definition: Hemoglobin <12 mg/dL in women or <14 mg/dL in men

Symptoms include fatigue, dyspnea on exertion, lightheadedness, dizziness, syncope, palpitations, angina, and claudication. **Signs** include tachycardia, pallor (especially of the sclera and mucous membranes), systolic ejection murmurs (from high flow), and signs of the underlying cause (e.g., jaundice in hemolytic anemia, positive stool guaiac in gastrointestinal [GI] bleed). Important clues in the history:

- **Medications:** Many medications can cause anemia through various mechanisms. The classic example is methyldopa, which causes red blood cell (RBC) antibodies and hemolysis (penicillins and sulfa drugs can do the same). Chloroquine and sulfa drugs cause hemolysis in glucose-6-phosphate dehydrogenase (G6PD) deficiency. Phenytoin causes megaloblastic anemia through interference with folate metabolism. Chloramphenicol, chemotherapeutic agents, and zidovudine cause aplastic anemia and bone marrow suppression.
- **Blood loss:** Trauma, surgery, melena, hematemesis, menorrhagia
- **Chronic diseases:** Liver disease, chronic kidney disease, and hypothyroidism are common causes of anemia of chronic disease. Also look for inflammatory and debilitating conditions, such as autoimmune diseases, infections, and cancer. Chronic conditions such as migraine headaches and osteoarthritis do not cause anemia of chronic disease (must be ongoing significant systemic inflammation).
- **Family history:** Hemophilia, thalassemia, G6PD deficiency, sickle cell disease, and so on
- **Alcoholism:** Anemia in people with alcoholism is often multifactorial and can be attributable to the direct toxic effects of alcohol, iron deficiency caused by GI bleeding, nutritional deficiencies (iron, folate, and vitamin B_{12} deficiencies), and anemia of chronic disease.
- Steps to diagnosing the cause of anemia:
1. Complete blood count (CBC) with differential and RBC indices. First and foremost, hemoglobin and hematocrit must be below normal. The mean corpuscular volume (MCV) tells you whether the anemia is microcytic (MCV <80 fl), normocytic (MCV 80–100 fl), or macrocytic (MCV >100 fl).
2. Peripheral smear. Classic findings (Table 12-1) can make for an easy diagnosis.
3. Reticulocyte index (RI). The RI should be greater than 2% with anemia; otherwise, the marrow is not responding properly. If the index is very high, think of hemolysis as the cause (the marrow is responding properly, so it is not the problem).

With these three parameters, you can make a reasonable differential diagnosis if the cause is not obvious (Box 12-1).

Clues to the presence of hemolytic anemia:
- Elevated lactate dehydrogenase (LDH)
- Elevated bilirubin (unconjugated as well as conjugated if the liver is working)
- Jaundice
- Low or absent haptoglobin (with intravascular hemolysis)
- Positive urobilinogen, bilirubin, or hemoglobin in the urine

Only conjugated bilirubin appears in the urine, and hemoglobin appears only when haptoglobin has been saturated, as in brisk intravascular hemolysis.

TABLE 12-1 Classic Findings of Anemia on Peripheral Smear

SMEAR FINDING	USUAL CAUSE
Acanthocytes, spur cells	Abetalipoproteinemia
Basophilic stippling	Lead poisoning
Bite cells	G6PD deficiency and other hemolytic anemias
Echinocytes, burr cells	Uremia
Heinz bodies	G6PD deficiency and α-thalassemia
Howell-Jolly bodies	Asplenia, splenic dysfunction
Hypersegmented neutrophils	Folate or vitamin B_{12} deficiency
Iron inclusions in RBCs of bone marrow	Sideroblastic anemia
Parasites inside RBCs	Malaria, babesiosis
Polychromasia	Reticulocytosis (consider hemolysis)
Rouleaux formation	Multiple myeloma
Schistocytes, helmet cells, fragmented RBCs	Intravascular hemolysis
Sickled cells	Sickle cell anemia
Spherocytes, elliptocytes	Hereditary spherocytosis or elliptocytosis
Target cells	Thalassemia, liver disease
Teardrop-shaped RBCs	Myelofibrosis

G6PD, glucose-6-phosphate dehydrogenase; RBC, red blood cell.

Box 12-1 Reticulocyte Indexing in the Diagnosis of Anemia

MICROCYTIC	NORMOCYTIC	MACROCYTIC
Normal to Elevated Reticulocyte Index		
Hemoglobinopathy Thalassemia	Acute blood loss Hemolytic (multiple causes) Medications (antibody causing)	None; all forms have a low RI
Low Reticulocyte Index		
Anemia of chronic disease (some) Iron deficiency Lead poisoning Sideroblastic anemia	Anemia of chronic disease (some) Aplastic anemia Cancer, dysplasia (e.g., myelophthisic anemia) Endocrine failure (thyroid, pituitary) Renal failure	Vitamin B_{12} deficiency Cirrhosis, liver disease Folate deficiency Medications (methotrexate, phenytoin)

RI, reticulocyte index

Microcytic Anemias

Iron-Deficiency Anemia

Iron deficiency (Fig. 12-1) is the most common cause of anemia in the United States. On CBC, the RBC is decreased, and the RDW is elevated. The primary screening test is ferritin. Also look for low iron, elevated total iron-binding capacity (TIBC; also known as transferrin), and low TIBC saturation. Rarely, patients have a craving for ice or dirt (pica) or Plummer-Vinson syndrome (esophageal web producing dysphagia, iron-deficiency anemia, and glossitis). In a patient older than 40 years, rule out colon cancer as a cause of chronic blood loss. Iron-deficiency anemia is common in women of reproductive age because of menstrual blood loss. The most definitive diagnostic test for iron-deficiency anemia is bone marrow stain looking for decreased iron stores, although this is seldom required in clinical practice.

Give iron supplements to all infants except full-term infants who are exclusively breastfed. Start iron supplementation at 4 to 6 months for full-term infants and at 2 months for preterm infants. Giving cow's milk before 1 year of age can cause anemia through GI bleeding. Iron supplements also are commonly given during pregnancy and lactation because of increased demand.

Treat iron-deficiency anemia by correcting the underlying cause, if possible, and prescribe oral iron supplementation for roughly 3 to 6 months to replete body iron stores.

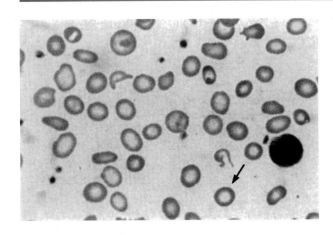

Figure 12-1 Peripheral blood smear showing iron-deficiency anemia: hypochromia (*arrow*), microcytosis, and poikilocytosis.

Thalassemia

Both thalassemia and iron deficiency cause microcytic, hypochromic anemia, but thalassemia must be differentiated from iron deficiency. Patients with thalassemia often have an elevated RBC, but the RDW is often normal to mildly increased. Iron levels are normal in thalassemia; iron is contraindicated because it can cause overload. Look for elevated hemoglobin A2 (β-thalassemia only) or hemoglobin F (β-thalassemia only), target cells, nucleated RBCs, radiography of the skull showing a "crew-cut" appearance, splenomegaly, and positive family history. Thalassemia is more common in blacks, Mediterraneans, and Asians.

Diagnosis is made by hemoglobin electrophoresis. There are four gene loci for the α-chain but only two for the β-chain. α-Thalassemia is symptomatic at birth or the fetus dies in utero (hydrops); β-thalassemia is not symptomatic until 6 months of age.

No treatment is required for minor thalassemia; patients often are asymptomatic because they are used to living at a lower level of hemoglobin and hematocrit. Thalassemia major is more dramatic and severe. Treat with as-needed transfusions and iron chelation therapy to prevent secondary hemochromatosis.

Lead Poisoning

Lead poisoning is classically seen in children and causes a hypochromic, microcytic anemia. With acute poisoning, look for vomiting, ataxia, colicky abdominal pain, irritability (aggressive behavior, behavioral regression), encephalopathy, cerebral edema, or seizures. Usually, however, poisoning is chronic and low level; look for pica (especially paint chips and dust in old buildings, which often still have lead paint), residence in an old or neglected building; basophilic stippling on peripheral smear, and an elevated venous blood lead level or free erythrocyte protoporphyrin. See Chapter 24, Pediatrics, for information on screening for lead poisoning.

Treat initially with decreased exposure (best strategy) as well as lead chelation therapy if needed. Use succimer in children and dimercaprol in adults; in severe cases, use dimercaprol plus ethylenediamine tetraacetic acid (EDTA) for children or adults.

Sideroblastic Anemia

Caused by defective heme synthesis. Test results show a microcytic, hypochromic anemia with elevated iron and ferritin levels and decreased TIBC (which distinguishes it from iron deficiency), polychromatophilic stippling, and the classic ringed sideroblast cell in the bone marrow. Sideroblastic anemia may be related to myelodysplasia or future blood dyscrasia. It may also be caused by certain drugs (e.g., isoniazid, chloramphenicol, alcohol). Manage supportively; in rare cases, the anemia responds to pyridoxine. Do not give iron!

Anemia of Chronic Disease

Anemia of chronic disease can be normocytic or microcytic. Look for diseases that cause chronic inflammation (rheumatoid arthritis, lupus erythematosus, cancer, tuberculosis), which leads to iron trapping in macrophages. Serum iron is low, but so is TIBC (thus, the percent saturation may be nearly normal). Serum ferritin is elevated (because ferritin is an acute-phase reactant, the level should be increased). Treat the underlying disorder to correct the anemia. Do not give iron!

Normocytic Anemias

Acute Blood Loss

Remember that immediately after blood loss, hemoglobin may be normal (takes a few hours to re-equilibrate). Look for pale cold skin, tachycardia, and hypotension. Transfuse if indicated even with a normal hemoglobin in the appropriate acute setting. Consider internal hemorrhage in the setting of trauma and abdominal aortic aneurysm in patients with a pulsatile abdominal mass.

Autoimmune Hemolytic Anemia

Autoimmune hemolytic anemia has several etiologies: lupus-like syndromes (or medications that cause lupus, e.g., procainamide, hydralazine, and isoniazid), drugs (classic is methyldopa; also penicillins, cephalosporins, sulfas, and quinidine), leukemia, lymphoma, or infection (classic is *Mycoplasma* spp.; also Epstein-Barr virus). Coombs test result is positive (presence of warm immunoglobulin G [IgG] antibodies against RBCs), and peripheral smear might reveal spherocytes because of incomplete macrophage destruction of RBCs. Treatment may include steroids, splenectomy, or both.

Sickle Cell Anemia

Peripheral smear gives it away (Fig. 12-2). Look for very high percentage of reticulocytes (8%–20%). Sickle cell anemia is almost always seen in blacks (8% are heterozygotes in the United States). Watch for classic manifestations of sickle cell disease:

○ Acute chest syndrome (mimics pneumonia)
○ Aplastic crises (caused by parvovirus B19 infection)
○ Autosplenectomy (increased infections with encapsulated bugs such as *Pneumococcus*, *Haemophilus*, and *Neisseria* spp.). The presence of Howell-Jolly bodies indicates a nonfunctioning spleen.
○ Bone pain (caused by bone infarcts; the classic example is avascular necrosis of the femoral or humeral head)
○ Dactylitis (hand–foot syndrome; classic initial manifestation in infants)
○ Renal papillary necrosis
○ Pigment cholelithiasis
○ Priapism
○ Splenic sequestration crisis
○ Stroke

Diagnosis is made by hemoglobin electrophoresis. Screening is done at birth, but symptoms usually do not appear until around 6 months of age because of lack of adult hemoglobin production. Treat with prophylactic penicillin until at least 5 years of age and perhaps longer (start as soon as the diagnosis is made), proper vaccination (including pneumococcal, meningococcal, and *Haemophilus influenzae* vaccines as well as yearly influenza vaccine), folate supplementation, early treatment of infections, and proper hydration.

A sickle cell crisis is characterized by severe pain in various sites caused by RBC sickling. Treat with oxygen, lots of intravenous (IV) fluids, and analgesics (including narcotics). Consider transfusions if symptoms or findings are severe.

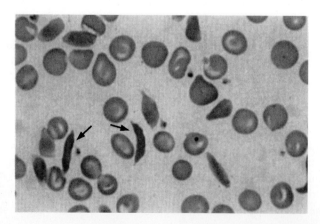

FIGURE 12-2 Sickle cell anemia. Sickled erythrocytes are prominent (*arrows*). Functional hyposplenia is indicated by the presence of a Howell-Jolly body (nuclear remnant in erythrocyte [center]).

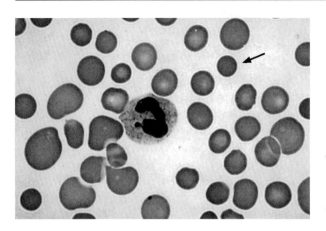

FIGURE 12-3 Hereditary spherocytosis. The peripheral smear reveals multiple fairly small red blood cells with intense staining and absent central pallor (*arrow*), which are called spherocytes. (*From Rubin R, Strayer DS, Rubin E (eds): Pathology, 6th ed. Philadelphia, Lippincott Williams & Wilkins, 2012, Figure 20-18, with permission.*)

Spherocytosis

Diagnosis is made from peripheral smear (Fig. 12-3), family history (autosomal dominant), splenomegaly, positive osmotic fragility test result, and an increased mean corpuscular hemoglobin concentration. Also look for reticulocytosis, hyperbilirubinemia, and a negative Coombs test result. Treatment often involves splenectomy. Give folic acid supplements. Remember that spherocytes may be seen in extravascular hemolysis (but the osmotic fragility test result is normal).

End-Stage Renal Disease

The kidneys make erythropoietin, so give erythropoietin in end-stage renal disease to correct the anemia. Make sure the patient dose not have an iron-deficiency anemia as well because this needs to be treated for erythropoietin to work. Patients with chronic renal failure develop a normocytic, normochromic anemia with a decreased reticulocyte count.

Aplastic Anemia

Aplastic anemia is usually idiopathic. It may be caused by chemotherapy or radiation, malignancy (especially acute leukemias), benzene, and medications (chloramphenicol, carbamazepine, phenylbutazone, sulfa drugs, zidovudine [AZT]). Look for decreased white blood cells (WBCs) and platelet count. Treat by stopping any possible causative medication. Patient might need antithymocyte globulin, colony-stimulating factors (e.g., erythropoietin, sargramostim, filgrastim, and pegfilgrastim), or bone marrow transplant.

Myelophthisic Anemia

Myelophthisic (or myeloplastic) anemia is usually caused by myelofibrosis or malignant invasion and destruction of bone marrow (most common cause). Look for marked anisocytosis (different size), poikilocytosis (different shape), nucleated RBCs, left shift in the granulocytes, and teardrop-shaped RBCs on the peripheral smear. A bone marrow biopsy is usually done and might reveal no cells (dry tap from fibrotic marrow in myelofibrosis) or malignant-looking cells.

Glucose-6-Phosphate Dehydrogenase Deficiency

X-linked recessive (males affected); most common in blacks and Mediterraneans. Look for sudden hemolysis or anemia after fava bean or drug exposure (antimalarials, salicylates, sulfa drugs) or after infection. Heinz bodies and "bite cells" may be seen on peripheral smear. Diagnosis is with an RBC enzyme assay (done when the patient is asymptomatic to avoid a false-negative result). Treat by avoiding precipitating foods and drugs (discontinue the triggering medication first).

Paroxysmal Nocturnal Hemoglobinuria

An intravascular hemolytic anemia and hypercoagulable state that may lead to aplastic anemia. Look for increased LDH and reticulocyte count and decreased haptoglobin level. Diagnose with flow cytometry. Treat with steroids, the monoclonal antibody eculizumab, or bone marrow transplant.

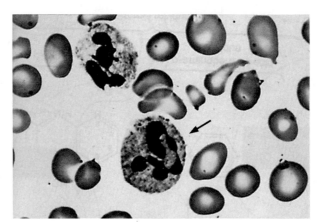

FIGURE   **12-4** Hypersegmented neutrophils (*arrow*) and large oval erythrocytes with poikilocytosis (irregular shape of red blood cells) seen in both folate and vitamin B$_{12}$ deficiencies. (*From Bonner H, Bagg A, Cossman J: The blood and the lymphoid organs. In Rubin E, Farber JL (eds): Pathology, 3rd edition. Philadelphia, Lippincott-Raven, 1999, pp. 1050–1151; with permission.)*

Macrocytic Anemias
Folate Deficiency

Folate deficiency (Fig. 12-4) is commonly seen in people with alcoholism (poor intake) and pregnant women (increased need). All women of reproductive age should take folate supplements to prevent neural tube defects in their offspring. Rare causes of folate deficiency include a poor diet (e.g., tea and toast), methotrexate, prolonged trimethoprim–sulfamethoxazole therapy, phenytoin, and malabsorption. Look for macrocytes and hypersegmented neutrophils with no neurologic signs or symptoms. Check folate level (serum or RBC). Treat with oral folate.

Vitamin B$_{12}$ Deficiency

Vitamin B$_{12}$ deficiency (see Fig. 12-4) is most commonly caused by pernicious anemia (antiparietal cell antibodies). Achlorhydria (no stomach acid secretion and elevated stomach pH), antiparietal cell or anti-intrinsic factor antibodies, and an elevated gastrin level generally confirm pernicious anemia as the cause of vitamin B$_{12}$ deficiency. Homocysteine is elevated in patients with vitamin B$_{12}$ and folate deficiencies; however, methylmalonic acid is elevated only with vitamin B$_{12}$ deficiency.

Vitamin B$_{12}$ deficiency can also result from gastrectomy, terminal ileum resection, diet (strict vegan), chronic pancreatitis, and *Diphyllobothrium latum* (fish tapeworm) infection. Look for neurologic deficiencies (loss of sensation, loss of position sense, paresthesias, ataxia, spasticity, hyperreflexia, positive Babinski sign, dementia), and glossitis. Check serum vitamin B$_{12}$. A nuclear medicine Schilling test can be helpful in cases with uncertain etiology. Treat with vitamin B$_{12}$ supplementation, usually via the parenteral (intramuscular) route because most patients cannot absorb the vitamin through the gut.

Miscellaneous rare causes of anemia:
- *Clostridium perfringens,* malaria, or babesiosis infection
- Endocrine failure (especially pituitary, liver, or thyroid)
- Hemolysis caused by microangiopathy (disseminated intravascular coagulation [DIC], thrombotic thrombocytopenic purpura [TTP], hemolytic uremic syndrome). Look for schistocytes and RBC fragments.
- Hypersplenism (always has splenomegaly and often low platelets and WBCs)
- Mechanical heart valves (which hemolyze RBCs)

TRANSFUSIONS

Transfusions are always based on clinical grounds. Treat the patient, not the lab value; there is no such thing as a trigger value for transfusion. Different blood components have different indications:
- **Whole blood:** Used only for rapid, massive blood loss or exchange transfusions (poisoning, TTP).
- **Packed RBCs:** Used instead of whole blood when the patient needs a transfusion.
- **Washed RBCs:** Free of traces of plasma, WBCs, and platelets; good for IgA deficiency and allergic or previously sensitized patients.

- **Platelets:** Given for symptomatic thrombocytopenia (usually <10,000/μL).
- **Granulocytes:** Rarely used for neutropenia with sepsis caused by chemotherapy (colony-stimulating factors such as filgrastim preferred).
- **Fresh-frozen plasma:** Contains all clotting factors; used for bleeding diathesis when one cannot wait for vitamin K to take effect (DIC, severe warfarin poisoning) or when vitamin K will not work (liver failure).
- **Cryoprecipitate:** Contains fibrinogen and factor VIII; used in von Willebrand disease and DIC.

The most common cause of a hemolytic blood transfusion reaction is lab error. Type O negative blood can be used when you cannot wait for blood typing or the blood bank does not have the patient's type. If a transfusion reaction occurs, the first step is to stop the transfusion! ABO mismatch can cause fever, hemolysis, DIC, and flank pain within 1 hour of transfusion. Patients with associated oliguria should be treated with IV fluids and diuresis (mannitol or furosemide). Massive transfusions can lead to bleeding diathesis from thrombocytopenia (look for oozing from puncture or IV sites) and citrate (calcium chelator). Hyperkalemia can also develop.

Types of transfusion reactions:

- **Allergic reaction** (urticaria, edema, dizziness, dyspnea, wheezing, anaphylaxis) from reaction to a (usually unknown) component in donor serum
- **Febrile reaction** (chills, fever, headache, back pain) from antibodies to WBCs
- **Hemolytic reaction** (anxiety or discomfort, dyspnea, chest pain, shock, jaundice) from antibodies to RBCs; usually occurs 2 to 10 days after transfusion

DISSEMINATED INTRAVASCULAR COAGULATION

DIC is most commonly caused by pregnancy and obstetric complications (50%), malignancy (30%), sepsis, and trauma (especially head trauma, prostate surgery, and snake bites). DIC usually manifests as bleeding diathesis. Look for the classic oozing or bleeding from puncture or IV sites, but patients might have thrombotic tendencies. Lab results reveal prolonged prothrombin time (PT), partial thromboplastin time (PTT), and bleeding time; positive D dimer and increased fibrin degradation products; thrombocytopenia; and decreases in fibrin and clotting factors (including factor VIII, which is normal in hepatic necrosis).

Treat the underlying cause (evacuate uterus; give antibiotics). Patients might need transfusions, fresh-frozen plasma, or (rarely) heparin (only in the presence of thrombosis).

EOSINOPHILIA AND BASOPHILIA

Causes of eosinophilia or increased eosinophil counts include:

- Idiopathic etiology
- Adrenal insufficiency
- Allergy
- Angioedema
- Atopy (allergic rhinitis, asthma, atopic dermatitis)
- Autoimmune diseases (e.g., lupus)
- Blood dyscrasias (especially lymphoma)
- Drug reactions
- Eczema
- Fungal infections
- IgA deficiency
- Immune disorders (Wiskott-Aldrich syndrome, hyper-IgE syndrome, IgA deficiency, thymoma)
- Loffler syndrome (pulmonary eosinophilia)
- Malignancies (lymphoma, leukemia, lung cancer, gastric cancer, pancreatic cancer, colon cancer, ovarian cancer)
- Parasitic infections

With basophilia, or an increased basophil count, think of allergies, neoplasm, or blood dyscrasia.

COAGULOPATHIES

The lupus anticoagulant can cause a prolonged PTT, but the patient has a tendency toward thrombosis. Look for associated lupus symptoms, positive Venereal Disease Research Laboratory or rapid plasma reagin test result for syphilis, or a history of miscarriages. Factor V Leiden; prothrombin G20210A gene mutation; hyperhomocysteinemia; elevated factor VIII level; and deficiencies in protein C, protein S, or antithrombin III can also cause an increased tendency toward thrombosis. Other causes of increased tendency toward thrombosis include antiphospholipid syndrome (lupus anticoagulant and anticardiolipin antibody), pregnancy, cancer, and estrogen-containing medications. Patients are treated with anticoagulant therapy to prevent deep venous thrombosis, pulmonary embolism, and other complications.

The differential diagnosis of the coagulopathies is given in Table 12-2.

Clotting tests: Use PT for extrinsic system (prolonged by warfarin), PTT for intrinsic system (prolonged by heparin but not affected by low-molecular-weight heparins), and bleeding time for platelet function. Causes of thrombocytopenia include:

- Alcohol
- Autoimmune disease
- Deficiencies (vitamin B_{12} or folate)
- DIC
- Hemolytic uremic syndrome
- Heparin (treat by first stopping heparin)
- Human immunodeficiency virus (HIV) infection
- Idiopathic thrombocytopenic purpura
- Medications (especially quinidine and sulfa drugs)
- Pancytopenia of any cause
- Splenic sequestration
- TTP

Bleeding from thrombocytopenia is in the form of petechiae, nosebleeds, and easy bruising.

 Do not give platelets to a patient with TTP or heparin-associated thrombocytopenia because doing so can cause thrombosis.

TABLE 12-2 Differential Diagnosis of Bleeding Disorders

DISEASE	PT	PTT	BT	PLATELET COUNT	RBC COUNT	OTHER
DIC	High	High	High	Low	Normal or low	Appropriate history, low factor VIII level
Hemophilia A or B	Normal	High	Normal	Normal	Normal	X-linked recessive; A = low factor VIII, B = low factor IX
Heparin	Normal	High	Normal	Normal or low	Normal	Watch for thrombocytopenia and thrombosis
ITP	Normal	Normal	High	Low	Normal	Watch for preceding URI
TTP	Normal	Normal	High	Low	Low	Hemolysis, CNS symptoms; treat with plasmapheresis; do not give platelets
Liver failure	High	Normal or high	Normal	Normal or low	Normal or low	Jaundice, normal factor VIII level; do not give vitamin K (ineffective)
Scurvy	Normal	Normal	Normal	Normal	Normal	Fingernail and gum hemorrhages, bone hemorrhages
von Willebrand disease	Normal	High	High	Normal	Normal	Autosomal dominant (look for family history)
Warfarin	High	Normal	Normal	Normal	Normal	Vitamin K antagonist (factors II, VII, IX, and X)

BT, bleeding time; CNS, central nervous system; DIC, disseminated intravascular coagulation; ITP, idiopathic thrombocytopenic purpura; PT, prothrombin time; PTT, partial thromboplastin time; RBC, red blood cell; TTP, thrombotic thrombocytopenic purpura; URI, upper respiratory infection.

Vitamin C deficiency (scurvy) can cause bleeding similar to that seen with low platelets (splinter and gum hemorrhages, petechiae); perifollicular and subperiosteal hemorrhages are unique to scurvy. Patients have a poor diet history (classic examples are hot dogs and soda or tea and toast diets), myalgias and arthralgias, and capillary fragility. Bleeding is caused by collagen dysfunction in the blood vessels. Treat with oral vitamin C. Easy bruising can also be caused by chronic steroid use, uremia (platelet dysfunction), and inherited tissue disorders (Ehlers-Danlos syndrome, Marfan syndrome).

End-stage renal disease can cause a coagulopathy with a normal platelet count because the platelets do not function properly. Look for a normal PTT and increased bleeding time. Treat with desmopressin (DDAVP).

QR CODE

The QR code includes three USMLE-style questions and answers. For more questions, redeem the PIN code on the inside cover for the Crush Step 2 question bank powered by USMLE Consult.

Please see the Introduction for instructions on how to access content using the QR codes.

Question

A 27-year-old G2P0 woman with a history of two miscarriages comes into the office with pain and swelling in her right leg. She denies other symptoms on thorough review of systems. An ultrasound scan reveals a blood clot in the right femoral vein. She is otherwise healthy, thin, and active; has no recent trauma or prolonged immobilization; and is not taking any medications or pills. Laboratory tests reveal the following:

Prothrombin time	Normal
Partial thromboplastin time	Slightly prolonged
Bleeding time	Normal
Hemoglobin	14 g/dL
Mean corpuscular volume	90 μm/cell
Platelet count	250,000/μL
VDRL syphilis test	Positive
HIV test	Negative

What is the most likely cause of this woman's blood clot?
(A) Syphilis-induced phlebitis
(B) Protein S deficiency
(C) Underlying malignancy
(D) Lupus anticoagulant
(E) Protein C deficiency

13 IMMUNOLOGY

HYPERSENSITIVITY

There are four types of hypersensitivity reactions: type I (anaphylactic), type II (cytotoxic), type III (immune complex mediated), and type IV (cell mediated [delayed]).

Type I (Anaphylactic)

Type I reaction is caused by preformed immunoglobulin E (IgE) antibodies, which cause release of vasoactive amines (e.g., histamine, leukotrienes) from mast cells and basophils. Examples are anaphylaxis (bee stings, food allergy [especially peanuts and shellfish], medications [especially penicillin and sulfa drugs], rubber glove allergy), atopy, hay fever, urticaria, allergic rhinitis, and some forms of asthma.

With chronic type I hypersensitivity (atopy, some asthma, allergic rhinitis), look for eosinophilia, elevated IgE levels, family history, and seasonal exacerbations. Patients also might have allergic shiners (bilateral infraorbital edema) and a transverse nasal crease (from frequent nose rubbing). Pale, bluish, edematous nasal turbinates with many eosinophils in clear, watery nasal secretions also are classic.

If patients have nasal polyps, do not give aspirin; you might precipitate a severe asthmatic attack.

True systemic anaphylaxis causes a dramatic and rapid change in status (e.g., flushing, itching, facial swelling, severe respiratory distress, hypotension, or shock) that classically occurs within seconds (intravenous [IV] drug) to minutes (oral) of exposure to medication or iodinated contrast. Patients can die within minutes. Treat immediately by securing the airway. Laryngeal edema can prevent intubation, in which case do a cricothyrotomy, if needed. Give subcutaneous (second choice is IV) epinephrine. Steroids are sometimes given for severe reactions, but they take hours to have an effect and are a secondary consideration, so they are not primary therapy in this setting.

C1 esterase inhibitor (complement) deficiency is a cause of hereditary angioedema. Patients have diffuse swelling of the lips, eyelids, and possibly the airway or bowel unrelated to any allergen exposure. The deficiency is autosomal dominant; look for a positive family history. C4 complement is low. Treat acutely as anaphylaxis; androgens are used for long-term treatment to increase liver production of C1 esterase inhibitor.

Skin testing might identify an allergen if it is not obvious.

Type II (Cytotoxic)

Type II reaction is caused by preformed IgG and IgM, which react with antigen and cause secondary inflammation. Examples are autoimmune hemolytic anemia (classic causes are methyldopa or penicillin or sulfa drugs) and other cytopenias caused by antibodies (e.g., idiopathic thrombocytopenic purpura), transfusion reactions, erythroblastosis fetalis (Rh incompatibility), Goodpasture syndrome (watch for linear immunofluorescence on kidney biopsy), myasthenia gravis, Graves disease, pernicious anemia, pemphigus, and hyperacute transplant rejection (as soon as the anastomosis is made at transplant surgery, the transplanted organ deteriorates in front of your eyes).

 With anemia caused by a type II hypersensitivity reaction, watch for a positive Coombs test result; in pregnancy, watch for a positive indirect Coombs test result.

Type III (Immune Complex–Mediated) Reaction

Type III (immune complex–mediated) reaction is caused by deposits of antigen–antibody complexes (usually in vessels) that cause an inflammatory response. Examples are serum sickness, lupus, rheumatoid arthritis, polyarteritis nodosa, chronic hepatitis, cryoglobulinemia, and glomerulonephritis.

Type IV (Cell-Mediated) Reaction

Type IV (cell-mediated [delayed]) reaction is caused by sensitized T lymphocytes, which release inflammatory mediators. Examples include tuberculosis skin test, contact dermatitis (especially poison ivy, nickel earrings, cosmetics, medications), chronic transplant rejection, and granulomas (e.g., sarcoidosis).

HUMAN IMMUNODEFICIENCY VIRUS AND ACQUIRED IMMUNODEFICIENCY SYNDROME

Initial seroconversion can manifest as a mononucleosis-type syndrome (fever, malaise, pharyngitis, rash, lymphadenopathy). Keep HIV seroconversion in the back of your mind as a differential diagnosis for any sore throat or Epstein-Barr virus–type presentation. Neonates can present with oral thrush, failure to thrive, and lymphadenopathy. Diagnosis is made with the enzyme-linked immunosorbent assay (ELISA), which, if the result is positive, should be confirmed with a Western blot test. Do all tests before you tell the patient anything! It takes 6 to 12 weeks for antibodies to develop in the majority of patients; antibodies are present by 6 months in 95% of patients. Therefore, if a patient comes to you for testing because of recent risk-taking behavior, you should retest the patient in 6 months if the initial test result is negative.

IMPORTANT POINTS

1. After the diagnosis of HIV infection has been made, the patient should get a CD4 count every 3 to 4 months. CD4 counts may be repeated every 6 months for patients who are adherent to therapy with sustained viral suppression and stable clinical status for more than 2 to 3 years.
2. Antiretroviral therapy should be started when the CD4 count falls below $350/mm^3$ (or sooner if there is a history of an AIDS-defining illness). Antiretroviral therapy also should be initiated in pregnant women, in patients with HIV-associated nephropathy, and in patients with hepatitis B coinfection.
3. When the CD4 count is less than $200/mm^3$, start prophylaxis for *Pneumocystis jiroveci* pneumonia (PCP). Use trimethoprim–sulfamethoxazole (TMP-SMX). If the patient is allergic to or intolerant of TMP-SMX, use dapsone or pentamidine.
4. When the CD4 count is less than $50/mm^3$, start prophylaxis for *Mycobacterium avium intracellulare* with azithromycin or clarithromycin; rifabutin is an alternative. Consider cryptococcal and candidal prophylaxis with fluconazole.
5. When the CD4 count is less than $200/mm^3$, the patient is automatically considered to have AIDS (even without opportunistic infections).
6. Give measles, mumps, and rubella (MMR) vaccine to HIV-positive patients if the CD4 count is above $200/mm^3$; this is the only live vaccine given to HIV patients.
7. Give pneumococcal, hepatitis B, inactivated polio vaccine, and annual influenza vaccines to all HIV-positive patients. Give a tetanus booster every 10 years.
8. Do an annual purified protein derivative (PPD) test for tuberculosis in HIV patients; get an annual chest radiograph if the patient is anergic.
9. Do not give oral polio vaccine to HIV-positive patients or their contacts.
10. Classic AIDS-associated malignancies include Kaposi sarcoma (due to human herpesvirus 8) and non-Hodgkin lymphoma (especially primary B-cell lymphomas of the central nervous system).

(Continued)

IMPORTANT POINTS—Cont'd

11. A positive India ink preparation of the cerebrospinal fluid indicates *Cryptococcus neoformans* meningitis.

12. Ring-enhancing lesions in the brain usually mean toxoplasmosis (Fig. 13-1) or lymphoma. Also consider cysticercosis (*Taenia solium*) in Latin American patients.

13. Other commonly seen HIV sequelae include wasting syndrome (progressive weight loss), dementia, peripheral neuropathies, thrombocytopenia, and loss of delayed hypersensitivity (type IV) on skin testing (anergy).

14. Give pregnant HIV-positive patients zidovudine (AZT or ZDV) and give infants zidovudine 6 weeks after birth. This protocol reduces mother-to-child transmission from roughly 25% to 8%. The infant can have a falsely positive HIV antibody test for 6 to 12 months because of maternal antibodies. Check DNA or RNA polymerase chain reaction test (or perform culture) to detect the virus directly. Cesarean section also can reduce transmission.

15. HIV-positive mothers should not breastfeed because they can transmit the disease to their infants through breast milk.

16. Use valganciclovir for cytomegalovirus retinitis; foscarnet or cidofovir are second-choice agents.

17. In any patient with HIV and pneumonia, think of PCP first, especially if the CD4 count is below $200/mm^3$ (although plain community-acquired pneumonia is probably more common). Look for severe hypoxia with normal radiographs or diffuse, bilateral interstitial and air-space infiltrates. Usually the patient has a dry, nonproductive cough. PCP may be detectable with silver stains (Wright-Giemsa, Giemsa, methenamine silver) of induced sputum; if not, bronchoscopy with bronchoalveolar lavage and brush biopsy can make the diagnosis if needed, but patients are generally treated empirically initially and, if response occurs, invasive testing is not needed. Treat with TMP-SMX; pentamidine is an alternative if the patient has a sulfa allergy.

18. Any adult patient with thrush should make you think of HIV, leukemia, or diabetes. Think of *Candida* infection in HIV patients with a sore throat.

19. Any young adult who presents with herpes zoster should make you consider HIV.

20. *Cryptosporidium* and *Isospora* spp. are diarrheal infections uniquely seen in HIV-positive patients.

21. For dirty needle sticks, do an HIV test and start highly active antiretroviral therapy (HAART) immediately. Repeat the HIV test in 6 weeks, 3 months, and 6 months.

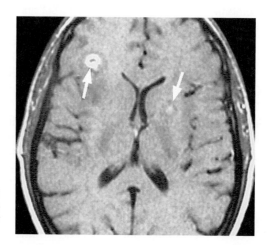

FIGURE 13-1 Toxoplasmosis in an immunosuppressed patient. Lesions on contrast-enhanced magnetic resonance image may be either ring enhancing (*left arrow*) or nodular (*right arrow*).

PRIMARY IMMUNODEFICIENCIES

Because primary immunodeficiencies are rare, your job is simply to recognize the classic case presentation.

○ **IgA deficiency:** The most common primary immunodeficiency. Look for recurrent respiratory and gastrointestinal (GI) infections. IgA is low, and IgG subclass 2 may be low. Do not give immunoglobulins; you might cause anaphylaxis caused by development of anti-IgA antibodies. Alternatively, in any patient who develops anaphylaxis after immunoglobulin exposure, you should think of IgA deficiency.

○ **X-linked agammaglobulinemia (Bruton agammaglobulinemia):** X-linked recessive disorder (i.e., affects male patients). B cells are low or absent; infections begin after 6 months when maternal antibodies disappear. There is a poor response to immunizations. Look for recurrent lung and sinus infections with *Streptococcus* and *Haemophilus* spp.

○ **DiGeorge syndrome:** Caused by hypoplasia of the third and fourth pharyngeal pouches. Look for hypocalcemia and tetany (from absent parathyroids) in the first 24 to 48 hours of life. Also look for absent or hypoplastic thymus, congenital heart defects, and typical facies. These patients are particularly susceptible to fungal and viral infections.

○ **Severe combined immunodeficiency (SCID):** May be autosomal recessive or X-linked. Many cases are caused by adenosine deaminase deficiency (autosomal recessive). Patients have B- and T-cell defects and severe infections in the first few months of life, and cutaneous anergy usually is present. Other signs include an absent or dysplastic thymus and lymph nodes.

○ **Wiskott-Aldrich syndrome:** X-linked recessive disorder that affects male patients. Look for classic triad: eczema, thrombocytopenia (look for bleeding), and recurrent infections (usually respiratory).

○ **Chronic granulomatous disease:** Usually an X-linked recessive disorder (i.e., male patients). Patients have a defect in nicotinamide adenine dinucleotide phosphate (NADPH) oxidase activity and thus get recurrent infections with catalase-positive organisms (e.g., *Staphylococcus aureus*, *Pseudomonas* spp.). The diagnosis is clinched if the question mentions deficient nitroblue tetrazolium (NBT) dye reduction by granulocytes (measures respiratory burst, which patients lack) or positive superoxide production testing. On the USMLE, if you see "CGD," then look for "NBT" in the answer.

○ **Chediak-Higashi syndrome:** Usually autosomal recessive. Look for giant granules in neutrophils and associated oculocutaneous albinism. The cause is a defect in microtubule polymerization.

○ **Complement deficiencies:** C5 through C9 deficiencies cause recurrent *Neisseria* infections; specific complement component is low.

○ **Chronic mucocutaneous candidiasis:** A cellular immunodeficiency specific for *Candida* spp. Patients have candidal thrush, scalp, skin, and nail infections and anergy to *Candida* spp. with skin testing. Hypothyroidism is often an associated finding. The rest of the immune function is intact; no other types of infection are present.

○ **Hyper IgE syndrome (Job-Buckley syndrome):** Patients get recurrent staphylococcal infections (especially of the skin) and have extremely high IgE levels. They also commonly have fair skin, red hair, and eczema.

○ **Hyper IgM syndrome:** Look for increased IgM and decreased IgG and IgA levels. There is a poor response to immunizations. These children are susceptible to *P. jiroveci*, sinopulmonary, and GI infections.

○ **Leukocyte adhesion defect:** Look for delayed separation of the umbilical cord, necrotic skin lesions, and early loss of teeth.

○ **Abnormal B-lymphocyte maturation:** Presents at 6 months of age after maternal antibodies disappear. These children are prone to bacterial infections.

QR CODE

The QR code includes two USMLE-style questions and answers. For more questions, redeem the PIN code on the inside cover for the Crush Step 2 question bank powered by USMLE Consult.

Please see the Introduction for instructions on how to access content using the QR codes.

Question

What condition should you suspect if a patient has an anaphylactic reaction to immunoglobulin therapy?
(A) Emphysema
(B) Leukemia
(C) IgA deficiency
(D) Severe combined immunodeficiency
(E) DiGeorge syndrome

14 INFECTIOUS DISEASE

GENERAL

Table 14-1 lists empiric treatment to use while waiting for test results. Table 14-2 lists empiric treatment for various bacteria.

Staining hints:

- ○ Gram-positive organisms are blue-purple; gram-negative organisms are red.
- ○ Gram-positive cocci in chains = streptococci
- ○ Gram-positive cocci in clusters = staphylococci
- ○ Gram-positive cocci in pairs (diplococci) = *Streptococcus pneumoniae*
- ○ Gram-negative coccobacilli (small rods) = *Haemophilus* spp.
- ○ Gram-negative diplococci = *Neisseria* (gonorrhea, septic arthritis, meningitis) or *Moraxella* spp. (lungs, sinusitis)
- ○ Gram-negative rod that is plump and has a thick capsule (mucoid appearance) = *Klebsiella* spp.
- ○ Gram-positive rods that form spores = *Clostridium, Bacillus* spp.
- ○ Pseudohyphae = *Candida* spp. (hyphae are a marker for the presence of fungi; Fig. 14-1)
- ○ Acid-fast organisms = *Mycobacterium* tuberculosis, *Nocardia* spp.
- ○ Gram-positive organism with sulfur granules = *Actinomyces* spp. (pelvic inflammatory disease in women who use intrauterine devices; rare cause of neck mass and cervical adenitis)
- ○ Silver-staining = *Pneumocystis jiroveci* and cat-scratch disease
- ○ Positive India ink preparation (thick capsule) = *Cryptococcus* spp.
- ○ Spirochete = *Treponema, Leptospira* spp. (both seen only on dark-field microscopy), *Borrelia* spp. (regular light microscope)
- ○ Catalase positive organisms = *Staphylococcus aureus, Serratia* spp., *Klebsiella* spp., *Aspergillus* spp.
- ○ Classic topics for infectious disease questions:
  - ○ Patient (perhaps a gardener) stuck with thorn: *Sporothrix schenckii* (a fungus). Treat with itraconazole, fluconazole, or oral potassium iodide.
  - ○ Aplastic crisis in sickle cell disease or other hemoglobinopathy: parvovirus B19
  - ○ Sepsis after splenectomy (or autosplenectomy in sickle cell disease): *S. pneumoniae, H. influenzae, N. meningitidis* (encapsulated bugs)
  - ○ Pneumonia in the Southwest (California, Arizona): *Coccidioides immitis;* treat with itraconazole, fluconazole, or amphotericin B (for severe disease)
  - ○ Pneumonia after cave exploring or exposure to bird droppings in Ohio and Mississippi River valleys: *Histoplasma capsulatum;* causes acute pulmonary symptoms, fever, malaise; treat with intravenous amphotericin B; lifelong itraconazole if HIV positive
  - ○ Pneumonia after exposure to a parrot or exotic bird: *Chlamydia psittaci*
  - ○ Fungus ball or hemoptysis after tuberculosis-induced cavitary disease: *Aspergillus* spp. Look for a "halo sign" on computed tomography (CT); treat with voriconazole
  - ○ Pneumonia in a patient with silicosis: tuberculosis
  - ○ Diarrhea after hiking or drinking from a stream: *Giardia lamblia;* cysts in stool; treat with metronidazole.
  - ○ Pregnant women with cats: *Toxoplasma gondii*; treat with spiramycin
  - ○ Vitamin B_{12} deficiency and abdominal symptoms: *Diphyllobothrium latum*
  - ○ Seizures with ring-enhancing brain lesion on CT: *Taenia solium* (cysticercosis) or toxoplasmosis; treat with albendazole or praziquantel, usually with steroids; consider anticonvulsants
  - ○ Bladder cancer (squamous cell) in Middle East and Africa: *Schistosoma haematobium*

Table 14-1 Empiric Therapy while Awaiting Culture and Sensitivity Results

CONDITION	MAIN ORGANISM(S)	EMPIRIC ANTIBIOTIC(S)
Bronchitis	Virus, *Haemophilus influenzae*, *Moraxella* spp.	Usually no benefit from antibiotics. May consider a macrolide or doxycycline.
Cellulitis	Streptococci, staphylococci	Cephalexin or dicloxacillin. Use clindamycin or trimethoprim–sulfamethoxazole if MRSA is suspected.
Endocarditis	Staphylococci, streptococci	Antistaphylococcal penicillin† (or vancomycin) + aminoglycoside
Meningitis (child or adult)	*Streptococcus pneumoniae*, *Neisseria meningitidis**	Cefotaxime or ceftriaxone + vancomycin
Meningitis (neonate)	Streptococci B, *Escherichia coli*, *Listeria* spp.	Ampicillin + aminoglycoside, third-generation cephalosporin that enters the CSF (cefotaxime)
Osteomyelitis	*Staphylococcus aureus*, *Salmonella* spp.	Oxacillin, cefazolin, vancomycin
Pneumonia (atypical)	*Mycoplasma, Chlamydia* spp.	Macrolide antibiotic, doxycycline
Pneumonia (classic)	*S. pneumoniae*, H. *influenzae*	Third-generation cephalosporin, azithromycin
Septic arthritis‡	*S. aureus*	Antistaphylococcal penicillin, vancomycin
	Gram-negative bacilli	Ceftazidime or ceftriaxone or cefotaxime
	Gonococci	Ceftriaxone or cefotaxime
Sepsis	Gram-negative organisms, streptococci, staphylococci	Third-generation penicillin or cephalosporin + aminoglycoside, imipenem
Urinary tract infection	*E. coli*	Trimethoprim-sulfamethoxazole, nitrofurantoin, amoxicillin, quinolones

**H. influenzae* type b is no longer as common a cause of meningitis in children because of widespread vaccination. In a child with no history of immunization, *H. influenzae* is the most likely cause of meningitis.
†Examples: dicloxacillin, methicillin.
‡Think of staphylococci if the patient is monogamous or not sexually active. Think of gonorrhea for younger adults who are sexually active.
CSF, cerebrospinal fluid.

Table 14-2 Empiric Antibiotics of Choice for Different Bugs*

BUG	ANTIBIOTIC	OTHER CHOICES
Bacteroides sp.	Metronidazole	Clindamycin
Borrelia spp.	Doxycycline (not recommended for children younger than 8 years old or pregnant or lactating women), amoxicillin, cefuroxime	Erythromycin
Chlamydia spp.	Azithromycin, doxycycline	Erythromycin, ofloxacin, levofloxacin
Enterococci	Penicillin or ampicillin + aminoglycoside	Vancomycin + aminoglycoside
Escherichia coli	Third-generation cephalosporin, fluoroquinolone	Aminoglycoside
Gonococci†	Ceftriaxone plus either doxycycline or azithromycin	
Haemophilus spp.	Second- or third-generation cephalosporin	Ampicillin
Klebsiella spp.	Third-generation cephalosporin, fluoroquinolone	Third-generation penicillin + aminoglycoside
Meningococcus	Cefotaxime or ceftriaxone	Penicillin G if proven to be penicillin susceptible
Mycobacterium tuberculosis	Isoniazid + rifampin + pyrazinamide + ethambutol	
Mycoplasma spp.	Macrolide	Doxycycline, fluoroquinolone (levofloxacin or moxifloxacin)
Pseudomonas spp.	Antipseudomonal penicillin (ticarcillin, piperacillin) + aminoglycoside	Ceftazidime, cefepime, aztreonam, imipenem, ciprofloxacin
Streptococci A or B	Penicillin, cephazolin	Erythromycin
Treponema spp.	Penicillin	Doxycycline
Streptococcus pneumoniae	Third-generation cephalosporin	Fluoroquinolone
Staphylococci	Antistaphylococcal penicillin	Vancomycin (MRSA)

*Always use culture sensitivities to guide therapy if available.
†With genital infections, treat for presumed *Chlamydia* coinfection with azithromycin or doxycycline.
MRSA, methicillin-resistant *Staphylococcus aureus*.

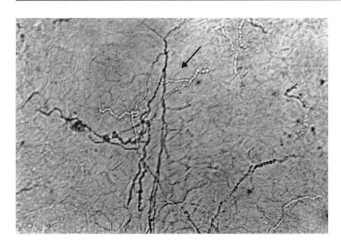

FIGURE 14-1 Hyphae in a potassium hydroxide (KOH) prep (*arrow*).

○ Worm infection in children: *Enterobius* spp. (positive tape test result, perianal itching that is worse at night); treat with mebendazole or albendazole

○ Fever, muscle pain, eosinophilia, and periorbital edema after eating raw meat: *Trichinella spiralis* (trichinosis)

○ Gastroenteritis in young children: rotavirus, Norwalk virus

○ Food poisoning after eating creams or dairy: *S. aureus* caused by preformed toxin

○ Food poisoning after eating reheated rice: *Bacillus cereus* caused by preformed toxin; antibiotics don't help

○ Food poisoning after eating raw seafood: *Vibrio parahaemolyticus*

○ Diarrhea after traveling to Mexico (Montezuma's revenge): *Escherichia coli*; treat with ciprofloxacin

○ Diarrhea after antibiotics: *Clostridium difficile* (Fig. 14-2); treat with oral metronidazole or vancomycin

○ Infant paralyzed after eating honey: *Clostridium botulinum* (toxin blocks acetylcholine release); bacteria colonizes the gut; causes constipation, poor feeding, hypotonia, neurogenic bladder

○ Genital lesions in children in the absence of sexual abuse or activity: molluscum contagiosum

○ Cellulitis after cat or dog bites: *Pasteurella multocida* (treat cat and dog bites with prophylactic amoxicillin-clavulanate)

○ Slaughterhouse worker with fever: *Brucella* spp.

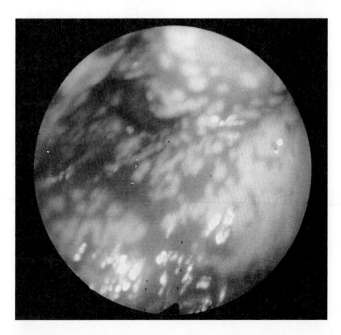

FIGURE 14-2 Colonoscopy reveals the classic "pseudomembranes" (the light-colored, 3- to 10-mm plaques scattered about the mucosa) of *Clostridium difficile* colitis.

○ Pneumonia after being in a hotel, near an air conditioner, or near a water tower: *Legionella pneumophila;* causes headache and gastrointestinal symptoms such as nausea, vomiting, diarrhea, and abdominal pain; treat with azithromycin or levofloxacin

○ Burn wound infection with blue-green color: *Pseudomonas* spp. (*S. aureus* is most common in the first week; no blue-green color)

PNEUMONIA

Look for classic clues to differentiate. The gold standard for diagnosis is sputum culture; do blood cultures, too, because bacteremia is common with pneumonia.

Common causes:

○ ***Streptococcus pneumoniae:*** Most common cause, especially in older adults. Look for a rapid onset of shaking chills after an upper respiratory infection; then fever, pleurisy, and productive cough (yellowish-green or rust-colored from blood). Radiographs show lobar consolidation (Fig. 14-3). White blood cell count is high, with a large percentage of neutrophils. Give vaccine to all children, patients older than 65 years, splenectomized patients, patients with sickle cell disease, immunocompromised patients (HIV, malignancy, organ transplant), and all patients with chronic disease (diabetes mellitus; cardiac, pulmonary, renal, or liver disease). Treat with a macrolide (e.g., azithromycin, clarithromycin), doxycycline, third-generation cephalosporin with a macrolide or doxycycline, or a fluoroquinolone with atypical coverage (e.g., levofloxacin, moxifloxacin).

○ ***Haemophilus influenzae:*** Now uncommon in children because of vaccination. Resembles *S. pneumoniae* clinically. Treat with ampicillin or amoxicillin or second- or third-generation cephalosporin if gram-negative coccobacilli are seen on sputum Gram stain.

○ ***Staphylococcus aureus:*** Causes hospital-acquired pneumonia and pneumonia in patients with cystic fibrosis (in addition to *Pseudomonas* spp.), intravenous (IV) drug abusers, and patients with chronic granulomatous disease (look for recurrent lung abscesses). Empyema and lung abscesses are relatively common. Culture results usually are positive.

○ **Gram-negative organisms:** *Pseudomonas* spp. classically are associated with cystic fibrosis; *Klebsiella* spp. is the classic cause in skid-row alcoholics and homeless persons (watch for the classic description of currant jelly sputum); enteric gram-negative organisms (e.g., *E. coli*) are common with aspiration, neutropenia, and hospital-acquired pneumonia. High mortality rate because of the type of patients affected and severity of pneumonia (abscesses common). Treat empirically with an antipseudomonal penicillin (e.g., ticarcillin, piperacillin) with or without a beta lactamase inhibitor (e.g., clavulanate, tazobactam). Alternatives include ceftazidime or ciprofloxacin.

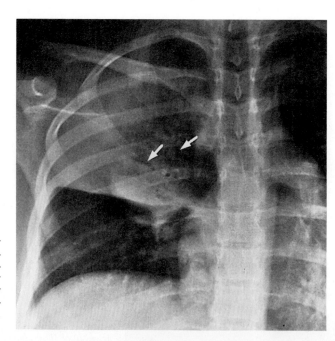

FIGURE 14-3 Alveolar lung disease—air bronchograms. Note the black, air-filled airways (*arrows*) surrounded by white, fluid-filled airspaces in this patient with right upper lobe pneumococcal pneumonia. The sharply defined lower margin of the area of pneumonia is produced by the minor, or horizontal, fissure.

○ *Mycoplasma* **spp.**: Most common in adolescents and young adults (the classic case is a college student who lives in a dorm and has sick contacts). Called "atypical" pneumonia because the clinical course is different from that of *S. pneumoniae*, with a long prodrome and gradual worsening of malaise, headaches, dry nonproductive cough, and sore throat. Chest radiography shows a patchy, diffuse bronchopneumonia (the radiograph classically looks terrible, although the patient does not feel that bad). Look for positive cold-agglutinin antibody titers (can cause hemolysis and anemia). The classic empiric treatment of atypical pneumonia is a macrolide antibiotic (e.g., azithromycin) or broad-spectrum fluoroquinolone (e.g., levofloxacin or moxifloxacin).

○ *Chlamydia pneumoniae:* Second only to *Mycoplasma* spp. as the cause of pneumonia in adolescents and young adults. It manifests similarly but has negative cold-agglutinin antibody titer results. Treat empirically with a macrolide antibiotic (azithromycin) or broad-spectrum fluoroquinolone (e.g., levofloxacin or moxifloxacin).

○ **Viral pneumonia:** Viruses commonly cause respiratory infections (respiratory syncytial virus, influenza, parainfluenza, adenovirus)

○ *Pneumocystis jiroveci* pneumonia (PCP) and cytomegalovirus (CMV): Always suspect in HIV-positive patients (especially those with CD4 counts <200/mm³) and other severely immunocompromised patients (e.g., organ transplant recipients taking immunosuppressants or patients on chemotherapy). PCP is more common; bronchoalveolar lavage often is required to obtain the diagnosis, though many treat empirically. PCP can be seen with silver stains and typically causes bilateral interstitial lung infiltrates. Treat with trimethoprim–sulfamethoxazole; the alternative is pentamidine. PCP prophylaxis should be started in HIV-positive patients when the CD4 count is below 200/mm³. CMV is characterized by intracellular inclusion bodies. Treat with ganciclovir; foscarnet is an alternative.

SYPHILIS

Screen with Venereal Disease Research Laboratory (VDRL) or rapid plasma reagin (RPR) test; if the result is positive, confirm with fluorescent treponemal antibody, absorbed (FTA-ABS) or microhemagglutination *Treponema pallidum* (MHA-TP) test. *T. pallidum* also can be seen with dark-field microscopy but not with a Gram stain. Screen all pregnant women with VDRL or RPR. Treatment is penicillin; use doxycycline for patients with penicillin allergy. Three stages of syphilis:

1. **Primary:** Look for painless chancre (Fig. 14-4) that resolves on its own within 8 weeks.
2. **Secondary:** Roughly 6 weeks to 18 months after infection; look for condyloma lata (Fig. 14-5), maculopapular rash (especially involving palms and soles of feet), and lymphadenopathy.
3. **Tertiary:** Now quite rare; it occurs years after the initial infection. Between secondary and tertiary stages is the latent phase, when the disease is quiet and asymptomatic. Look for gummas (granulomas in many different organs), neurologic symptoms and signs (neurosyphilis, Argyll Robertson pupil, dementia, paresis, tabes dorsalis, Charcot joints), and thoracic aortic aneurysms.

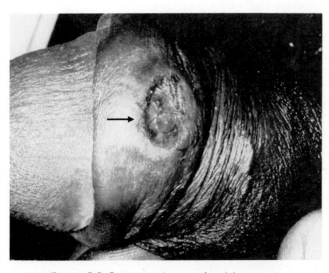

FIGURE 14-4 Primary chancre of syphilis (*arrow*).

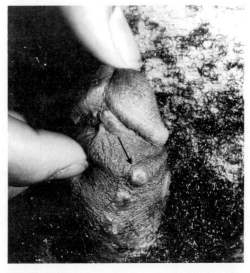

FIGURE 14-5 Condyloma lata of the penis (*arrow*).

Watch for false-positive VDRL or RPR results in patients with lupus erythematosus. For other sexually transmitted diseases, see Chapter 11, Gynecology.

 Remember the presentation of congenital syphilis: It is initially asymptomatic in neonates. Early signs and symptoms include cutaneous lesions on the palms and soles, anemia, and rhinorrhea. Late signs and symptoms include frontal bossing, Hutchinson teeth, and saddle nose.

ENDOCARDITIS

There are two clinical types of endocarditis, acute (fulminant, most commonly caused by *S. aureus*) and subacute (insidious onset, most commonly caused by *Streptococcus viridans*). Look for general signs of infection (e.g., fever, tachycardia, malaise) plus new-onset heart murmur, embolic phenomena (stroke and other infarcts), Osler nodes (painful nodules on tips of fingers), Roth spots (round retinal hemorrhages with white centers), splinter hemorrhages under the fingernails, and septic shock (more dramatic with acute than subacute disease). Osler nodes and Roth spots are caused by an immune vasculitis. Diagnosis of endocarditis is made by blood cultures. Echocardiography may be able to visualize valve vegetations.

Empiric treatment is begun with wide-spectrum antibiotics until culture and sensitivity results are known. A third-generation penicillin or cephalosporin plus aminoglycoside is a reasonable choice.

Patients more likely to be affected include IV drug abusers (who develop right-sided lesions, although left-sided lesions are much more common in the general population) and patients with abnormal heart valves (prosthetic valves, rheumatic valvular disease, or congenital heart defects such as ventricular septal defect or tetralogy of Fallot).

MENINGITIS

The highest incidence of meningitis is seen in neonates; more than 75% of cases are seen in patients younger than 2 years. Thus, the decision about when to do a lumbar tap is difficult because such patients often do not have classic physical findings (Kernig and Brudzinski signs). Look for lethargy, hyper- or hypothermia, poor tone, bulging fontanelle, vomiting, photophobia, altered consciousness, and signs of generalized sepsis (hypotension, jaundice, respiratory distress). Seizures may be seen, but simple febrile seizures also are possible if the patient is between 5 months and 6 years old and has a fever above 102°F in the absence of other signs of meningitis. If seizures occur in the presence of other signs of meningitis or sepsis, proceed to supportive measures, lumbar puncture, and broad-spectrum antibiotics.

The most common neurologic sequela of meningitis is hearing loss. All patients need formal hearing evaluation after a bout of meningitis; vision testing also is recommended. Other sequelae include mental retardation, motor deficits or paresis, epilepsy, and learning and behavioral disorders.

Common causes of community-acquired meningitis in children and adults: *S. pneumoniae* and *N. meningitidis*. *H. influenzae* type B is now much less common in children because of widespread vaccination. Treat with vancomycin and ceftriaxone.

IMPORTANT POINTS

1. Mumps and measles are possible causes of aseptic (nonbacterial or culture-negative) meningitis. The best prevention is immunization.
2. Watch for neonatal herpes encephalitis (Fig. 14-6) if the mother has herpes simplex lesions at the time of the infant's birth. Look for mention of temporal lobe abnormalities on a CT or magnetic resonance imaging scan of the head. Give IV acyclovir.
3. If meningitis is caused by *Neisseria* spp., give all contacts rifampin, ciprofloxacin, ceftriaxone, or azithromycin as prophylaxis.
4. For cerebrospinal fluid findings in meningitis, see Chapter 18, Neurology.

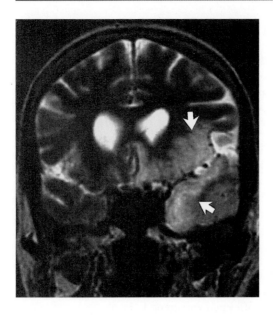

FIGURE 14-6 Magnetic resonance image of herpes encephalitis.

PEDIATRIC RESPIRATORY INFECTIONS

See Chapter 24, Pediatrics.

RABIES

In the United States, rabies is usually caused by bites from bats, skunks, raccoons, or foxes. Vaccination has virtually eliminated dog rabies. The incubation period is usually around 1 to 2 months. Classic symptoms are hydrophobia (fear of water because of painful swallowing) and central nervous system signs (paralysis). After a bite, take these steps:

1. Local wound treatment: Cleanse thoroughly with soap; do not cauterize or suture the wound. Amoxicillin–clavulanate is often given for cellulitis prophylaxis.
2. Observe the animal. If possible, capture and observe a dog or cat to see if it develops rabies. If a wild animal (bat, skunk, raccoon, fox) is caught, it should be killed and the tissue examined for rabies.
3. Prophylaxis with rabies immunoglobulin and vaccine:
○ If a captured or killed animal has rabies, definitely give rabies immunoglobulin and vaccinate the patient.
○ If a wild animal (bat, skunk, raccoon, fox only) that bites is not captured (so rabies testing on the animal is not possible), give rabies immunoglobulin and vaccinate the patient.
○ In the United States, if a dog or cat bites and escapes, prophylaxis and a vaccine generally are not required *unless* the animal acted strangely or bit the patient without provocation *and rabies is prevalent in the area (rare)*. In developing countries where dog rabies is more prevalent, a biting dog should be considered rabid if not available for testing and observation.
○ Rabbits and other small rodents (rats, mice, squirrels, chipmunks) almost never have rabies, so prophylaxis and vaccination usually are not required. Consultation with local health authorities is advised.

STREPTOCOCCAL INFECTION

Enterococcus Faecalis

Enterococcus faecalis are normal bowel flora. *E. faecalis* causes endocarditis, urinary tract infection, and sepsis. For endocarditis, treat with a cell wall active agent (ampicillin, vancomycin) and an aminoglycoside (gentamicin). For vancomycin-resistant enterococci (VRE), treat with linezolid.

Streptococcus Agalactiae

Streptococcus agalactiae (group B strep) is famous as the most common cause of neonatal meningitis and sepsis. It is acquired from the maternal birth canal, in which it is part of the normal flora. Expectant mothers are cultured for group B strep, and if it is present around the time of delivery, prophylactic penicillin or ampicillin is given to the mother to prevent meningitis in the newborn.

Streptococcus Pneumoniae

Streptococcus pneumoniae is the common cause of pneumonia, otitis media, meningitis, sinusitis, and sepsis.

Streptococcus Pyogenes

Streptococcus pyogenes (strep A) causes several important infections.

Pharyngitis

Look for sore throat with fever, tonsillar exudate, enlarged tender cervical nodes, and leukocytosis. Streptococcal throat culture confirms the diagnosis, but the rapid "strep test" is commonly used for convenience. Avoid treating on the boards without confirming the diagnosis. Elevated antistreptolysin O (ASO) and anti-DNase titers also are used retrospectively when needed (rheumatic fever, poststreptococcal glomerulonephritis). Treat with penicillin to avoid rheumatic fever and scarlet fever.

○ **Rheumatic fever:** Diagnosis is made by history of streptococcal pharyngitis and Jones criteria. The major criteria include migratory polyarthritis, carditis, chorea, erythema marginatum, and subcutaneous nodules. The minor criteria include elevated erythrocyte sedimentation rate, C-reactive protein, white blood cell count, and ASO titer; prolonged PR interval on electrocardiogram; and arthralgia. The diagnosis of rheumatic fever requires a history of streptococcal pharyngitis plus at least one major criterion. Treat with aspirin; steroids are used for severe carditis (e.g., congestive heart failure).

○ **Scarlet fever:** Some untreated cases progress to scarlet fever if the streptococcal species produces erythrogenic toxin. Symptoms include red flush in skin (which blanches with pressure, classically with circumoral pallor), truncal rash, strawberry tongue, and late skin desquamation. Kawasaki syndrome is another cause for this set of symptoms.

○ **Poststreptococcal glomerulonephritis:** Occurs most commonly after a streptococcal skin infection, but it can occur after pharyngitis. The patient presents with a history of streptococcal infection (by a nephritogenic strain) 1 to 3 weeks earlier and an abrupt onset of hematuria, proteinuria (mild, not in nephrotic range), red blood cell casts, hypertension, edema (especially periorbital), and elevated blood urea nitrogen and creatinine. Treat supportively: control blood pressure and use diuretics for severe edema. Unlike scarlet and rheumatic fever, glomerulonephritis cannot be prevented by treating streptococcal infections with antibiotics.

Skin Infections

Skin infections often occur after a break in the skin because of trauma, scabies, or insect bite. Watch for development of poststreptococcal glomerulonephritis.

○ **Impetigo:** Maculopapules; vesicopustules or bullae; or honey-colored, crusted lesions. Staphylococci are a more common cause than streptococci. Definitely think of staphylococci if a furuncle or carbuncle is present; think of streptococci if glomerulonephritis occurs. Infection is contagious; watch for sick contacts. Treat empirically with antistaphylococcal penicillin (e.g., dicloxacillin), cephalexin, or clindamycin.

○ **Erysipelas:** A superficial cellulitis that is red, shiny, swollen, and tender; may be associated with vesicles or bullae, fever, and lymphadenopathy. Treated the same as impetigo, although erysipelas may require parenteral therapy.

○ **Cellulitis:** Involves subcutaneous tissues (deeper than erysipelas). Streptococci are the most common cause, but staphylococci also may be implicated. Treat empirically with antistaphylococcal penicillin or vancomycin to cover both. If *Pseudomonas* spp. are suspected (diabetic foot ulcers, burns, severe trauma), treat with broad-spectrum penicillin plus an aminoglycoside. If *Pasteurella multocida* is suspected (after dog or cat bites), treat with IV ampicillin. If *Vibrio vulnificus* is suspected (fishermen or those with other salt-water exposure), treat with tetracycline.

○ **Necrotizing fasciitis:** Progression of cellulitis to necrosis and gangrene, crepitus, and systemic toxicity (tachycardia, fever, hypotension). Often multiple organisms (aerobes and anaerobes) are involved. Treat with IV fluids, incision and drainage or debridement, and broad-spectrum antibiotics (broad-spectrum penicillin or cephalosporin plus an aminoglycoside).

Endometritis or Puerperal Fever

Endometritis is postdelivery fever and uterine tenderness. Treat with clindamycin plus gentamicin after getting local cultures.

Streptococcus Viridans

Streptococcus viridans causes subacute endocarditis and dental caries (*Streptococcus mutans*).

STAPHYLOCOCCAL INFECTION

S. aureus is a common cause of various infections:
○ Abscess: especially in the breast after breastfeeding or in the skin after a furuncle
○ Cellulitis
○ Endocarditis: especially in drug users
○ Food poisoning: preformed toxin
○ Furuncle or carbuncle
○ Impetigo
○ Osteomyelitis: most common cause except in patients with sickle cell disease
○ Pneumonia: often forms lung abscess or empyema
○ Scalded skin syndrome: preformed toxin that affects younger children, who often start with impetigo and then desquamate (Fig. 14-7)
○ Septic arthritis
○ Toxic shock syndrome: preformed toxin, classically in a woman who leaves a tampon in place too long and develops hypotension, fever, and a rash that desquamates
○ Wound infections
○ *Staphylococcus epidermidis*: IV catheter infections, infections of prosthetic implants (heart valves, vascular grafts), and sepsis
○ *Staphylococcus saprophyticus*: common cause of urinary tract infection; treat empirically with standard urinary tract infection antibiotics

 Health care workers who are chronic staphylococcus nasal carriers can cause nosocomial infections. Treat the carrier with antibiotics.

 With all staph infections, treat abscesses with incision and drainage, other infections with antistaphylococcal penicillin (e.g., methicillin, dicloxacillin). Use vancomycin, clindamycin, or trimethoprim–sulfamethoxazole if methicillin-resistant Staphylococcus aureus (MRSA) is known or suspected. MRSA is a rapidly growing problem.

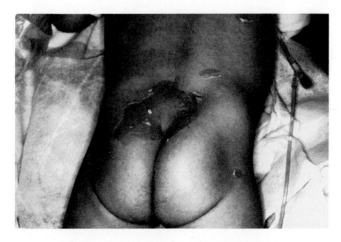

Figure 14-7 Staphylococcal scalded skin syndrome.

TUBERCULOSIS

Remember the following treatment recommendations:

○ An exposed adult with a negative purified protein derivative (PPD) skin test result does not require treatment.
○ An exposed child younger than 5 years old with a negative PPD result should be given isoniazid (INH) for 3 months and then be given a repeat PPD.
○ Prophylaxis for PPD conversion (negative to positive result) but no active disease is INH for 9 months.
○ Active pulmonary disease or positive culture result is treated using quadruple therapy with INH, rifampin, pyrazinamide, and ethambutol for 2 months and then INH and rifampin for 4 months in most patients.

IMPORTANT POINTS

1. Multidrug-resistant strains are an increasing problem and require four-drug therapy in most circumstances.
2. If the patient is noncompliant, directly observed therapy (someone watches the patient take medications every day) is recommended.
3. Consider supplementation with vitamin B_6 (pyridoxine) for patients on INH or watch for signs of deficiency, such as neuropathy, confusion, angular chelitis, or a seborrheic dermatitis-like rash.
4. Watch for liver dysfunction in patients on therapy.

QR CODE

The QR code includes three USMLE-style questions and answers. For more questions, redeem the PIN code on the inside cover for the Crush Step 2 question bank powered by USMLE Consult.
    Please see the Introduction for instructions on how to access content using the QR codes.

Question

A 21-year-old woman comes to the office complaining of sore throat, rash, and fatigue. The sore throat and fatigue began roughly 8 days ago, accompanied by a subjective fever (temperature not recorded). Three days before this visit, the patient visited an urgent care center and was given amoxicillin for her symptoms. A "rash" subsequently developed. The patient denies any drug allergies and remembers taking penicillin several years ago without having a problem. Her sore throat and fatigue did not improve with the amoxicillin. Vital signs are as follows:

Temperature	99.6°F
Blood pressure	126/82 mm Hg
Pulse rate	88 beats/min
Respirations	14 breaths/min

On examination, the patient has a maculopapular rash on her trunk and marked pharyngeal erythema. What is the most likely cause of the patient's symptoms?

(A) *Streptococcus agalactiae* infection
(B) Epstein-Barr virus
(C) *Streptococcus pyogenes* infection
(D) *Staphylococcus aureus* infection
(E) Allergic reaction to amoxicillin

HYPERTENSION

Screening

Screening for hypertension should be done roughly every 2 years, starting at the age of 3 years. Whenever a patient comes in for any kind of medical visit or hospitalization, it is standard practice to measure the blood pressure. The current accepted cut-off value is 140/90 mm Hg (lower in children). A blood pressure of 145/75 mm Hg or 115/95 is still considered hypertension (isolated systolic hypertension or isolated diastolic hypertension, respectively) and should be treated if it persists. Systolic and diastolic hypertension both decrease life expectancy. Hypertension is not diagnosed until *two separate measurements on two separate occasions are* above 140/90 mm Hg (except in pregnancy, when preeclampsia may be the cause of hypertension and waiting for a return visit could be devastating). Also, if hypertension is severe (>210 mm Hg systolic, >120 mm Hg diastolic, or end-organ effects), immediate treatment with medication is warranted. Initial drug treatment for hypertension is listed in Table 15-1.

Evaluation

Basic studies and evaluation in a new hypertensive patient include urinalysis, chemistry panel 7, electrocardiogram (EKG), hemoglobin and hematocrit, and a lipid panel. Do *not* treat hypertension until you have a diagnosis (hypertension on two separate visits)! However, if asked, institute conservative (i.e., nonpharmacologic) measures and address associated comorbidities (e.g., obesity, diabetes) after the first abnormal measurement. Conservative measures include dietary changes (i.e., low salt, low fat, low calorie), reduced smoking and alcohol intake, weight loss, and exercise. For stage I hypertension, it is reasonable to give a 1- to 2-month trial of lifestyle modifications before starting medication. In patients with stage II hypertension or those with diabetes or renal disease, early pharmacologic treatment is often preferred.

There are a few important exceptions to the "start conservative and remeasure" strategy, however, and more aggressive approaches are gaining favor. Patients with hypertensive urgency or emergency require more immediate treatment, as do pregnant women with hypertension (see below for a discussion of these three conditions).

Treatment

There are five first-line agents for treating hypertension: thiazide diuretics (preferred agent in patients without additional comorbidities or indications), angiotensin-converting enzyme (ACE) inhibitors, angiotensin-receptor blockers (ARBs), β-blockers, and calcium channel blockers. Which one you choose is often based on comorbidities (Table 15-2).

For **pregnant patients,** use hydralazine, labetalol, or α-methyldopa. Remember that in patients with preeclampsia, magnesium sulfate ($MgSO_4$) lowers blood pressure. For side effects of hypertension medications (high yield), see Chapter 25, Pharmacology.

Hypertensive urgency occurs when blood pressure is above 200/120 mm Hg without symptoms. Hypertensive emergency is defined as blood pressure above 200/120 mm Hg with symptoms or evidence of end-organ damage. Evidence of end-organ damage includes acute left ventricular failure, unstable angina, myocardial infarction, and encephalopathy (e.g., headaches, mental status changes, vomiting, blurred vision, dizziness, papilledema). Hypertensive urgencies and emergencies are an exception to the rule of measuring blood pressure two times before treating! Hypertensive urgency

Table 15-1 Initial Drug Treatment for Hypertension*

SYSTOLIC BLOOD PRESSURE (MM HG)	DIASTOLIC BLOOD PRESSURE (MM HG)	CLASSIFICATION†	INITIAL DRUG TREATMENT
<120	<80	Normal	None
120–139	80–89	Prehypertension	None unless compelling indications‡
140–159	90–99	Stage 1 hypertension	Thiazides preferred. Use other agents for comorbidities or combination treatment (see Table 15-2).
≥160	≥100	Stage 2 hypertension	Two-drug combination for most patients. Thiazide diuretic plus ACE inhibitor or ARB or β-blocker, or calcium channel blocker.

*Note: All patients should make lifestyle modifications.
†Classification is based on the worse number (e.g., 168/60 mm Hg is considered stage II hypertension even though diastolic pressure is normal).
‡Compelling indications are diabetes and chronic kidney disease. Such patients should be treated with a goal of less than 130/80 mm Hg.
ACE, angiotensin-converting enzyme; ARB, angiotensin receptor blocker.

Table 15-2 Indications and Contraindications for Antihypertensive Medication

DRUG CLASS	USE IN PATIENTS WITH	AVOID IN PATIENTS WITH
ACE inhibitors	Heart failure, diabetes, acute coronary syndrome or unstable angina, acute or prior MI, high risk of coronary artery disease or stroke, chronic kidney disease	Pregnancy, angioedema, renovascular hypertension (can cause renal failure)
Aldosterone receptor blockers (e.g., spironolactone, eplerenone)	Heart failure, prior MI	Hyperkalemia, pregnancy
ARBs (e.g., losartan, irbesartan)	Heart failure, diabetes, chronic kidney disease	Pregnancy, renovascular hypertension (can cause renal failure)
β-Blockers	Stable angina, acute coronary syndrome or unstable angina, acute or prior MI, high risk of coronary artery disease, atrial tachycardia or fibrillation, thyrotoxicosis (short term), essential tremor, migraines	Asthma, COPD, heart block, sick sinus syndrome
Calcium channel blockers	Raynaud syndrome, atrial tachyarrhythmias	Heart block, sick sinus syndrome, congestive heart failure (all related to central-acting agents), pregnancy
Thiazides	Heart failure, diabetes, high risk of coronary artery disease or stroke, osteoporosis	Gout, electrolyte disturbances (e.g., hyponatremia), pregnancy

ACE, angiotensin-converting enzyme; ARB, angiotensin-receptor blocker; COPD, chronic obstructive pulmonary disease; MI, myocardial infarction.

typically is treated orally with furosemide, clonidine, or captopril. There are many treatment options for hypertensive emergency, but intravenous (IV) nitroprusside, nitroglycerin, labetalol, and nicardipine are the most common.

Note *Nitroprusside dilates arteries and veins. Nitroglycerin is a venodilator only. Hydralazine, α1=antagonists, and calcium channel blockers are arterial dilators only. Venodilators reduce preload, and arterial dilators reduce afterload. Nitroprusside does both.*

Note *Lowering blood pressure lowers risk for stroke (hypertension is the most important stroke risk factor), heart disease, myocardial infarction, renal failure, atherosclerosis, and dissecting aortic aneurysm. Coronary disease is the most common cause of death among untreated hypertensive patients. Don't forget to treat isolated systolic or diastolic hypertension if it persists.*

Secondary Hypertension

Clues to **secondary hypertension** include onset before age 30 years or after age 55 years and other suggestive history or lab values. In a young woman, the most common cause is birth control pills (discontinue them). The next most common cause in younger women is renovascular hypertension caused by fibromuscular dysplasia; a renal bruit may be present on exam. Use magnetic resonance angiogram (MRA) or computed tomography (CT) for diagnosis (ultrasound and nuclear medicine screening tests for renovascular hypertension are also used), and treat with angioplasty and stenting. In a young man, think of excessive alcohol intake or "exotic" conditions (pheochromocytoma, Cushing syndrome, Conn syndrome, polycystic kidney disease). In elderly patients with new-onset hypertension, think of renovascular hypertension caused by atherosclerosis. Look for a renal bruit or a patient who develops acute renal failure after being given an ACE inhibitor. If you suspect secondary hypertension (95% of cases of hypertension are essential, primary, or idiopathic), remember the following hints and tests to order:

○ **Pheochromocytoma:** Urinary catecholamines (vanillylmandelic acid, metanephrines) and/or plasma unfractionated metanephrines plus intermittent severe hypertension, dizziness, confusion, and the classic triad of diaphoresis, headache, and tachycardia.

○ **Polycystic kidney disease:** Flank mass, family history, elevated creatinine, and elevated blood urea nitrogen. Autosomal dominant polycystic kidney disease is the more common form. Autosomal recessive polycystic kidney disease is usually diagnosed in infancy.

○ **Cushing syndrome:** Look for stigmata of Cushing syndrome (moon facies, truncal obesity, buffalo hump, abdominal striae, menstrual irregularities, glucose intolerance, poor wound healing, osteoporosis, depression, or psychosis). Diagnose using a dexamethasone suppression test or 24-hour urine cortisol level.

○ **Renovascular hypertension:** Renal angiography is the diagnostic gold standard, but MRA, CT angiography, and duplex ultrasonography are more commonly used because they are less invasive. An ACE inhibitor nuclear medicine scan is not used for screening but can be used to assess the hemodynamic significance of a stenotic lesion. For the purposes of the USMLE, if there is a bruit on exam (Fig. 15-1), treat with angioplasty and stenting.

○ **Conn syndrome:** Caused by an aldosterone-secreting adrenal neoplasm. High aldosterone level, **low renin** level, hypernatremia, hypokalemia, metabolic alkalosis, or an adrenal mass on CT are hallmarks.

○ **Coarctation of the aorta:** upper extremity hypertension only, unequal pulses, brachial-femoral delay, and rib notching on radiography; associated with **Turner syndrome**. Diagnosed with MRA or angiography.

DIABETES

Screening

Universal screening is generally *not recommended*. Screening is more accepted, but not uniformly, in patients who are obese (body mass index >25 kg/m²), are older than 45 years, are members of certain subgroups (black, American Indian, Hispanic), or have diabetes risk factors such as family history in a first-degree relative, habitual physical inactivity, gestational diabetes, hypertension, or dyslipidemia.

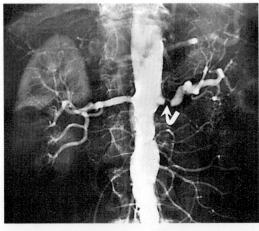

FIGURE 15-1 Conventional renal angiogram revealing a high-grade, proximal left renal artery atherosclerotic-type stenosis (*arrow*) and associated atherosclerotic irregularity in the abdominal aorta. Fibromuscular dysplasia usually occurs in the midrenal artery, has a beaded appearance, and usually occurs without other evidence of atherosclerosis (i.e., in young patients).

Signs and Symptoms

Classic presenting signs and symptoms of diabetes mellitus (DM) are fatigue, polydipsia, polyuria, polyphagia, and weight loss. Acanthosis nigricans can often be appreciated. In women, vaginal discharge caused by monilial infection can be the initial complaint. A diagnosis of diabetes is made by a fasting plasma glucose of 126 mg/dL or greater (after an overnight fast of 8 hours), a random glucose (no fasting) of 200 mg/dL or greater, or a hemoglobin A1C (HbA1c) level of 6.5% or greater. If the patient has classic symptoms, one measurement is enough to confirm a diagnosis, but in an asymptomatic patient, repeat the test. An oral glucose tolerance test is commonly used in pregnancy; otherwise, it is rarely used for the diagnosis of diabetes. Differences between type 1 DM (T1DM) and type 2 DM (T2DM) are shown in Table 15-3.

Treatment

The **goal of treatment** is to keep postprandial glucose below 180 mg/dL, fasting glucose 70 to 130 mg/dL, and HbA1c below 7.0%. Stricter control results in too many episodes of hypoglycemia (look for symptoms of sympathetic discharge and mental status changes), which can cause brain damage in the long term. Good glucose control, however, delays or prevents nearly all of the complications of diabetes.

The treatment of T1DM requires insulin. Intensive insulin therapy is recommended for most patients with T1DM and should be started as early as possible after the diagnosis is made. There are many different intensive therapy regimens, but they all include a basal insulin (intermediate- or longer acting insulin or continuous subcutaneous insulin infusion) plus adjustable doses of premeal insulin (short-acting insulin or rapid-acting insulin analogs). Although intensive insulin therapy has clear benefits, the main drawbacks are hypoglycemic episodes and weight gain.

Patients with T2DM who are overweight should be encouraged to lose weight because it may reduce glucose levels by reducing insulin resistance. Medications are usually needed to treat T2DM, and the most current guidelines encourage starting medications at the time of diagnosis. Oral agents are usually tried first, typically beginning with metformin. Other agents include insulin secretagogues (glipizide, glimepiride, nateglinide, glyburide, repaglinide), thiazolidinediones (rosiglitazone, pioglitazone), alpha-glucosidase inhibitors (acarbose, miglitol), incretin mimetics (exenatide), incretin enhancers (saxagliptin, sitagliptin), and amylin analogues (pramlintide).

A combination of metformin plus an insulin secretagogue (e.g., a sulfonylurea) is common. Many people with type 2 diabetes eventually require insulin, and insulin may be required early if the blood glucose or HbA1c levels are significantly elevated. Current recommendations encourage the use of insulin earlier in the course of the disease than was previously recommended.

TABLE 15-3 Differences between Type 1 and Type 2 Diabetes Mellitus		
FEATURE	**TYPE 1**	**TYPE 2**
Age at onset	Most commonly <30 y	Most commonly >30 y*
Associated body habitus	Thin	Obese
Develop ketoacidosis	Yes	No
Develop hyperosmolar state	No	Yes
Level of endogenous insulin	Low to none	Normal to high (insulin resistance)
Twin concurrence	<50%	>50%
HLA association	Yes	No
Response to oral hypoglycemics	No	Yes
Antibodies to insulin	Yes (at diagnosis)	No
Risk of diabetic complications	Yes	Yes
Islet cell pathology	Insulitis (loss of most β cells)	Normal number but with amyloid deposits

HLA, human leukocyte antigen.
*Be aware, however, of the "epidemic" of type 2 diabetes in those younger than 30 years, including children and adolescents, which is partly attributable to the obesity epidemic.

IMPORTANT POINTS

1. Remember the importance of C peptide in distinguishing between too much exogenous insulin (low C peptide with accidental overdose in a patient with diabetes or in a patient with factitious disorder) and an insulinoma (high C peptide). C peptide is produced when the body makes insulin but is absent in prescription insulin preparations.

2. Because IV contrast agents can precipitate acute renal failure in diabetic patients and patients with renal insufficiency, use iodinated contrast for imaging studies only when absolutely necessary. To prevent renal damage, make sure a patient with kidney disease or diabetes is well hydrated before using contrast agents. Acetylcysteine and bicarbonate may decrease the risk of contrast nephropathy in high-risk patients.

3. Diabetic ketoacidosis is traditionally seen in patients with T1DM but is becoming more common in T2DM. It is sometimes the patient's first manifestation of the disease. Look for Kussmaul breathing (deep, rapid respirations), hyperglycemia, dehydration, metabolic acidosis, and increased ketones in the serum and urine. Treatment involves fluids, IV regular insulin, and aggressive potassium and phosphorus replacement. Do not use bicarbonate unless the pH is below 7. Search for the cause, which usually is noncompliance with insulin therapy or infection. Death occurs without treatment.

4. Nonketotic hyperglycemic hyperosmolar state is seen in patients with T2DM. Hyperglycemia and increased serum osmolarity are present in the absence of ketones and acidosis. Treatment involves IV fluids (first initial choice), IV insulin, and electrolyte replacement. Mortality rate is high, especially if mental status changes are present at the time of diagnosis.

Complications

Long-term complications of DM that happen in both T1DM and T2DM include:

○ **Atherosclerosis:** Coronary artery disease, peripheral vascular disease (claudication, atrophy), myocardial infarction, and stroke.

○ **Retinopathy:** Diabetes is the leading cause of blindness in the United States for persons younger than the age of 50 years. When retinopathy is proliferative, treat with panretinal laser photocoagulation to prevent progression and blindness. All patients with diabetes should be seen once a year (initially) by an ophthalmologist to monitor for retinal changes.

○ **Nephropathy:** Diabetes is the leading cause of end-stage renal disease requiring hemodialysis. ACE inhibitors and ARBs help prevent nephropathy.

○ **Increased risk of infections** as a consequence of vascular insufficiency; peripheral neuropathy; and the effects of hyperglycemia on neutrophil chemotaxis and adhesion, phagocytosis, opsonization, and cell-mediated immunity.

○ **Neuropathy** (see later)

○ **Foot ulcers, infections, and gangrene:** Diabetes is the most common cause of nontrauma amputations. Amputation is usually required because of tissue necrosis caused by some combination of diabetes-induced vascular disease, neuropathy, and immune dysfunction or infection. Patients should wear comfortable, properly fitting shoes with socks and should regularly inspect their feet. Most cases of foot gangrene in diabetics begin as a callous, blister, or ulcer.

○ **Peripheral neuropathy** (autonomic and sensory) causes many problems in patients with diabetes:

  ○ Gastroparesis (early satiety, nausea). Treat with motility enhancers such as metoclopramide.

  ○ Charcot joints (joints deform because of lack of sensation; patient puts too much stress on joints and might not feel injury or stress)

  ○ Impotence from autonomic neuropathy as well as peripheral vascular disease

  ○ Cranial nerve palsies, especially cranial nerves III, IV, and VI. Patients present with diplopia and extraocular muscle paralysis. These usually resolve spontaneously within a few months.

  ○ Orthostatic hypotension caused by a lack of effective sympathetic innervation; when the patient stands up, the heart rate and vascular tone do not increase appropriately to maintain blood pressure

  ○ "Silent" myocardial infarction (because of neuropathy, there is no chest pain)

TABLE 15-4 Insulin Preparations and Use

INSULIN PREPARATION	ONSET (H)	PEAK (H)	DURATION (H)	WHEN TO USE
ULTRA RAPID ACTING				
Insulin aspart	<0.25	1–3	3–5	Right before meals
Insulin lispro	0.25–0.5	0.5–2.5	3–5	Right before meals
Insulin glulisine	0.2–0.5	1.5–2.5	3–4	Right before meals
RAPID ACTING				
Regular insulin	0.5–1	2–4	5–8	Inpatients (can be given IV), 0.5–1 h before a meal for outpatients
INTERMEDIATE TO LONG ACTING				
NPH insulin	2–3	4–12	12–20	Generally part of standard regimens that mix with shorter acting insulin (e.g., 70/30 or 50/50 of NPH/regular)
LONG ACTING				
Insulin glargine	1.5–4	None	24+	Provides basal insulin level; supplement with short-acting insulin
Insulin detemir	3–4	3–9	Dose dependent; 6–23 hours	Provides basal insulin level

IV, intravenous; NPH, neutral protamine Hagedorn.

Insulin

Know how to use different preparations of insulin, especially lispro, **regular, neutral protamine Hagedorn** (NPH), glargine, and detemir insulin (Table 15-4). Patients with T1DM generally require insulin 0.5 to 1.0 U/kg of body weight per day, although initial requirements are often less than this because of a small amount of residual endogenous insulin production. In T2DM, insulin is often started as a basal insulin (start at 10 U or 0.2 U/kg of body weight of NPH or a long-acting insulin analog at bedtime), often given in addition to metformin. Requirements ultimately may be greater than 1 U/kg per day because of insulin resistance.

○ If the patient has high (low) 7 AM glucose, increase (decrease) NPH insulin at dinner the night before.
○ If the patient has high (low) noon glucose, increase (decrease) morning regular insulin or increase (decrease) before-breakfast lispro or aspart insulin.
○ If the patient has high (low) 5 PM glucose, increase (decrease) morning NPH or increase (decrease) before-lunch lispro or aspart insulin.
○ If the patient has high (low) 9 PM glucose, increase (decrease) dinnertime regular insulin or increase (decrease) before-dinner lispro or aspart insulin.

Somogyi Effect versus Dawn Phenomenon

The *Somogyi effect* is the body's reaction to hypoglycemia. If too much NPH or other longer acting insulin preparation is given at dinnertime, the 3 AM glucose level will be low (hypoglycemia). The body reacts by releasing stress hormones, which cause the 7 AM glucose level to be high. The treatment is to *decrease* the evening insulin dose. The *dawn phenomenon* is hyperglycemia caused by normal early AM growth hormone secretion. The 7 AM glucose is high without 3 AM hypoglycemia (glucose is normal or high at 4 AM). The treatment is to *increase* the evening insulin dose.

Compliance

Follow compliance by checking the HbA1c level, which is an accurate measure of overall control for the previous 3 months. Patients are not afraid to alter their home test numbers to please their doctors, and this is the way to catch them. Strive for a level less than 7%.

Surgery

For surgery, patients with diabetes (and without diabetes) are allowed nothing by mouth (NPO). Give one-third to one-half of the normal insulin dose, then monitor glucose closely through surgery and postoperatively, using 5% dextrose in water (D_5W) and IV regular insulin to maintain glucose control.

Medications

Chlorpropamide (rarely used) can cause the syndrome of inappropriate secretion of antidiuretic hormone (SIADH). Patients with T1DM are not helped by oral medications. Remember that β-blockers can prevent many of the physical manifestations of hypoglycemia (tachycardia, diaphoresis), thereby also preventing early detection, but treatment benefits might outweigh the risks (e.g., after a myocardial infarction).

CHOLESTEROL

Measure a fasting lipoprotein profile (total cholesterol, low-density lipoprotein [LDL] cholesterol, high-density lipoprotein [HDL] cholesterol, and triglycerides) every 5 years (unless abnormal) starting at age 20 years. Consider earlier and more aggressive screening for obese patients and patients with a family history of hypercholesterolemia.

 Lipoprotein analysis involves measuring total cholesterol, HDL, and triglycerides. LDL can then be calculated from the formula LDL = Total cholesterol − HDL − (Triglycerides/5).

Total cholesterol goal is less than 200 mg/dL; greater than 240 mg/dL is considered high. Normal triglyceride level is less than 150 mg/dL; greater than 200 is considered high. LDL is usually the main player for treatment decisions; interventions at various LDL levels are given in Table 15-5. Look for xanthelasma (Fig. 15-2), corneal arcus in younger patients (this is a normal variant in elderly individuals), lipemic-looking serum, and obesity as markers of possible **familial hypercholesterolemia.** Family members should be tested. Also look for pancreatitis with no risk factors (e.g., no alcohol, no gallstones) as a marker for familial hypertriglyceridemia.

TABLE 15-5 LDL Cholesterol Levels and Interventions

NO CHD RISK FACTORS	≥2 CHD RISK FACTORS*	KNOWN CAD OR EQUIVALENT†	VERY HIGH RISK‡	INTERVENTION
LDL <160 mg/dL	LDL <100 mg/dL	LDL <100 mg/dL	LDL <70 mg/dL	None (meets goal)
LDL 160–189 mg/dL	LDL 100–129 mg/dL		LDL 70–99 mg/dL	Diet ± medications§
LDL >190 mg/dL	LDL >130 mg/dL	LDL >100 mg/dL	LDL >100 mg/dL	Medications (+ diet)

*Risk factors for coronary heart disease (CHD) are listed in the text.
†CHD equivalents include diabetes mellitus, peripheral arterial atherosclerotic disease, symptomatic carotid artery disease, and abdominal aortic aneurysm.
‡"Very" high-risk patients are those with coronary heart disease (CAD) who have a heart attack, diabetes, or other severe and poorly controlled risk factors (e.g., metabolic syndrome, heavy smoking).
§"Diet" includes general lifestyle modifications such as eating less and healthier, decreasing alcohol intake, exercising, and so on. The trend is toward more aggressive intervention, so you will not be faulted for initiating medications at these gray-area LDL levels, particularly in higher risk people.

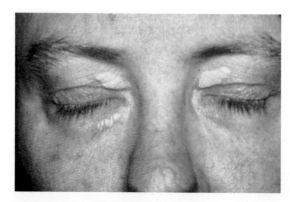

Figure 15-2 Patient with xanthelasma in all four lids. *(From Tasman W, Jaeger EA: The Wills Eye Hospital Atlas of Clinical Ophthalmology, 2nd ed. Philadelphia, Lippincott Williams & Wilkins, 2001, Figure 10.39, with permission.)*

Be aware of **secondary causes of hyperlipidemia**, including uncontrolled DM, hypothyroidism, uremia, the nephrotic syndrome, obstructive liver disease, excessive alcohol intake (increases triglycerides), obesity, and medications (oral contraceptives, isotretinoin, glucocorticoids, thiazides, and β-blockers).

Atherosclerosis caused partly by hyperlipidemia is involved in about half of all deaths in the United States and one-third of deaths between ages 35 and 65 years. Atherosclerosis is the most important cause of permanent disability and accounts for more hospital days than any other illness. (Translation: *Understand atherosclerosis for the boards.*)

Risk Factors

The decision to treat hyperlipidemia depends largely on a patient's coronary heart disease risk factors. These risk factors include:

○ Age (men ≥45 years, women ≥55 years or with premature menopause and no estrogen replacement therapy)
○ Family history of premature coronary heart disease (CHD; defined as definite myocardial infarction or sudden death in father or other first-degree male relative younger than 55 years or mother or other first-degree female relative younger than 65 years)
○ Cigarette smoking
○ Hypertension (≥140/90 mm Hg or on antihypertensive medications)
○ Low HDL (<40 mg/dL) (note, however, that HDL = 60 mg/dL is considered to be protective and negates one risk factor)

Diabetes is a risk factor but is not used or counted in determining the number of risk factors when deciding cholesterol treatment because diabetes is considered a coronary artery disease (CAD) equivalent and warrants immediate aggressive treatment by itself.

LDL and total cholesterol are risk factors for CHD, but do not count them in deciding whether to treat high cholesterol. Male sex is a risk factor because men develop coronary heart disease earlier than women (but postmenopausal women quickly catch up with age-matched men). However, male sex is not counted when calculating the number of risk factors because it is incorporated into age as a risk factor.

C-reactive protein (CRP) and homocysteine are hot topics right now, but elevated CRP and homocysteine are not considered major risk factors for coronary artery disease (according to the Third Report of the National Cholesterol Education Panel, Adult Treatment Panel III). Obesity and a type A personality (think of the hard-driving attorney) are weaker risk factors, as are stress and physical inactivity. Hypertriglyceridemia alone is not a significant risk factor but in association with high cholesterol causes more coronary heart disease than high cholesterol alone. For Step 2 boards, use only the definite risk factors mentioned in the previous question (especially when deciding how to treat a patient with high cholesterol) but keep these other factors in mind.

Treatment

Give lower-risk patients 3 to 6 months to try lifestyle modifications (exercise and decreased calories, cholesterol, saturated fats, alcohol, and smoking) before initiating drug therapy. If the patient has coronary artery disease or a coronary artery disease equivalent (e.g., diabetes, peripheral vascular disease) and the LDL mg/dL is 100 or above, medication therapy is indicated.

 High HDL is protective against atherosclerosis and is increased by exercise, estrogens, and moderate alcohol intake (one or two drinks per day) but not by high alcohol intake. HDL is decreased by smoking, androgens, progesterone, and hypertriglyceridemia.

After the decision to start medications has been made, **first-line agents** are HMG-CoA reductase inhibitors (statins); watch for rare but potentially serious side effects such as hepatotoxicity and rhabdomyolysis (muscle damage). Second-line agents include niacin (poorly tolerated but effective, particularly to raise HDL), ezetimibe (selectively inhibits the intestinal absorption of cholesterol), and bile acid–binding resins (e.g., cholestyramine).

SMOKING

Smoking is the single most significant source of preventable morbidity and premature death in the United States. Whenever you are not sure which risk factor to eliminate, smoking is a safe guess.

IMPORTANT POINTS

1. Smoking is the best risk factor to eliminate to prevent heart disease–related deaths (responsible for 30%–45% of such deaths in the United States). Risk decreases by 50% within 1 year of quitting and by 15 years after quitting, the risk is the same as someone who has never smoked.

2. Smoking increases the risk of the following cancers: lung (85%–90% of cases), oral cavity (90% of cases), esophagus (70%–80% of cases), larynx, pharynx, bladder (30%–50% of cases), kidney (20%–30% of cases), pancreas (20%–25% of cases), cervix, stomach, colon, and rectum.

3. Chronic obstructive pulmonary disease is often a result of smoking. Emphysema almost always is caused by smoking (unless the patient is very young or has no smoking history, in which case you should consider α_1-antitrypsin deficiency). Although the changes of emphysema are irreversible, the risk of death still decreases after smoking cessation.

4. When parents smoke, children are at increased risk for asthma and upper respiratory infections, including otitis media. Secondhand smoke is also a risk factor for lung cancer and other lung disease.

5. Smoking retards healing of peptic ulcer disease, and cessation stops Buerger disease (Raynaud symptoms in a young male smoker).

6. Smoking by pregnant women increases the risk of low birth weight, prematurity, spontaneous abortion, stillbirth, and infant mortality.

7. Smoking cessation preoperatively is the best way to decrease the risk of postoperative pulmonary complications, especially if it is stopped at least 8 weeks before surgery.

8. Do *not* give birth control pills to women older than 35 years who smoke (or women younger than 25 who smoke ≥15 cigarettes per day). The risk of thromboembolism is increased sharply in women who smoke and take birth control pills.

9. The antidepressant bupropion, varenicline, and nicotine preparations (e.g., patch, gum, nasal spray, lozenge) can help some people quit smoking.

ALCOHOL

Alcohol is involved in roughly 50% of fatal car accidents, 67% of drownings and homicides, 70% to 80% of deaths in fires, and 35% of suicides. Alcohol abuse is the most common cause of cirrhosis and esophageal varices, and it increases the risk of the following cancers: oral cavity, larynx, pharynx, esophagus, liver, and lung. It also may be associated with gastric, colon, pancreatic, and breast cancer.

Alcoholic hepatitis:

○ In alcoholic hepatitis, the ratio of aspartate aminotransferase (AST; also known as serum glutamate oxaloacetate transaminase [SGOT]) to alanine aminotransferase (ALT; also known as serum glutamate pyruvate transaminase [SGPT] is at least 2:1, although both may be elevated.

○ Other causes of hepatitis usually are associated with the opposite ratio or equal elevation of both AST and ALT.

○ In acute alcoholic hepatitis, treatment consists of supportive care and in severe cases, glucocorticoids.

○ In chronic alcoholic hepatitis, treatment consists of adequate nutrition, prevention of complications, and of course abstinence from alcohol.

Wernicke vs. Korsakoff syndromes:

○ Wernicke syndrome is an acute encephalopathy characterized by ophthalmoplegia, nystagmus, ataxia, or confusion. It can be fatal but often is reversible with thiamine.

○ Korsakoff syndrome is a chronic psychosis characterized by **anterograde amnesia** (inability to form memories) and **confabulation** (lying). Korsakoff syndrome is generally irreversible and is thought to be caused by damage to the mamillary bodies and thalamic nuclei.

○ Both conditions are caused by thiamine deficiency.

Alcohol withdrawal can be fatal (1%–5% mortality rate if delirium tremens are present). Treat on an inpatient basis with benzodiazepines (e.g., chlordiazepoxide, lorazepam); barbiturates are rarely used. Gradually taper the dose over days.

Withdrawal stages and symptoms:

1. **Acute withdrawal syndrome**, 12 to 48 hours after the last drink. Symptoms include tremors, sweating, hyperreflexia, and seizures ("rum fits").
2. **Alcoholic hallucinosis**, 24 to 72 hours after the last drink. Symptoms include hallucinations (auditory, visual, or both) and illusions without autonomic symptoms.
3. **Delirium tremens**, usually 2 to 7 days after the last drink; involves hallucinations and illusions commonly involving insects, confusion, poor sleep, and autonomic lability (sweating, increased pulse and temperature). It occasionally is fatal. Fatality usually is associated with this stage.

See Box 15-1 for stigmata of chronic liver disease in alcoholics, Box 15-2 for classic laboratory findings of liver disease in alcoholics and Box 15-3 for diseases and conditions caused by alcohol abuse.

BOX 15-1 STIGMATA OF LIVER DISEASE IN PATIENTS WITH ALCOHOLISM

Abdominal wall varices (caput medusae)

Esophageal varices

Hemorrhoids (internal)

Jaundice

Ascites

Palmar erythema

Gynecomastia

Dupuytren contractures

Terry nails (white proximal nail, reddened distal nail)

Testicular atrophy

Encephalopathy

Asterixis

Scleral icterus

Edema

Spider angiomas

Fetor hepaticus

BOX 15-2 CLASSIC LABORATORY FINDINGS OF LIVER DISEASE IN PATIENTS WITH ALCOHOLISM

Anemia (classically macrocytic)

Hyperbilirubinemia

Thrombocytopenia

Prolonged prothrombin time

Hypoalbuminemia

BOX 15-3 DISEASES AND CONDITIONS CAUSED BY ALCOHOL ABUSE

Gastritis

Pancreatitis (acute or chronic)

Hepatitis

Wernicke and Korsakoff syndrome

Rhabdomyolysis

Peripheral neuropathy (via thiamine deficiency and a direct effect)

Rhabdomyolysis (acute or chronic)

Cerebellar degeneration (ataxia, past-pointing)

Mallory-Weiss tears

Fatty change in the liver

Cirrhosis

Dilated cardiomyopathy

The best treatment for alcoholism is Alcoholics Anonymous or another support group. Disulfiram also may be tried (patients get sick when they drink because of aldehyde dehydrogenase enzyme inhibition).

Metronidazole and certain cephalosporins can cause a disulfiram-like reaction in those who drink alcohol.

Alcohol is a definite teratogen. Recognize **fetal alcohol syndrome**, which includes mental retardation, microcephaly, microphthalmia, short palpebral fissures, midfacial hypoplasia (including a smooth philtrum and a thin vermilion border of the upper lip), and cardiac defects. No amount of alcohol consumption can be considered safe during pregnancy. An estimated one in 1000 births may be affected by fetal alcohol syndrome, which is the *most common cause* of preventable mental retardation.

Incidence

Alcohol abuse is more common in men. Roughly 10% to 15% of the U.S. population abuses alcohol. Alcoholism has a heritable component and is especially passed from fathers to sons.

IMPORTANT POINTS

1. Severe alcoholics commonly develop aspiration pneumonia with enteric or oral flora bugs such as *Klebsiella* spp. (currant-jelly sputum), anaerobes, *Escherichia coli*, streptococci, and staphylococci.
2. Give thiamine before glucose in a patient with alcoholism; if you give them in the reverse order, you can precipitate Wernicke encephalopathy as thiamine is consumed during glucose metabolism.
3. People with alcoholism develop just about every type of vitamin and mineral deficiency because of poor nutrition. Especially common are deficiencies of folate, magnesium, and thiamine. Low potassium, low sodium, and elevated uric acid (resulting in gout) also occur.
4. Alcohol can precipitate hypoglycemia (but give thiamine first).
5. Bleeding varices are treated with stabilization first (IV fluids and blood if needed). If indicated, correct clotting factor deficiencies with fresh-frozen plasma, fresh blood, and vitamin K. Next, upper endoscopy is performed to determine the cause of the upper gastrointestinal bleed (there are many possibilities in a patient with alcoholism). If varices are identified on endoscopy, sclerotherapy of the veins is attempted with cauterization, banding, or vasopressin. The mortality rate is high, and rebleeding is common, especially early. If you must choose, try a transjugular intrahepatic portosystemic shunt (TIPS) over an open surgical portacaval shunt for more definitive management. Open surgical shunt procedures are now rarely performed (splenorenal is the most physiologic shunt type).
6. Varices with no history of bleeding are treated with nonselective β-blockers (propranolol, nadolol, timolol) to relieve portal hypertension, provided that there is no contraindication to the use of β-blockers.

ACID-BASE STATUS

You must know how to interpret an **arterial blood gas** result when given pH, O_2, CO_2, and bicarbonate. Here are good basic hints:
○ pH tells you whether you are dealing with acidosis or alkalosis as the primary event. The body will compensate as much as it can (secondary event).
○ Look at the CO_2. If it is high, the patient either has respiratory acidosis (pH <7.4) or is compensating for metabolic alkalosis (pH >7.4). If CO_2 is low, the patient either has respiratory alkalosis (pH >7.4) or is compensating for metabolic acidosis (pH <7.4).

○ Look at the bicarbonate. If it is high, the patient either has metabolic alkalosis (pH >7.4) or is compensating for respiratory acidosis (pH <7.4). If bicarbonate is low, the patient either has metabolic acidosis (pH <7.4) or is compensating for respiratory alkalosis (pH >7.4). Common causes of different primary disturbances:

○ **Respiratory acidosis:** Chronic obstructive pulmonary disease, asthma, drugs (opioids, benzodiazepines, barbiturates, alcohol, and other respiratory depressants), chest wall problems (paralysis, pain), and sleep apnea

○ **Respiratory alkalosis:** Anxiety or hyperventilation, aspirin or salicylate overdose

○ **Metabolic acidosis:** Ethanol, diabetic ketoacidosis, uremia, lactic acidosis (sepsis, shock, bowel ischemia), methanol or ethylene glycol poisoning, aspirin or salicylate overdose, diarrhea, and carbonic anhydrase inhibitors

○ **Metabolic alkalosis:** Diuretics (except carbonic anhydrase inhibitors), vomiting, volume contraction, antacid abuse or milk-alkali syndrome, and hyperaldosteronism

○ **Salicylate (aspirin) overdose** causes two primary disturbances, respiratory alkalosis and metabolic acidosis. Look for coexisting tinnitus, hypoglycemia, vomiting, and a history of "swallowing several pills." Alkalinization of the urine (with bicarbonate) speeds excretion.

○ **In certain patients with chronic lung disease,** pH may be alkaline during the day (classic in patients with sleep apnea) because they breathe better when they are awake. In addition, just after an episode of bronchitis or similar respiratory disorder, the metabolic alkalosis that usually compensates for respiratory acidosis is no longer compensatory and becomes the primary disturbance (elevated pH and bicarbonate).

Treatment

Do *not* use bicarbonate to treat low pH unless the pH is below 7 and other measures have failed (always try IV fluids and correction of underlying cause first).

Beware the patient with asthma whose blood gas goes from alkalotic to normal. The patient might be about to crash and need intubation. The pH is initially high in patients with asthma because they are eliminating carbon dioxide. If the patient tires and does not breathe appropriately, carbon dioxide will begin to increase, and the pH will begin to normalize. Eventually, the patient becomes acidotic and requires emergent treatment, which includes β_2 agonists, steroids, and oxygen. Prepare for elective intubation.

ELECTROLYTE DISTURBANCES

Hyponatremia

Signs and symptoms of hyponatremia are lethargy, mental status changes (confusion, disorientation), anorexia, seizures, cramps, and coma. The first step in determining the cause of true hyponatremia is to look at the volume status (Box 15-4).

BOX 15-4 CAUSES OF HYPONATREMIA BY VOLUME STATUS		
HYPOVOLEMIC	**EUVOLEMIC**	**HYPERVOLEMIC**
Dehydration	Syndrome of inappropriate secretion of antidiuretic hormone	Congestive heart failure
Diuretics		Nephrotic syndrome
Diabetes mellitus or diabetic ketoacidosis	Psychogenic polydipsia Oxytocin use	Cirrhosis Toxemia
Addison disease		Renal failure
Hypoaldosteronism		

IMPORTANT POINTS

1. SIADH commonly results from head trauma, surgery, meningitis, small-cell lung cancer, painful states (e.g., trauma, postoperative state), pulmonary infections (pneumonia, tuberculosis), opioids, or chlorpropamide. Treatment is water restriction. Occasionally, when refractive to conservative management, patients with SIADH are treated with demeclocycline (a tetracycline that causes nephrogenic diabetes insipidus [DI]).

2. With Addison disease and hypoaldosteronism, potassium is classically elevated, and blood pressure is low.

3. Treat hypovolemic hyponatremia with saline. Treat euvolemic and hypervolemic hyponatremia with free water restriction and possibly diuretics for hypervolemia.

4. Never correct hyponatremia rapidly because you can cause brainstem damage (central pontine myelinolysis). Hypertonic saline is used only when the patient has seizures because of hyponatremia and even then only briefly and cautiously. *Normal saline is a better choice 99 times out of 100 for board purposes.* Serum sodium concentration correction should not exceed 10 to 12 mEq/L in the first 24 hours or 18 mEq/L in the first 48 hours. In chronic severe symptomatic hyponatremia, the rate of correction should not exceed 0.5 to 1.0 mEq/L/hr.

5. Spurious (false) hyponatremia is caused by hyperglycemia, hyperlipidemia, and severe hyperproteinemia. In these instances, the total-body sodium is normal even though the lab value is low. Do not give the patient extra salt or saline. When glucose exceeds 200 mg/dL, sodium decreases by 1.6 mEq/L for each increase of 100 mg/dL in glucose.

6. In a surgical patient, the most common cause of hyponatremia is inappropriate or excessive fluid administration, but don't forget adrenal insufficiency as a possible cause. Iso-osmotic hyponatremia may occur when nonconductive glycine or sorbitol flushing solutions are administered during transurethral resection of the prostate or bladder or during hysteroscopic or laparoscopic irrigation.

7. Oxytocin administration can cause hyponatremia (ADH-like effect) in pregnant women.

Hypernatremia

Signs and symptoms are similar to those of hyponatremia: confusion, mental status changes, hyperreflexia, seizures, and coma. Common causes:

○ Dehydration
○ Inability to drink (paralysis, dementia)
○ Diuretics
○ Diabetes insipidus (pituitary or nephrogenic)
○ Diarrhea
○ Renal disease (e.g., isosthenuria from sickle cell disease)
○ Iatrogenic administration of excessive salt

Hypokalemia and hypercalcemia also cause an impairment in renal concentrating ability that can mimic diabetes insipidus.

Treatment of hypernatremia involves water replacement. Often the patient is so dehydrated that normal saline is initially used until the patient is hydrated and hemodynamically stable. Then the patient may be switched to half-normal saline (0.45% NaCl) if still hypernatremic. Five percent dextrose in water (D_5W) should *not* be used.

Central versus nephrogenic diabetes insipidus:

○ Central DI responds to vasopressin (DDAVP); nephrogenic DI does not.
○ Nephrogenic DI can be caused by medications (lithium, demeclocycline, methoxyflurane, and amphotericin B) and is treated with a low-salt, low-protein diet; thiazide diuretic (paradoxical effect); and nonsteroidal antiinflammatory drugs (indomethacin).
○ Central DI can be caused by tumor, trauma, or sarcoidosis, although it is often idiopathic.

Hypokalemia

Hypokalemia causes **muscle weakness,** including weakness of smooth muscles. The patient might have an ileus or hypotension. Muscle weakness can lead to paralysis and ventilatory failure. Electrocardiographic (EKG) findings include loss of T wave or T-wave flattening, the presence of **U waves,** premature ventricular and atrial contractions, and ventricular and atrial tachyarrhythmias.

Changes in pH can cause changes in serum potassium (alkalosis causes hypokalemia; acidosis causes hyperkalemia). For this reason, bicarbonate is given to severely hyperkalemic patients. Normalization of deranged pH most likely will correct the potassium derangement automatically (no need to give or restrict potassium).

IMPORTANT POINTS

1. The heart is particularly sensitive to hypokalemia when the patient is taking digitalis. Potassium should be watched carefully in all patients taking digitalis, especially if they also take diuretics (common).
2. Do *not* replace potassium too quickly! The best method of replacement is oral, but if potassium must be given IV, do not exceed 20 mEq/hr. Monitor the EKG if potassium must be given quickly because potentially fatal arrhythmias may develop.
3. If hypomagnesemia is present, it is difficult to correct the hypokalemia unless you also correct the hypomagnesemia. When magnesium is low, the body cannot retain potassium effectively. Therefore, if hypokalemia persists even after administration of significant amounts of potassium, check the magnesium level.

Hyperkalemia

If the patient is asymptomatic and the EKG is normal, but the lab result points to hyperkalemia, you should wonder whether the specimen was hemolyzed. Hemolysis causes a **false hyperkalemia.** Repeat the test.

Signs and symptoms can include weakness or paralysis, but the most important (and most tested) effects are cardiac. **EKG changes** (in order of increasing potassium value) include tall, peaked T waves (Fig. 15-3); widening of the QRS complex; PR interval prolongation; loss of P waves; and a sine wave pattern. Arrhythmias include asystole and ventricular fibrillation.

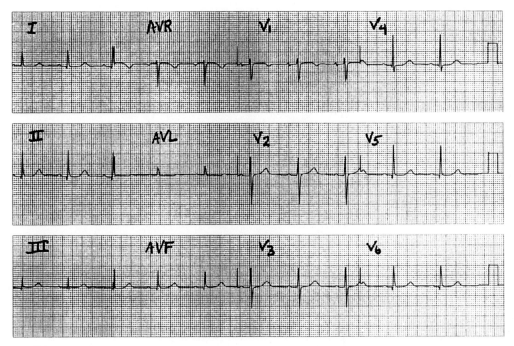

FIGURE 15-3 Mild hyperkalemia. Note the tall, peaked T waves, most prominent in V2–V5. No other abnormalities are present.

Common causes:

○ Renal failure (acute or chronic)
○ Severe tissue destruction (potassium is released from the cells of the damaged tissue)
○ Hypoaldosteronism (e.g., hyporeninemic hypoaldosteronism in diabetes)
○ Medications (potassium-sparing diuretics, β-blockers, nonsteroidal antiinflammatory drugs, ACE inhibitors, and ARBs). Try stopping all implicated medications.
○ Adrenal insufficiency (also associated with low sodium and low blood pressure)

Get an EKG first to look for cardiotoxicity. The **best therapy** for hyperkalemia is decreased oral potassium intake, sodium polystyrene resin (Kayexalate), and loop or thiazide diuretics. If, however, potassium is very high (>6.5 mEq/L) or cardiac toxicity is apparent (more than peaked T waves), immediate IV therapy is needed. First give calcium gluconate, which is cardioprotective, even though it does not change potassium levels. Then give sodium bicarbonate (alkalosis causes potassium to shift inside cells) and glucose with insulin, which also forces potassium inside cells. β2 agonists (albuterol) also may be used in severe cases. If the patient has renal failure or initial treatment is ineffective, prepare to institute dialysis emergently.

 Sodium bicarbonate, insulin with glucose, and β2 agonists only cause transient intracellular shifts of potassium and do not decrease total-body potassium. Further treatment with diuretics or binding resins are thus necessary.

Hypocalcemia

Hypocalcemia produces **neurologic findings**, the most tested of which is tetany. Tetany is evidenced by tapping on the facial nerve at the angle of the jaw to elicit contraction of the facial muscles (Chvostek sign) or applying a tourniquet or blood pressure cuff and inflating it to elicit hand muscle (carpopedal) spasms (Trousseau sign). Other symptoms are depression, encephalopathy, dementia, laryngospasm, and convulsions or seizures. EKG shows **QT interval prolongation** (Fig. 15-4).

Low albumin levels can cause hypocalcemia. If the calcium is low, first check the albumin level or the ionized or free calcium level to make sure "true" hypocalcemia is present. For every 1-g/dL decrease in albumin below 4 g/dL, correct the calcium by adding 0.8 mg/dL to the given calcium value.

Common causes of hypocalcemia:

○ DiGeorge syndrome (tetany shortly after birth, absent thymic shadow)
○ Renal failure (because of the kidney's role in vitamin D metabolism)
○ Hypoparathyroidism (watch for postthyroidectomy patients; all four parathyroids might have been accidentally removed)

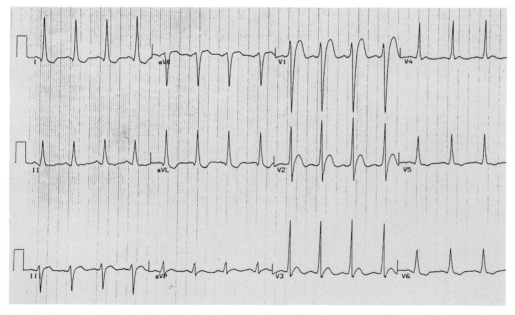

FIGURE 15-4 Hypocalcemia. Note the QT interval of 0.46 sec (normally ≤0.42 sec for the heart rate of 65 beats/min). No other electrocardiographic abnormalities are present.

○ Vitamin D deficiency
○ Pseudohypoparathyroidism (short fingers, short stature, mental retardation, and normal levels of parathyroid hormone [PTH] with end-organ unresponsiveness to PTH)
○ Acute pancreatitis
○ Renal tubular acidosis

IMPORTANT POINTS

1. Hypoproteinemia (i.e., low albumin) of any etiology can cause hypocalcemia because the protein-bound fraction of calcium is decreased. In this instance, however, the patient is asymptomatic because the ionized (unbound, physiologically active) fraction of calcium (which can be ordered and measured as a specific test) is unchanged (no treatment needed).
2. Hypomagnesemia of any cause makes it difficult to correct the hypocalcemia until the hypomagnesemia is also corrected.
3. Rickets and osteomalacia are the skeletal effects of vitamin D deficiency in children and adults, respectively.
4. Alkalosis can cause symptoms similar to hypocalcemia because of effects on the ionized fraction of calcium (alkalosis causes calcium to shift intracellularly). This scenario is most common with hyperventilation and anxiety syndromes in which the patient eliminates too much carbon dioxide, becomes alkalotic, and develops perioral and extremity tingling. Treat by correcting the pH and the underlying problem.
5. Phosphorus and calcium levels usually go in opposite directions, and derangements in one can cause problems with the other. In renal failure, therefore, you should not only raise calcium (with vitamin D and calcium supplements) but also restrict phosphorus.

Hypercalcemia

Hypercalcemia is **usually asymptomatic** and discovered by routine lab tests. *When symptoms are present,* remember "bones, stones, groans, and psychiatric overtones" (bone changes such as osteopenia or pathologic fractures; kidney stones and polyuria; abdominal pain, anorexia, constipation, ileus, nausea, vomiting; and depression, psychosis, delirium, and confusion). EKG shows **QT interval shortening** (Fig. 15-5).

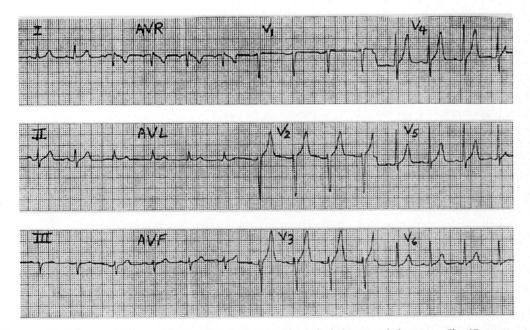

FIGURE 15-5 Electrocardiogram showing hypercalcemia with marked QT interval shortening. The ST segment is almost absent. (*From Carabello BA, Gazes PC: Cardiology Pearls, 2nd ed. Philadelphia, Hanley & Belfus, 2000.*)

Common causes:

○ Hyperparathyroidism (most common cause in outpatients)
○ Malignancy (most common cause in inpatients)
○ Multiple myeloma
○ Vitamin A or D intoxication
○ Sarcoidosis
○ Thiazide diuretics
○ Familial hypocalciuric hypercalcemia (look for low urinary calcium, which is rare with hypercalcemia)
○ Immobilization

Hyperproteinemia of any etiology can cause hypercalcemia because of an increase in the protein-bound fraction of calcium, but the patient is asymptomatic because the ionized (unbound) fraction (which can be measured and ordered directly as a separate test) is unchanged.

Treatment: First give IV fluids. When the patient is well hydrated, give furosemide to cause calcium diuresis (thiazides are *contraindicated* because they increase serum calcium levels). Other treatments include phosphorus administration (use oral phosphorus; IV is rarely used because it is dangerous), calcitonin, bisphosphonates (e.g., etidronate, which is also used in Paget disease), plicamycin, or prednisone (especially for malignancy-induced hypercalcemia). These measures are all temporary until definitive treatment for the underlying cause of hypercalcemia can be achieved.

Severe prolonged hypercalcemia can cause nephrocalcinosis, urolithiasis, and renal failure from calcium salt deposits in the kidneys. It may also result in bone disease secondary to loss of calcium.

Other Electrolyte Disturbances and Fluid Administration

Magnesium Disturbances

Hypomagnesemia is seen most often in people with alcoholism because of wasting through the kidneys. Signs and symptoms, which include EKG changes and tetany, are similar to those of hypocalcemia. Hypomagnesemia is notorious because it makes hypokalemia and hypocalcemia difficult to correct. Treat with oral replacement.

Hypermagnesemia is classically iatrogenic (pregnant patients treated with magnesium sulfate for preeclampsia) on the boards, but it is often caused by renal failure. Patients being treated with magnesium sulfate should be monitored carefully because the physical findings of hypermagnesemia are progressive. The initial sign is decreased deep tendon reflexes; then hypotension and respiratory depression occur sequentially.

Treatment includes stopping magnesium sulfate treatment if it is being given (first step) and providing supportive treatment (intubate if necessary), IV hydration, furosemide, and dialysis as a last resort.

Phosphorus Disturbances

Hypophosphatemia is seen primarily in patients with diabetic ketoacidosis and in patients with alcoholism. Signs and symptoms are neuromuscular disturbances (encephalopathy, weakness), rhabdomyolysis (especially in alcoholics), and anemia with white blood cell and platelet dysfunction.

Hyperphosphatemia is seen almost always in patients with renal failure. Treat with phosphate restriction, dialysis, and possibly phosphate-binding resins (calcium carbonate [$CaCO_3$]).

Fluid Administration

Give hypovolemic patients normal saline or Ringer lactate even if they are hypernatremic.

Maintenance fluid in NPO patients is usually 5% dextrose in half-normal saline (0.45% NaCl). In pediatric patients, use 5% dextrose in one-fourth (0.225% NaCl) or one-third (0.3% NaCl) normal saline because of renal differences. Hypokalemia can develop acutely in normal NPO patients if intermittent potassium supplements are not given (e.g., 10 mEq or 20 mEq KCl in the first liter of IV fluid each day, assuming that the baseline potassium level is normal).

VITAMINS AND MINERALS

Signs and symptoms of vitamin and mineral deficiencies and toxicities are shown in Table 15-6.

TABLE 15-6 Signs and Symptoms of Vitamin and Mineral Deficiencies and Toxicities

MICRONUTRIENT	SIGNS AND SYMPTOMS OF DEFICIENCY	SIGNS AND SYMPTOMS OF TOXICITY
Vitamins		
Vitamin A	Night blindness, scaly rash, xerophthalmia (dry eyes), Bitot spots (debris on conjunctiva), increased infections	Pseudotumor cerebri, bone thickening, teratogenicity
Vitamin D	Rickets, osteomalacia, hypocalcemia	Hypercalcemia, nausea and vomiting, renal toxicity
Vitamin E	Anemia, peripheral neuropathy, ataxia	Necrotizing enterocolitis (infants)
Vitamin K	Hemorrhage, prolonged prothrombin time	Hemolysis (kernicterus)
Vitamin B_1 (thiamine)	Wet beriberi (high-output cardiac failure), dry beriberi, (peripheral neuropathy), Wernicke and Korsakoff syndromes	
Vitamin B_2 (riboflavin)	Cheilosis, angular stomatitis, dermatitis	
Vitamin B_3 (niacin)	Pellagra (dementia, dermatitis, diarrhea), stomatitis	
Vitamin B_6 (pyridoxine)	Peripheral neuropathy, cheilosis, stomatitis, convulsions in infants, microcytic anemia, seborrheic dermatitis	Peripheral neuropathy (only B vitamin with toxicity)
Vitamin B_{12} (cobalamin)	Megaloblastic anemia *plus* neurologic symptoms	
Folic acid	Megaloblastic anemia *without* neurologic symptoms	
Vitamin C	Scurvy (hemorrhages—skin petechiae, bone, gums; loose teeth; gingivitis), poor wound healing, hyperkeratotic hair follicles, bone pain (from periosteal hemorrhages)	
Minerals		
Iron	Microcytic anemia, koilonychia (spoon-shaped fingernails)	Hemochromatosis
Iodine	Goiter, cretinism, hypothyroidism	Can cause myxedema
Fluorine	Dental caries (cavities)	Fluorosis with mottling of teeth and bone exostoses
Zinc	Hypogeusia (decreased taste), rash, slow wound healing	
Copper	Menkes disease (X-linked, kinky hair, and mental retardation)	Wilson disease
Selenium	Cardiomyopathy and muscle pain	Loss of hair and nails
Manganese		"Manganese madness" in miners of ore
Chromium	Impaired glucose tolerance	

IMPORTANT POINTS

1. Deficiency of fat-soluble vitamins (A, D, E, K) is often attributable to malabsorption (e.g., cystic fibrosis, cirrhosis, celiac disease, duodenal bypass, bile duct obstruction, pancreatic insufficiency, chronic giardiasis, inflammatory bowel disease). In such patients, parenteral supplements may be needed, but try high-dose oral supplements first.

2. People with alcoholism can have just about any deficiency, but watch for folate, thiamine, phosphorus, and magnesium deficiencies.

3. Vitamin B_{12} deficiency is most commonly caused by pernicious anemia, in which antiparietal cell antibodies destroy the ability to secrete intrinsic factor. Conditions associated with pernicious anemia include hypothyroidism, type 1 diabetes, and vitiligo. Schilling

(Continued)

test is used to diagnose the cause of B$_{12}$ deficiency. The tapeworm *Diphyllobothrium latum*, removal of the ileum, and inflammatory bowel disease also cause B$_{12}$ deficiency.

4. Isoniazid causes B$_6$ (pyridoxine) deficiency, especially in young people. Patients taking isoniazid are often given prophylactic B$_6$ supplements.

5. Anticonvulsants (especially phenytoin), methotrexate, and trimethoprim can cause folate deficiency.

6. Vitamin A is teratogenic, and any female patient given one of the vitamin A analogues as treatment for acne (e.g., isotretinoin) *must* have a negative pregnancy test result before medication is started and *must* be put on some form of birth control and counseled about the risks of teratogenicity if pregnancy occurs. Offer periodic pregnancy tests.

7. Rickets causes interesting physical findings, including craniotabes (poorly mineralized skull and bones that feel like a ping-pong ball), rachitic rosary (costochondral beading with small, round masses on anterior rib cage), delayed fontanelle closure, bossing of the skull, kyphoscoliosis, bowlegs, and knock knees. Bone changes first appear at the lower ends of the radius and ulna (seen on radiographs).

8. *Vitamin K is given to all newborns* as prophylaxis against hemorrhagic disease of the newborn. Vitamin K is needed for the synthesis of factors II, VII, IX, and X as well as proteins C and S. Chronic liver disease (cirrhosis) can cause prolongation of the prothrombin time and international normalized ratio (INR) because of inability to synthesize clotting factors even in the presence of adequate vitamin K. Treat with fresh-frozen plasma in this case because vitamin K is ineffective in the setting of severe liver disease.

9. Vitamin K deficiency may result from prolonged therapy with broad-spectrum antibiotics. These medications eliminate the normal gut bacteria that synthesize much of the vitamin K required daily.

10. Folate supplements should be taken by sexually active women of reproductive age to reduce the risk of neural tube defects in the fetus. The maximal benefit often occurs before the woman knows she is pregnant.

SHOCK

Definition: Shock is a state in which blood flow to and perfusion of peripheral tissues is inadequate to sustain life. Although not included in a rigid definition of shock for board purposes, associated findings include hypotension, oliguria or anuria, cool or clammy skin, mental status changes, and metabolic acidosis. Tachycardia is also usually present.

Pragmatically speaking, there are three main clinical types of shock:

○ Hypovolemic
○ Cardiogenic
○ Distributive (includes septic shock, neurogenic shock, anaphylactic shock, and toxic shock syndrome)

Your job is to figure out why the patient is in shock while keeping him or her alive with the ABCs (airway, breathing, circulation). Give fluids and, if appropriate, inotropes or vasoconstrictors while you're thinking. Positive signs include increases in blood pressure and fluid output. Place a Foley catheter to ensure accurate monitoring of urine output. If the patient does not respond to a fluid bolus and you are given the choice, use invasive hemodynamic monitoring (Swan-Ganz catheter) to help make diagnostic and therapeutic decisions. Hemodynamic parameters of shock are shown in Table 15-7.

Associated findings help to differentiate the etiology of shock:

○ **Hypovolemic shock:** History of fluid loss (hemorrhage, diarrhea, vomiting, sweating, diuretics, inability to drink water). The patient has cold, clammy skin and looks pale. Fluid loss may be internal, as with a ruptured abdominal aortic or thoracic aneurysm; with pancreatitis; after surgery; or with obstruction or infarction of the spleen, pancreas, or bowel. Other signs include orthostatic hypotension, tachycardia, sunken eyes, tenting of the skin, and a sunken fontanelle (in babies).

TABLE 15-7 Hemodynamic Parameters of Shock

TYPE OF SHOCK	CO	PCWP	SVR	SVO₂
Hypovolemic*	Low	Low	High	Low
Cardiogenic	Low	High	High	Low
Septic (early)	High	Low	Low	High
Neurogenic	Low	Low	Low	Low

*Also the parameters for late septic shock.

CO, cardiac output; PCWP, pulmonary capillary wedge pressure; SVO_2, systemic venous oxygen saturation; SVR, systemic vascular resistance.

○ **Cardiogenic shock:** History of myocardial infarction, chest pain, congestive heart failure, or several risk factors for coronary artery disease. Most patients have cold, clammy skin and look pale. Distended neck veins and pulmonary congestion (on exam and radiography) are usually present. Patients usually need diuretics—IV fluid can make them worse!

○ **Neurogenic shock:** History of severe central nervous system trauma or bleed; flushed skin. Heart rate may be normal.

○ **Septic shock:** Fever, changes in white blood cell count (leukocytosis unless the patient is on chemotherapy or has an immunosuppressive condition such as AIDS), skin that is flushed and warm to the touch, and extremes of age. Use broad-spectrum antibiotics after "pan culturing" the patient (get blood, sputum, and urine cultures plus others if history and physical exam dictate).

○ **Anaphylaxis:** Onset of hives, pruritus, flushing, or swelling of mucous membranes (e.g., lips) over minutes to hours after exposure to a known or possible allergen. **Anaphylactic shock** is different than anaphylaxis and involves respiratory compromise, reduced blood pressure, or symptoms of end-organ dysfunction such as syncope. It may include gastrointestinal symptoms such as nausea, vomiting, diarrhea, or abdominal pain. Look for bee stings, peanuts, and shellfish and for penicillins, sulfas, and other medications. Treat with epinephrine and fluids, administer O_2, and intubate if necessary (do a tracheostomy or cricothyroidotomy if laryngeal edema prevents intubation). Antihistamines help only when the reaction is mild. Use corticosteroids when the reaction is prolonged or severe (not first-line drugs for treatment of anaphylaxis). Monitor all patients for at least 6 hours after the initial reaction.

○ **Pulmonary embolus:** Look for risk factors for deep vein thrombosis (Virchow triad: endothelial damage, stasis, hypercoagulable state), history of recent delivery (amniotic fluid embolus), history of recent travel on an airplane or train, oral contraceptive use, fractures (fat emboli), deep vein thrombosis (positive Homan sign with painful, swollen leg), and recent surgery (especially orthopedic or pelvic surgery). Patients are often asymptomatic but may have tachycardia, chest pain, tachypnea, shortness of breath, parasternal heave, right-axis shift on EKG, and positive ventilation–perfusion (V/Q) scan or CT pulmonary angiogram. Heparinize to prevent further clotting and emboli. If severe hemodynamic compromise occurs, treatment with thrombolytics or interventional radiology may be required.

○ **Pericardial tamponade:** Classic is a history of stab wound in left chest with distended neck veins on exam. Do pericardiocentesis emergently in the setting of shock. Remember Beck triad for cardiac tamponade: diminished arterial blood pressure, jugular venous distension, and distant muffled heart sounds.

○ **Toxic shock syndrome:** The classic patient is a woman of reproductive age who leaves a tampon in place too long. Look for skin desquamation. Caused by *Staphylococcus aureus* toxin.

○ **Addisonian crisis:** The classic patient is a postoperative patient who has a history of chronic steroid use but received no extra steroids perioperatively. Hyponatremia and hyperkalemia are usually present. Treat with steroids.

Note ABCs (airway, breathing, circulation) come first. Patients in shock often need heroic measures to survive. Intubate if necessary, keep the patient NPO, and avoid narcotics if possible (mental status changes are often an important clue to impending doom). Monitor EKG, vital signs, Swan-Ganz parameters, urine output, arterial blood gases (ABGs), chest radiographs, hemoglobin, and hematocrit.

TABLE 15-8 Action of Medications on Adrenergic Receptors

RECEPTOR	PRIMARY SITES OF ACTION OF MEDICATIONS	AGONIST ACTION
α_1	Norepinephrine, epinephrine, phenylephrine, dobutamine	Smooth muscle contraction (increased force of heart contraction)
α_2	Epinephrine > norepinephrine	Smooth muscle constriction and neurotransmitter inhibition
β_1	Epinephrine, norepinephrine, dobutamine, dopamine, isoproterenol	Increase in rate and force heart contraction
β_2	Epinephrine, norepinephrine, dobutamine, isoproterenol	Smooth muscle relaxation (vasodilation)
Dopamine receptor	Dopamine	Smooth muscle relaxation (dilates renal blood vessels)

 Most patients in shock need fluid. The standard bolus is 10 to 20 mL/kg of normal saline (roughly 1–2 L infused as fast as it will go). After the bolus, reassess the patient to determine whether the bolus helped. Do not be afraid to bolus twice if the first bolus has no effect. Of course, you must watch for fluid overload, which can cause congestive heart failure.

Understand IV medications and their use to support blood pressure:

○ **Dobutamine:** β_1-agonist used to increase cardiac output by increasing contractility (it is the ICU equivalent of digoxin)
○ **Dopamine:** Affects dopamine receptors at low doses and results in selective vasodilation (the traditional use for renal perfusion is questionable). Higher doses have β_1-agonist effects to increase contractility. Highest doses have α_1-agonist effects and cause vasoconstriction. Some authorities debate this differential effect, but it might still come up on boards.
○ **Norepinephrine:** Used for its α_1-agonist effects; given in hypotension to increase peripheral resistance so that perfusion to vital organs can be maintained. Also has β-agonist effects.
○ **Phenylephrine:** Used for its α_1-agonist effects. It is similar to norepinephrine but has no β effects.
○ **Epinephrine:** Used for cardiac arrest and anaphylaxis for its α and β effects
○ **Isoproterenol** is used for its β_1 and β_2 effects in hypovolemic, septic, and cardiogenic shock.
○ **Milrinone and amrinone:** Phosphodiesterase inhibitors used in refractory heart failure (*not* first-line agents) because they have a positive inotropic effect via potentiation of cyclic adenosine monophosphate (cAMP), but they cannot be used in hypotensive patients.

For shock in the setting of trauma, see trauma section in Chapter 8, General Surgery.

Table 15-8 provides a summary of medication effects on adrenergic receptors. Remember that norepinephrine primarily activates α receptors, and epinephrine primarily activates β receptors.

QR CODE

The QR code includes three USMLE-style questions and answers. For more questions, redeem the PIN code on the inside cover for the Crush Step 2 question bank powered by USMLE Consult.

Please see the Introduction for instructions on how to access content using the QR codes.

Question

A 35-year-old woman comes to the office complaining of numbness and tingling in the fingers of both of her hands and around her mouth. When the nurse takes her blood pressure, the patient's hand closes involuntarily and starts to have painful spasms. The nurse removes the blood pressure cuff and attempts to take the blood pressure from the other arm, and the same thing happens. Which of the following is correct concerning this woman's condition?

(A) Electrocardiogram probably will show QT interval shortening.
(B) You should ask about a recent history of thyroid surgery.
(C) She most likely has Graves disease.
(D) Voluntary hyperventilation may improve symptoms.
(E) The patient requires high-dose corticosteroids.

16 LABORATORY MEDICINE

ELECTROLYTES

○ Hyperkalemia may be caused by a hemolyzed blood sample (consider rechecking the lab result if it doesn't make sense), rhabdomyolysis (caused by high intracellular potassium concentration), or renal failure.

○ Alkalosis can cause hypokalemia and symptoms of hypocalcemia (perioral numbness, tetany) because of cellular shift; acidosis can cause hyperkalemia by the same mechanism. Correction of the acid–base status will correct the potassium and calcium derangements.

○ Pseudohyponatremia may be caused by hyperglycemia, hyperproteinemia, or hyperlipidemia; these forms of pseudohyponatremia will correct with correction of the glucose, lipid, or protein levels.

○ Correcting hyponatremia aggressively (especially with hypertonic saline [3%]) can cause brainstem damage (osmotic myelinolysis, or central pontine myelinolysis).

○ Hypokalemia and hypocalcemia may be caused by hypomagnesemia. You cannot correct the hypokalemia until you correct the hypomagnesemia.

○ Watch for hypophosphatemia and hypokalemia in diabetic ketoacidosis.

ENZYMES

○ Increased levels of amylase and lipase may be caused by sources other than the pancreas (salivary glands, gastrointestinal tract, renal failure, ruptured tubal pregnancy), but elevation of both in the same patient with abdominal pain is almost always caused by pancreatitis. Lipase is more specific to the pancreas than amylase.

○ Alkaline phosphatase can be elevated by biliary disease, bone disease, or pregnancy. If the elevation is attributable to biliary disease, γ-glutamyl transpeptidase (GGT) or 5-nucleotidase (5-NT) also should be elevated. Both values, however, remain normal in bone disease and pregnancy.

○ Elevated creatine kinase (CK) may be attributable to muscle injury (striated or myocardial), drugs (HMG-CoA reductase inhibitors), or burns (CK-MB is more specific for cardiac muscle).

OTHER

○ Hypothyroidism can cause elevated cholesterol.

○ Blood urea nitrogen-to-creatinine ratio greater than 15 usually implies dehydration.

○ Positive results on the rapid plasma reagin or Venereal Disease Research Laboratory (VDRL) test for syphilis may be caused by systemic lupus erythematosus.

○ In patients with isosthenuria and hyposthenuria—the inability to concentrate urine—think of diabetes insipidus or sickle cell disease or trait. The specific gravity of urine and serum is the same, classically 1.010.

○ The erythrocyte sedimentation rate (ESR) is a worthless test in pregnancy; ESR is elevated by pregnancy itself. Blood urea nitrogen (BUN) and creatinine are decreased significantly in pregnancy after the first trimester. A high-normal BUN or creatinine level can mean renal disease in pregnancy because the glomerular filtration rate increases during pregnancy.

○ Elevated levels of the binding protein can cause elevation of the total concentration of a substance without elevating the free or active portion of that substance, which is rarely important clinically and doesn't need treatment (e.g., elevated thyroid hormone with elevation of thyroid-binding globulin levels; decrease in calcium levels caused by decreased albumin levels). Check the free, unbound, or active portion of the substance of interest or order the associated carrier or binding protein level to make sure you don't fall for this one. In the case of calcium levels, the free calcium level is rarely given on the USMLE Step 2. Be sure you know how to correct the calcium level using the albumin:
  ○ Corrected calcium = (0.8 × (Normal albumin − Serum albumin)) + Serum calcium
  ○ In this formula, the normal albumin is 4.

QR CODE

The QR code includes three USMLE-style questions and answers. For more questions, redeem the PIN code on the inside cover for the Crush Step 2 question bank powered by USMLE Consult.
    Please see the Introduction for instructions on how to access content using the QR codes.

Question

A 55-year-old woman is scheduled to undergo a cholecystectomy for symptomatic gallstones, and you are asked to provide preoperative clearance. The patient has no significant medical history, and a routine physical examination done 1 year ago was within normal limits. Family history is significant for a father who died of lung cancer. The patient is currently taking no medications. A review of systems and physical examination are within normal limits other than mild obesity. Routine laboratory tests reveal the following:

Hemoglobin	14 g/dL
Mean corpuscular	88 μm/cell volume
Sodium	140 mEq/L
Potassium	7.9 mEq/L
Chloride	105 mEq/L
CO_2	26 mEq/L
BUN	8 mg/dL
Creatinine	0.9 mg/dL
Total bilirubin	0.5 mg/dL (reference range, 0.1–1 mg/dL)
Indirect bilirubin	0.4 mg/dL (reference range, 0.1–0.8 mg/dL)

Electrocardiogram and chest radiograph are within normal limits. Which of the following is true regarding the patient's potassium level?
(A) It likely is attributable to intrinsic renal disease.
(B) It likely is attributable to a problem within the adrenal glands.
(C) You should call the laboratory and ask about hemolysis of the specimen.
(D) It most likely represents early multiple myeloma.
(E) Urgent treatment is needed.

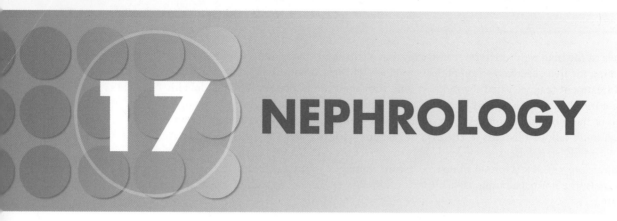

17 NEPHROLOGY

ACUTE RENAL FAILURE

Symptoms of acute renal failure (ARF) include fatigue, nausea, vomiting, anorexia, shortness of breath, and mental status changes. Signs include a progressive rise in creatinine and blood urea nitrogen (BUN), metabolic acidosis, hyperkalemia, altered mental status, and hypervolemia (rales, elevated jugular venous pressure, edema, and dilutional hyponatremia). There are three categories: prerenal, postrenal, and renal.

Prerenal

The most common example is hypovolemia (dehydration, hemorrhage). Look for a BUN-to-creatinine ratio higher than 20 and signs of hypovolemia (e.g., tachycardia, weak pulse, depressed fontanelle). Give intravenous (IV) fluids, blood, or both. Other prerenal causes are sepsis (treat the sepsis and give IV fluids), heart failure (give inotropes and diuretics), liver failure (hepatorenal syndrome; treat with midodrine, octreotide and supportive care), and renal artery stenosis.

Postrenal

Urine is blocked from being excreted at some point distal to the kidneys (ureters, prostate, urethra). The most common example is benign prostatic hyperplasia (BPH). The patient is a man older than 50 years with BPH symptoms (e.g., hesitancy, dribbling), and ultrasonography reveals bilateral hydronephrosis. Treat with catheterization (suprapubic catheterization if necessary) to relieve obstruction and prevent further renal damage; then consider surgery (transurethral prostatectomy [TURP]). Malignancy of the bladder, cervix, or bowel is another cause. Nephrolithiasis is a rare cause because stones have to be bilateral to cause renal failure. Also consider retroperitoneal fibrosis, especially with a history of methysergide use.

Renal

Acute tubular necrosis is the most common type. Examples of renal causes:
- **Glomerulonephritis:** Poststreptococcal glomerulonephritis is the classic example on board exams. It is usually seen in children with a history of upper respiratory infection or strep throat 1 to 3 weeks earlier. They present with edema, hypervolemia, hypertension, hematuria, and oliguria. Red blood cell casts on urinalysis clinch the diagnosis. Treat supportively.
- **Goodpasture syndrome:** Caused by antiglomerular basement membrane antibodies (linear immunofluorescence pattern on renal biopsy), which also react with and damage the lungs. Look for a young male patient with hemoptysis, dyspnea, and renal failure. Treat initially with cyclophosphamide. Methotrexate or azathioprine is used for maintenance.
- **Intravenous contrast:** Do not give to diabetic patients or renal patients if you can avoid it; you can precipitate ARF. If you must give it, give lots of hydration. Also consider using oral acetylcysteine on the day before and the day of contrast administration.
- **Lupus erythematosus:** Look for malar rash and arthritis. Renal failure is a major cause of morbidity and mortality in patients with lupus.
- **Myoglobinuria or rhabdomyolysis:** From strenuous exercise (e.g., marathon), alcohol, burns, muscle trauma, heat stroke, or neuroleptic malignant syndrome. Muscle breaks down and plugs up the renal filtration system. Look for very high levels of creatine phosphokinase. Treat with hydration and diuretics.
- **Toxins and medications:** Chronic nonsteroidal antiinflammatory drug use (may cause acute tubular necrosis or papillary necrosis), cyclosporine, aminoglycosides, methicillin, or chemotherapeutic agents (e.g., cisplatin).

○ **Wegener granulomatosis:** A vasculitis that affects the lungs and kidneys; patients typically present after age 40 years. Look for nasal involvement (bloody nose, nasal perforation) or hemoptysis and pleurisy as presenting symptoms. Patients have positive antineutrophil cytoplasm antibody (ANCA) titer results. Treat with cyclophosphamide and steroids. Methotrexate is an alternative.

○ **Immunoglobulin A (IgA) nephropathy (Berger disease):** The most common glomerulonephritis worldwide. Caused by deposition of IgA antibodies in the glomerulus. If deposition is systemic, it is known as Henoch-Schönlein purpura (HSP). Look for hematuria shortly after an upper respiratory infection. It is associated with liver failure, celiac disease, rheumatoid arthritis, reactive arthritis (formerly called Reiter disease), ankylosing spondylitis, and HIV infection. Treatment ranges from observation to steroids, cyclosporine, azathioprine, and mycophenolate mofetil.

○ **Membranoproliferative glomerulonephritis:** Caused by deposits in the glomerular mesangium and basement membrane that activate complement. A tram-tracking appearance is seen under electron microscopy.

○ **Cryoglobulinemia:** Cryoglobulins, immune complex proteins that become insoluble at low temperatures, can deposit in the kidneys and cause ARF. It is associated with multiple myeloma, Waldenstrom macroglobulinemia, and hepatitis C. Extrarenal symptoms include hyperviscosity syndromes, purpura, arthralgias, and myalgias. Treatment involves managing the underlying condition. Steroids, plasmapheresis, and cytotoxic agents are used for severe disease.

○ **Multiple myeloma:** Causes renal failure from tubular damage caused by excretion of light chains, also known as Bence Jones proteins. Can induce renal failure from hypercalcemia and amyloidosis. Renal failure in Waldenstrom macroglobulinemia, a similar condition, is rare and usually linked to amyloidosis or cryoglobulinemia.

○ **Minimal change disease:** Causes nephritic syndrome in young children (peak incidence at ages 2–3 years). No pathologic changes are seen under light microscopy. Under electron microscopy, a loss of podocytes is seen. The disease is highly responsive to steroids.

○ **Membranous glomerulonephritis:** A common progressive disease affecting patients between 30 and 50 years of age. Most cases are idiopathic, but it has also been linked to autoimmune conditions, infections, drugs, and malignancies. It is caused by circulating immune complexes. Under microscopy, subepithelial immunoglobulin-containing deposits are seen along the glomerular basement membrane. Treatment involves immunosuppressive agents.

 In all cases of ARF, dialysis may be required. Remember the acronym AEIOU for indications for dialysis: **a**cidosis (roughly, pH <7.25), **e**lectrolyte abnormalities (hyperkalemia), **i**ngestions (e.g., salicylates, methanol, barbiturates), **o**verload (heart failure), and **u**remic encephalopathy.

NEPHROTIC SYNDROME

Nephrotic syndrome is characterized by proteinuria (>3.5 g/day), hypoalbuminemia, edema (classic example is morning periorbital edema), and hyperlipidemia and lipiduria. In children, the nephrotic syndrome is usually caused by minimal change disease (also called lipoid nephrosis; effaced podocyte foot processes on electron microscopy), often after an infection. Measure 24-hour urine protein to clinch the diagnosis and treat with steroids. Causes in adults include diabetes mellitus, hepatitis B, amyloidosis, lupus, and drugs (gold, penicillamine, captopril).

NEPHRITIC SYNDROME

Nephritic syndrome includes oliguria, azotemia (rising BUN and creatinine), hypertension, and hematuria. Patients might have some proteinuria but not in the nephrotic range. The classic cause is poststreptococcal glomerulonephritis. Red blood cell casts on urinalysis are classic.

CHRONIC RENAL FAILURE

Any of the causes of ARF can cause chronic renal failure (CRF) if the insult is severe or prolonged. The majority of cases of CRF are caused by diabetes mellitus (number one cause of CRF) and hypertension. Another classic cause is polycystic kidney disease (multiple cysts in the kidney); look for a positive family history (usually autosomal dominant; autosomal recessive form presents in children), hypertension, hematuria, palpable renal masses, berry aneurysms in the circle of Willis, and cysts in liver and other organs. Metabolic derangements caused by CRF:

○ **Anemia:** From lack of erythropoietin (synthetic erythropoietin can correct)
○ **Anorexia, nausea, and vomiting:** From build-up of toxins
○ **Azotemia:** High BUN and creatinine
○ **Bleeding:** Caused by disordered platelet function; patients can have prolonged bleeding time test
○ **Central nervous system disturbances:** Mental status changes and even convulsions or coma from toxin build-up
○ **Fluid retention:** Can cause hypertension, edema, congestive heart failure, and pulmonary edema
○ **Hyperkalemia:** Watch for electrocardiographic changes
○ **Hypocalcemia or hyperphosphatemia:** Vitamin D production is impaired; bone loss leads to renal osteodystrophy
○ **Increased susceptibility to infection:** Caused by decreased cellular immunity
○ **Metabolic acidosis**
○ **Skin pigmentation and pruritus:** Skin turns yellowish-brown and itches; caused by metabolic byproducts
○ **Uremic pericarditis:** Classically causes an audible friction rub

Treatment: Regular hemodialysis (usually 3 times/week), water-soluble vitamins (which are removed during dialysis), phosphate restriction and binders (calcium carbonate, calcium acetate, or sevelamer), erythropoietin, and hypertension control. The only cure is renal transplant.

URINARY TRACT INFECTION

Urinary tract infections (UTIs) are much more common in female patients except in the neonatal and early pediatric period. They are usually caused by *Escherichia coli* (less often by *Staphylococcus saprophyticus* and *Proteus, Pseudomonas, Klebsiella, Enterobacter, Enterococcus* spp. or other enteric organisms). Patients who acquire UTIs in the hospital or from a chronic, indwelling Foley catheter are more likely to have organisms other than *E. coli*.

Look for urgency, dysuria, suprapubic or low back pain, and low-grade fever. The gold standard for diagnosis is urine culture (at the least, get a midstream sample; best is a catheterized sample or suprapubic tap). Urinalysis shows white blood cells, bacteria, positive leukocyte esterase, or positive nitrite. Treat with trimethoprim–sulfamethoxazole, amoxicillin, nitrofurantoin, ciprofloxacin, or first-generation cephalosporin for about 5 days.

IMPORTANT POINTS

1. In pediatric patients, UTI is a cause for concern because it may be the presenting symptom of a genitourinary malformation. The most common examples are vesicoureteral reflux (VUR) and posterior urethral valves. Urine culture should be obtained. Order an ultrasonography and either a voiding cystourethrogram (VCUG) or radionuclide cystogram (RNC) to evaluate the urinary tract in any child 2 months to 2 years with a first UTI. Recommendations for imaging in older children are less clear cut, but imaging should be considered for any child with recurrent UTIs or pyelonephritis.
2. In elderly patients, UTI is one of the most common causes of altered mental status.
3. Conditions that promote urinary stasis (prostate hyperplasia, pregnancy, stones, neurogenic bladder, VUR) or bacterial colonization (indwelling catheter, fecal incontinence, surgical instrumentation) predispose patients to UTI. They also predispose patients to ascending UTI (pyelonephritis) and to bacteremia and sepsis.
4. Asymptomatic bacteriuria is treated in pregnancy (high risk of progression to pyelonephritis). In nonpregnant patients, asymptomatic bacteriuria should not be treated.

PYELONEPHRITIS

Pyelonephritis usually results from an ascending UTI and is caused by *E. coli* (>80% of cases). Patients present with high fever, shaking chills, costovertebral angle tenderness or flank pain, or UTI symptoms. Urinalysis and urine and blood cultures establish the diagnosis. Computed tomography (CT) can detect complications such as abscess. Treat on an inpatient basis with intravenous antibiotics while awaiting culture results (e.g., fluoroquinolone or extended-spectrum penicillin or cephalosporin).

KIDNEY AND HEMATOLOGIC DISORDERS IN CHILDREN

See Chapter 24, Pediatrics.

RENAL STONES

Renal stones (nephrolithiasis) manifest with severe, intermittent, unilateral flank or groin pain. Most stones (85%) show up on abdominal radiographs and are composed of calcium, but CT is now the standard diagnostic method (detects >95% of stones and more accurately localizes them; avoids contrast as needed with intravenous pyelography). Most cases are idiopathic and should be treated with lots of hydration and pain control (to see if the stone will pass). If the stone does not pass, it needs to be removed surgically (preferably endoscopically) or by lithotripsy.

Underlying causes of stones:

- ○ **Hypercalcemia:** From hyperparathyroidism or malignancy (metastases or squamous cell lung cancer secreting parathyroid hormone)
- ○ **Infection:** From ammonia-producing bugs (*Proteus*, *Staphylococcus* spp.); look for Staghorn calculi (Fig. 17-1)
- ○ **Hyperuricemia:** Uric acid stones are associated with gout and leukemia treatment (allopurinol and intravenous fluids can be given before chemotherapy as preventive measures)
- ○ **Cystinuria and aminoaciduria:** Suspect this hereditary cause if the stone is made of cystine or you are presented with a patient who repetitively forms stones.

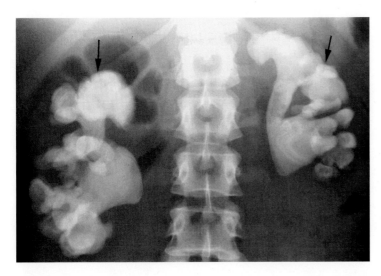

FIGURE 17-1 Radiograph of bilateral Staghorn calculi (*arrows*).

QR CODE

The QR code includes three USMLE-style questions and answers. For more questions, redeem the PIN code on the inside cover for the Crush Step 2 question bank powered by USMLE Consult.
   Please see the Introduction for instructions on how to access content using the QR codes.

Question

Which of the following does NOT increase the risk of forming calcium stones in the kidney?
(A) Hyperoxaluria
(B) Hypercalcemia
(C) Hyperparathyroidism
(D) Thiazide diuretics
(E) Hypercalciuria

18 NEUROLOGY

NEUROLOGY TESTS

Lumbar puncture is most commonly indicated for suspected meningitis or a sterile inflammatory central nervous system (CNS) disorder (e.g., multiple sclerosis, Guillain-Barré syndrome). Table 18-1 shows the classic findings in various conditions. Also used for the diagnosis of subarachnoid hemorrhage when the head computed tomography (CT) scan results are negative.

IMPORTANT POINTS

1. Do not perform lumbar puncture in patients with acute head trauma or signs of intracranial hypertension (e.g., papilledema) until you have a negative computed tomography or magnetic resonance imaging result. You might cause uncal herniation and death.
2. Tuberculosis and fungal meningitis have low glucose (<50 mg/dL) with high cells (>100/μL), which are predominantly lymphocytes. Watch for a positive India ink preparation for *Cryptococcus* spp.

Nerve conduction velocities are slowed by demyelination (Guillain-Barré syndrome, multiple sclerosis). Repetitive stimulation can assess fatigability. Myasthenia gravis is characterized by *increasing* fatigue with stimulation; Eaton-Lambert syndrome is characterized by *decreasing* fatigue with stimulation.

Electromyography (EMG) measures the electrical (contractile) properties of muscle. Lower motor neuron lesions are associated with fasciculations and fibrillations at rest. When the disease is in the muscle itself, no electrical activity is seen at rest (which is normal), but amplitude is decreased with contraction of the muscle.

STROKE AND TRANSIENT ISCHEMIC ATTACK

Stroke

Cerebrovascular disease (stroke, cerebrovascular accident) is the most common cause of neurologic disability in the United States and the third leading cause of death. Ischemia from atherosclerosis is by far the most common cause of stroke; other classic causes include atrial fibrillation with resultant clot formation and emboli to the brain and septic emboli from endocarditis. A stroke can also be hemorrhagic, such as with an intracranial hemorrhage. Look for symptoms of numbness, weakness, paralysis, aphasia, confusion, visual disturbances, loss of coordination, and headache. You should start by obtaining an emergent head CT because it can tell you if the stroke is ischemic or hemorrhagic (Fig. 18-1). When the CT result is negative (and you have the resources), consider getting a magnetic resonance imaging (MRI) scan because it is much more sensitive for ischemic stroke.

Treatment of stroke depends on the etiology and the patient. Start by assessing and stabilizing the ABCs (airway, breathing, circulation) and providing supportive care such as supplemental oxygen

TABLE 18-1 Classic Cerebrospinal Fluid Findings in Different Conditions*

CONDITION	CELLS/μL†	GLUCOSE (MG/DL)	PROTEIN (MG/DL)	PRESSURE (MM H₂O)
Normal	0–3 (L)	50–100	20–45	100–200
Bacterial meningitis	**>1000 (PMN)**	<50	Around 100	>200
Viral or aseptic meningitis	>100 (L)	Normal	Normal or slightly increased	Normal or slightly increased
Pseudotumor cerebri	**Normal**	Normal	Normal	**>200**
Guillain-Barré syndrome	**0–100 (L)**	**Normal**	**>100**	Normal
Cerebral hemorrhage‡	**Bloody (RBC)**	Normal	>45	>200
Multiple sclerosis§	Normal or slightly increased (L)	Normal	Normal or slightly increased	Normal

*Note: Bold type highlights the most important considerations for each disorder.
†Main cell type is put in parenthesis after the number.
‡Think of subarachnoid hemorrhage, but the same findings also can occur after an intracerebral hemorrhage.
§On electrophoresis of cerebrospinal fluid, look for oligoclonal bands caused by increased immunoglobulin G production and an increased level of myelin basic protein during active demyelination.
CSF, cerebrospinal fluid; L, lymphocytes; PMN, polymorphonuclear neutrophil; RBC, red blood cell.

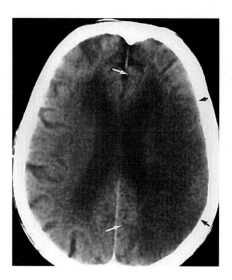

FIGURE 18-1 Large left middle cerebral artery infarct, nonhemorrhagic (*black arrows*) on computed tomography (CT). The sulci have been obliterated by swelling. Note sparing of the brain supplied by the left anterior and posterior cerebral arteries (*white arrows*).

and intravenous (IV) fluids. For an ischemic stroke, you can restore the vessel patency by either direct means (clot retrieval devices) or tissue plasminogen activator (t-PA) can be given up to 3 hours of the onset of symptoms (and ≤4.5 hours of the onset of symptoms with additional minor exclusions such as age older than 80 years). Table 18-2 lists contraindications for t-PA. Do not treat blood pressure acutely in patients with ischemic stroke because their condition can actually deteriorate if the blood pressure is lowered. However, if the hypertension is extreme (systolic blood pressure ≥220 mm Hg or diastolic blood pressure ≥120 mm Hg), the blood pressure can be lowered cautiously by about 15% in the first 24 hours. For a hemorrhagic stroke, supportive care is the best we have.

Transient Ischemic Attack

Transient ischemic attack is a focal neurologic deficit that lasts minutes to hours and then resolves spontaneously; it is often a precursor to stroke. The classic presentation is ipsilateral blindness (amaurosis fugax) or unilateral hemiplegia, hemiparesis, weakness, or clumsiness. Get a carotid duplex ultrasonography scan to look for stenosis. For long-term therapy, use aspirin or other antiplatelet medications (e.g., clopidogrel), carotid endarterectomy (if carotid stenosis is >70%–99%), or both. Risk factor modification, such as smoking cessation and better management of comorbid conditions such as diabetes and hypertension, is also important.

The signs and symptoms can indicate the location of a CNS lesion (Table 18-3).

TABLE 18-2 Contraindications for Tissue Plasminogen Activator
Active intracranial hemorrhage
Intracranial or intraspinal injury within 3 months
Stroke or serious head injury within 3 months
History of intracranial hemorrhage
Uncontrolled hypertension (>185/110 mm Hg) at the time of treatment
Active internal bleeding
Intracranial neoplasm, arteriovenous malformation, or aneurysm

TABLE 18-3 Localizing a Stroke or Other Central Nervous System Lesion	
SYMPTOM OR SIGN	**THINK OF THIS AREA**
Decreased or no reflexes or fasciculations	Lower motor neuron lesion (or possibly a muscle problem)
Hyperreflexia	Upper motor neuron lesion (spinal cord or brain)
Apathy, inattention, uninhibited/labile affect	Frontal lobes
Broca (motor) aphasia	Dominant frontal lobe*
Wernicke (sensory) aphasia	Dominant temporal lobe*
Memory impairment, aggression, hypersexuality	Temporal lobes
Inability to read, write, name, or do math	Dominant parietal lobe*
Ignoring one side of the body, difficulty in dressing	Nondominant parietal lobe*
Visual hallucinations or illusions	Occipital lobes
CNs III and IV	Midbrain
CNs V, VI, VII, and VIII	Pons
CNs IX, X, XI, and XII	Medulla
Ataxia, dysarthria, nystagmus, intention tremor, dysmetria, scanning speech	Cerebellum
Resting tremor, chorea	Basal ganglia
Hemiballismus	Subthalamic nucleus

* The left hemisphere is dominant in more than 95% of the population (99% of right-handed people and 60%–70% of left-handed people).
CN, cranial nerve; CNS, central nervous system.

CRANIAL NERVE LESIONS

The **olfactory nerve (cranial nerve [CN] I)** is rarely important clinically. Kallmann syndrome is anosmia plus hypogonadism caused by deficiency of gonadotropin-releasing hormone.

Optic (CN II), oculomotor (CN III), trochlear (CN IV), and abducens (CN VI) lesions are discussed in Chapter 22.

The **trigeminal nerve (CN V)** innervates the muscles of mastication and facial sensation (including the afferent limb of the corneal reflex). Patients may have trigeminal neuralgia (tic douloureux), which is characterized by unilateral shooting pains in the face in older adults and is often triggered by activity (e.g., brushing teeth). Treat with carbamazepine, gabapentin, or other antiepilepsy medication. If the patient is young or female or the disease is bilateral, consider multiple sclerosis and other possible causes, such as tumor or stroke.

The **facial nerve (CN VII)** innervates muscles of facial expression, taste in the anterior two-thirds of the tongue, the skin of the external ear, the lacrimal and salivary glands (except parotid gland), and the stapedius muscle. Differentiate between *upper* motor neuron lesions (the forehead is spared on the affected side, and the cause is usually stroke or tumor) and *lower* motor neuron lesions (the forehead is involved on the affected side, and the cause is usually Bell palsy or tumor) of the facial nerve.

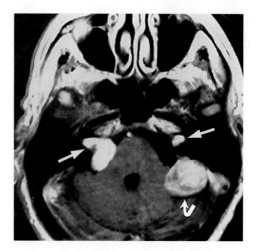

Figure 18-2 Contrast-enhanced axial magnetic resonance image of bilateral acoustic neuromas (*straight arrows*) in a patient with neurofibromatosis type 2. A posterior fossa meningioma (*curved arrow*) is also present.

In the case of Bell palsy, patients may be unable to close the eye; give artificial tears to prevent corneal ulceration. Some physicians treat with acyclovir (underlying herpes virus reactivation is a common cause) and/or prednisone; both are variably effective. Patients with Bell palsy can get hyperacusis (things sound much louder than they are) because of stapedial muscle paralysis. If CNs VII and VIII are affected, think of possible cerebellopontine angle tumor (e.g., acoustic neuroma or schwannoma, especially in neurofibromatosis).

The **vestibulocochlear nerve (CN VIII)** is for hearing and balance. Lesions cause deafness, tinnitus, and vertigo. In children, think of meningitis as a cause. In adults, think of toxins and medications (aspirin, aminoglycosides, loop diuretics, cisplatin), tumors (with CN VII co-involvement, think of acoustic neuroma, Fig. 18-2), or stroke.

The **glossopharyngeal nerve (CN IX)** innervates the pharyngeal muscles and mucous membranes (afferent limb of gag reflex), parotid gland, taste in the posterior third of the tongue, skin of the external ear, and carotid body and sinus. Look for loss of gag reflex and loss of taste in the posterior third of the tongue.

The **vagus nerve (CN X)** innervates the muscles of the palate, pharynx, larynx (efferent limb of gag reflex), taste buds in the base of the tongue, abdominal viscera, and skin of the external ear. Look for hoarseness, dysphagia, and loss of gag or cough reflex. If the cause is not a stroke or brainstem tumor, think of peripheral tumors, especially Pancoast left lung tumors or thoracic aortic aneurysms, which affect the peripheral left recurrent laryngeal nerve *only*.

The **spinal accessory nerve (CN XI)** innervates the sternocleidomastoid and trapezius muscles. With a CN XI lesion, the patient has trouble turning the head to the side opposite the lesion, and the ipsilateral shoulder droops.

The **hypoglossal nerve (CN XII)** innervates the muscles of the tongue. With a CN XII lesion, a protruded tongue deviates to the side of the lesion.

DELIRIUM AND DEMENTIA

Table 18-4 shows the differential diagnosis for delirium and dementia.

TABLE 18-4 Differential Diagnosis of Delirium and Dementia		
FEATURE	**DELIRIUM**	**DEMENTIA**
Onset	Acute and dramatic	Chronic and insidious
Common causes	Illness, toxin, withdrawal	Alzheimer disease, multi-infarct dementia, HIV/AIDS
Reversible	Usually	Usually not
Attention	Poor	Usually unaffected
Arousal level	Fluctuates	Normal

AIDS, acquired immunodeficiency syndrome; HIV, human immunodeficiency virus.

IMPORTANT POINTS

1. Both delirium and dementia can feature hallucinations, illusions, delusions, memory impairment (usually global in delirium, but remote memory is spared in early dementia), orientation difficulties (time, place, person), and sundowning (worsened symptoms at night). The deficits in delirium are waxing and waning, but with dementia the deficits are constant with slow progression over time.
2. In elderly adults, watch for pseudodementia, which is caused by depression and is reversible with treatment.
3. Treatable causes of dementia include vitamin B_{12} deficiency, hyperhomocysteinemia, endocrine disorders (especially thyroid and parathyroid), uremia, hypercalcemia, syphilis, brain tumors, and normal-pressure hydrocephalus. Treatment of Parkinson syndrome also can reverse dementia if it is present.
4. Watch for thiamine deficiency in people with alcoholism as the cause of delirium (Wernicke encephalopathy, which classically manifests with ataxia, ophthalmoplegia, nystagmus, and confusion). If untreated, it can progress to Korsakoff syndrome (memory loss with confabulation; usually irreversible).

For **delirious or unconscious patients in the emergency department** with no history of trauma, think first of hypoglycemia (give glucose), opioid overdose (give naloxone), and thiamine deficiency (give thiamine before giving glucose in people suspected of having alcoholism). Other common causes are alcohol, illicit drugs, prescription medications, diabetic ketoacidosis, stroke, and epilepsy or postictal state.

DIZZINESS AND VERTIGO

Vertigo is defined as the sensation of spinning movement. It is important to differentiate true vertigo from simple lightheadedness. There are multiple causes of vertigo:

○ **Benign paroxysmal positional vertigo:** The most common cause of vertigo. Caused by loose calcium debris moving in the semicircular canals. Patients complain of a brief (seconds) spinning sensation with head movement or looking up. The Dix-Hallpike maneuver is used for diagnosis. The Epley maneuver (or modified Epley maneuver) is used for treatment. These maneuvers involve a series of movements designed to move the loose debris in the semicircular canals to an area where they will not cause symptoms.
○ **Vestibular neuritis** (vestibular neuronitis or labyrinthitis): A viral or postviral inflammation of CN VIII. Look for the rapid onset of severe vertigo after a viral illness. Symptoms usually last 1 to 2 days only, with a gradual return to normal function. Steroids can be used to improve recovery.
○ **Meniere disease:** A disease in which there is excessive endolymphatic fluid pressure. Patients have episodic vertigo lasting minutes to hours. Look for these key symptoms: tinnitus, hearing loss (especially low frequency), and a sensation of ear fullness. Diagnosis is by audiometry and electronystagmography. Noninvasive treatments include diuretics (hydrochlorothiazide, acetazolamide) and decreasing salt intake.
○ **Cerebellar infarction or hemorrhage:** Patients complain of sudden onset intense vertigo. Look for associated cerebellar signs such as ataxia to differentiate this from vestibular neuritis. Diagnosis is by noncontrast CT to rule out bleeding and MRI to diagnose infarction. Because the posterior fossa is a small compartment, patients with cerebellar hemorrhage are at risk for increased intracranial pressure and herniation, so surgical decompression may be required.
○ **Perilymphatic fistula:** Look for episodic vertigo and hearing loss with straining (e.g., sneezing, lifting, coughing). There may be a history of head trauma. CT scan may show fluid in the region of the round window. Treatment includes bed rest, head elevation, and avoidance of activity. Refractory cases require surgery.
○ Other causes: Multiple sclerosis, migraines, head trauma

The symptoms of vertigo can be treated with **antihistamines** (meclizine, diphenhydramine), **benzodiazepines** (alprazolam, lorazepam, diazepam), and **antiemetics** (metoclopramide, ondansetron, prochlorperazine). These medications are used for cases such as vestibular neuritis in which the patient has extreme vertigo for extended periods of time.

HEADACHE

Causes of headache:
- **Tension headaches:** Most common cause. Look for a long history of headaches and stress plus a feeling of tightness or stiffness, usually frontal or occipital and bilateral. Patients may also complain of bandlike pain. Treat with stress reduction and acetaminophen or nonsteroidal antiinflammatory drugs (NSAIDs).
- **Cluster headaches:** Unilateral, severe, tender; occur in clusters. Look for associated symptoms such as unilateral lacrimation, ptosis, rhinorrhea, and conjunctival injection. These headaches are more common in men and usually last a short period of time (15 minutes–3 hours). Oxygen might abort an attack acutely; otherwise, treat with triptans.
- **Migraine headache:** Look for aura, photophobia, nausea and vomiting, and a positive family history. Patients might have neurologic symptoms during attacks; attacks usually begin between ages 10 and 30 years. Medications used for the acute treatment of migraines include NSAIDs, triptans, ergotamine, and antiemetics. Prophylaxis can be achieved with β-blockers, tricyclic antidepressants, topiramate, valproic acid, and calcium channel blockers.
- **Tumor or mass:** Look for associated neurologic symptoms and signs of intracranial hypertension (papilledema; nausea or vomiting, which may be projectile; and mental status changes or ataxia). The classic headache occurs every day and is worse in the morning. Watch for a headache that wakes the patient from sleep. Headaches from an intracranial mass get worse with a Valsalva maneuver, exertion, or sex. Order a CT with contrast or MRI.
- **Pseudotumor cerebri:** Can mimic tumor or mass; both cause intracranial hypertension, papilledema, and daily headaches that classically are worse in the morning and may be accompanied by nausea and vomiting. Found in young obese women, who are unlikely to have a brain tumor; CT and MRI results are negative. Pseudotumor cerebri can cause permanent vision loss. Treatment is usually supportive, including cerebrospinal fluid (CSF) removal periodically or with a permanent CSF shunt; weight loss usually helps. Large doses of **vitamin A,** tetracyclines, and withdrawal from corticosteroids are possible causes of pseudotumor cerebri.
- **Meningitis:** look for fever, Brudzinski or Kernig sign, and positive CSF findings (see Table 18-1). Treatment depends on age:
  - Younger than 1 month: Ampicillin + cefotaxime + vancomycin. Ampicillin is to cover for *Listeria* spp. and the vancomycin is to cover for methicillin-resistant *Staphylococcus aureus* (MRSA) if you suspect it is present.
  - 1 month to 50 years: Vancomycin + ceftriaxone. The vancomycin again is to cover for MRSA if you suspect it.
  - In the case of meningococcal meningitis, give prophylaxis to all household contacts and all health care workers exposed to bodily fluids. Use rifampin or ciprofloxacin.
- **Subarachnoid hemorrhage:** "Worst headache" of the patient's life—a sudden onset, severe headache, usually caused by an aneurysm rupture or trauma. If the bleed is large enough, you may be able to see it on a noncontrast head CT. However, if the head CT results are negative but you suspect the patient has a subarachnoid hemorrhage, perform a lumbar puncture because CT scans are not good enough at picking up a subarachnoid bleed. Acutely, a subarachnoid hemorrhage can be managed with endovascular coiling or embolization. If these are not available, treatment is supportive. Always remember to assess and stabilize the ABCs. If the patient is stable, order a CT angiogram, magnetic resonance angiogram, or traditional angiogram in an attempt to identify and localize the causative aneurysm.
- **Extracranial causes:** Eye pain (optic neuritis, eyestrain from refractive errors, iritis, glaucoma), middle ear pain (otitis media, mastoiditis), sinus pain (sinusitis), oral cavity pain (toothache), herpes zoster with CN involvement, and nonspecific headache (malaise from any illness)

MYASTHENIA GRAVIS

Myasthenia gravis is an autoimmune disease in which there are autoantibodies against the postsynaptic acetylcholine receptors. It usually manifests in women between ages 20 and 40 years. Look for ptosis, diplopia, and general muscle fatigability, especially toward the end of the day.

Diagnosis is made with the Tensilon test. Injection of edrophonium (Tensilon), a short-acting anticholinesterase, improves muscle weakness. Watch for associated thymomas; most patients improve after removal of the thymus, which can be part of standard treatment. Antibodies to acetylcholine receptors are usually present in the serum. EMG reveals jitter in muscle fibers, and repetitive nerve stimulation reveals declining amplitude of response over time.

Chronic medical treatment consists of long-acting anticholinesterase inhibitors (pyridostigmine), immunotherapy (glucocorticoids, mycophenolate, azathioprine, and cyclosporine), and thymectomy. Acute severe crisis is treated with plasmapheresis or IV immunoglobulin (IVIG).

EATON-LAMBERT SYNDROME

Eaton-Lambert syndrome is a paraneoplastic syndrome (classically seen with small cell lung cancer) characterized by muscle weakness, with sparing of the extraocular muscles (whereas myasthenia gravis almost always has prominent involvement of extraocular muscles). Eaton-Lambert syndrome has a different mechanism of disease (impaired release of acetylcholine from nerves) and a different response to repetitive nerve stimulation (myasthenia gravis worsens and Eaton-Lambert syndrome improves).

IMPORTANT POINTS

1. Do not forget organophosphate poisoning as a cause for myasthenia-like muscle weakness. Usually it occurs with agricultural exposure. Symptoms of parasympathetic excess also are present (e.g., miosis, excessive bronchial secretions, urinary urgency, diarrhea). Edrophonium causes worsening of the muscle weakness. Treatment is with atropine and pralidoxime.

2. Aminoglycosides in high doses can cause myasthenia-like muscle weakness and prolong the effects of muscle blockade in anesthesia.

NEUROMUSCULAR AND MOVEMENT DISORDERS

Amyotrophic Lateral Sclerosis

Amyotrophic lateral sclerosis (Lou Gehrig disease) is an idiopathic degeneration of both upper and lower motor neurons that is more common in men. The mean age at onset is 55 years. The key is to notice a combination of upper motor neuron lesion signs (spasticity, hyperreflexia, positive Babinski sign) and lower motor neuron lesion signs (fasciculations, atrophy, flaccidity) in the same patient. Treatment is supportive, but 50% of patients die within 3 years of onset.

Cerebellar Disorders

In children, think of brain tumor (cerebellar astrocytoma, medulloblastomas), hydrocephalus (enlarging head in infants younger than 6 months, possibly caused by Arnold-Chiari or Dandy-Walker syndrome), Friedreich ataxia (starts between ages 5 and 15 years; autosomal recessive; look for areflexia, loss of vibration or position sense, and cardiomyopathy), or ataxia–telangiectasia (progressive cerebellar ataxia, oculocutaneous telangiectasias, and immune deficiency).

In adults, think of alcoholism, tumor, ischemia or hemorrhage, or multiple sclerosis. Look for symptoms of cerebellar dysfunction, including ataxia, dysmetria (overshooting or undershooting an intended position with movement), dysarthria, intention tremor, and dysdiadochokinesia (difficulty with rapid alternating movements).

Floppy Baby Syndrome

Infantile hypotonia or flaccidity can be caused by two disorders:

○ **Werdnig-Hoffmann disease:** Autosomal recessive degeneration of anterior horn cells in the spinal cord and brainstem (lower motor neurons). Most infants are hypotonic at birth, and all are affected by 6 months of age. Look for a positive family history and a long and slowly progressive course of disease. Treatment is supportive.

○ **Infant botulism:** Look for sudden onset and a history of honey ingestion (or other home-canned foods). Diagnosis is made by finding *Clostridium botulinum* toxin or organisms in the feces. Treat on an inpatient basis with close monitoring of respiratory status. Patients might need intubation for respiratory muscle paralysis. Spontaneous recovery usually occurs within 1 week.

Guillain-Barré Syndrome

Look for history of mild infection or immunization roughly 1 week before onset of symmetric, distal weakness, paralysis, or mild paresthesias with loss of deep tendon reflexes in affected areas. As the ascending paralysis and weakness progress, respiratory paralysis can occur in severe cases. The hallmark of the disease is that motor function is affected but sensation is intact or only minimally impaired. Patients must be watched carefully; usually spirometry is used to follow inspiratory ability. Intubation may be required for patients with poor inspiratory effort because of respiratory muscle weakness. Diagnosis depends on clinical signs and symptoms, analysis of CSF (usually normal except for *markedly increased protein*), and nerve conduction velocities (slowed). The disease usually stops spontaneously. Plasmapheresis reduces the severity and length of disease. Do *not* use corticosteroids; you might make the patient worse.

Huntington Disease

Huntington disease is an autosomal dominant condition that usually begins at 35 to 50 years of age. Look for choreiform movements (irregular, spasmodic, involuntary movements of the limbs or facial muscles) and progressive intellectual deterioration, dementia, and psychiatric disturbances. Atrophy of the caudate nucleus may be seen on CT or MRI. Triplet repeat disorders such as Huntington disease demonstrate **anticipation**, in which the severity of disease increases with each successive generation. Anticipation also often involves the manifestations of disease starting earlier in life with each successive generation. Treatment is supportive; antipsychotics might help.

Muscular Dystrophy

Muscular dystrophy is most commonly due to **Duchenne muscular dystrophy**, an X-linked recessive disorder of dystrophin that usually manifests in boys ages 3 to 7 years. Look for muscle weakness, markedly elevated creatine kinase, and pseudohypertrophy of the calves (caused by fatty and fibrous infiltration of the degenerating muscle). IQ often is less than normal. Gowers sign is classic (in trying to rise from a prone position, the patient walks the hands and feet toward each other). Muscle biopsy establishes the diagnosis. Treatment is supportive. Most patients die by age 20 years.

Other muscular dystrophies:

○ **Becker muscular dystrophy:** This is also an X-linked recessive dystrophin disorder, but is milder than Duchenne. Onset usually is in young adulthood.
○ **Myotonic dystrophy:** An autosomal dominant disorder that manifests between 20 and 30 years of age. Myotonia (inability to relax muscles) classically manifests as an *inability to relax the grip* (an inability to release a handshake). Look for coexisting mental retardation, baldness, and testicular or ovarian atrophy. Treatment is supportive and includes genetic counseling. Diagnosis is clinical.
○ **Mitochondrial myopathies (e.g., Lever hereditary optic atrophy):** These are interesting because they are inherited mitochondrial defects (passed only from mother to offspring; male carriers cannot transmit). The key phrase is "ragged red fibers" on biopsy specimen. Ophthalmoplegia usually is present.

Do not forget the rare glycogen storage diseases (autosomal recessive) as a cause of muscle weakness (especially McArdle disease, a deficiency in glycogen phosphorylase that is relatively mild and manifests with weakness and cramping after exercise because of buildup of lactic acid).

Parkinson Disease

Signs are the classic tetrad of slowness or poverty of movement, muscle rigidity (lead pipe and cogwheel), resting pill-rolling tremor (which disappears with movement and sleep), and postural instability (shuffling gait and festination). Patients also might have dementia and depression. The mean age of onset is around 60 years. The cause is loss of dopaminergic neurons, especially in the substantia nigra, which projects to the basal ganglia; the result is decreased dopamine in the basal ganglia. Drug therapy, which aims to increase dopamine, includes dopamine precursors (levodopa with carbidopa), dopamine agonists (bromocriptine, apomorphine, pergolide, pramipexole, and ropinirole), monoamine oxidase-B inhibitors (selegiline), COMT (catechol-O-methyl transferase) inhibitors (entacapone and tolcapone), anticholinergics (trihexyphenidyl and benztropine), and amantadine.

 Antipsychotics can cause Parkinson-like symptoms in schizophrenics. Treat with anticholinergics (benztropine, trihexyphenidyl). Diphenhydramine also works because it has anticholinergic properties.

Tremor and Chorea

Resting tremor is generally caused by basal ganglia disease (chorea), intention tremor is caused by cerebellar disease, and hemiballismus (random, violent, unilateral flailing of the limbs) is caused by a lesion in the subthalamic nucleus. Besides Parkinson disease, a resting tremor may be caused by hyperthyroidism, anxiety, drug withdrawal or intoxication, or a benign (essential) hereditary tremor (usually autosomal dominant; look for a positive family history and use β-blockers to reduce the tremor). Also watch for Wilson disease (hepatolenticular degeneration secondary to copper deposition) and asterixis (outstretched hands flap slowly and involuntarily) in patients with liver or kidney failure.

SEIZURES

Five main types of seizures are tested on the boards (although there are others):
- **Simple partial (local, focal) seizures:** These may be motor (e.g., Jacksonian march), sensory (e.g., hallucinations), or psychiatric (cognitive or affective symptoms). The key point is that consciousness is *not* impaired. Treat with carbamazepine, lamotrigine, oxcarbazepine, or levetiracetam.
- **Complex partial (psychomotor) seizures:** Complex partial seizures are any simple partial seizure followed by impairment of consciousness. Patients perform purposeless movements and can become aggressive if restraint is attempted (people who get in fights or kill people are *not* having a seizure!). The first-line agents are valproate, lamotrigine, and levetiracetam.
- **Absence (petit mal) seizures:** These *never* begin after the age of 20 years. They are brief (10–30 seconds' duration), generalized seizures in which the main manifestation is loss of consciousness, often with eye or muscle flutterings. The classic description is a child in a classroom who stares off into space in the middle of a sentence (the child is not daydreaming but having a seizure) and then 20 seconds later resumes the sentence. There is no postictal state (an important differential point). The first-line agents are ethosuximide and valproate.
- **Tonic–clonic (grand mal) seizures:** The classic seizures that can have an aura; tonic muscle contraction is followed by clonic contractions, usually lasting 2 to 5 minutes. Patients often have incontinence and a postictal state (drowsiness, confusion, headache, muscle soreness). Look for tongue biting as well. Treat with valproate, lamotrigine, or levetiracetam.
- **Febrile seizures:** Between the ages of 5 months and 5 years old, children might have a seizure because of fever. The key is not the absolute temperature but the rate of rise in the temperature. Look for a parent who says, "He didn't have a fever this morning!" The seizure is usually short in duration (<1–2 minutes) and of the tonic–clonic, generalized type. Often, no specific seizure treatment is required. Treat the underlying cause of the fever, if possible, and give acetaminophen. Such children do *not* have epilepsy, and the chances of their getting it are just barely higher than in the general population's. Make sure that affected children do not have meningitis, tumors, or other serious cause of seizure. The board question will give clues in the case description if you are expected to pursue workup for a serious condition. There is a mnemonic to remember the characteristics of febrile seizures: the 5 Fs:
  - **F**ive months to **f**ive years
  - **F**ebrile
  - Non**f**ocal (they are generalized seizures)
  - **F**amily history (patients may have a family history of febrile seizures)
  - Lasts less than **f**ifteen minutes

If you have a febrile pediatric patient with a seizure that does not match these characteristics, you should be very concerned that the seizure is the result of a secondary cause, and you should work them up.

Secondary seizure disorder may be caused by:
○ Mass (tumor, hemorrhage)
○ Metabolic disorder (**hypoglycemia**, **hyponatremia**, hypoxia, phenylketonuria)
○ Toxins (lead, cocaine, carbon monoxide)
○ Drug withdrawal (**alcohol**, benzodiazepines, barbiturates, too-rapid anticonvulsant withdrawal)
○ Cerebral edema (severe or malignant hypertension; also watch for pheochromocytoma)
○ Eclampsia
○ CNS infections (meningitis, encephalitis, toxoplasmosis, cysticercosis)
○ Trauma
○ Stroke

Treatment: For all seizures, secure the airway and, if possible, roll the patient onto his or her side to prevent aspiration if not yet intubated. In secondary seizures of *any* etiology, treat the underlying disorder and use diazepam or phenytoin acutely to control the seizure.

Status epilepticus: Defined as a continuous seizure lasting longer than 5 to 10 minutes or frequent clinical seizures without an interictal return to baseline. These can occur spontaneously or result from withdrawing anticonvulsants too rapidly. Start treatment with IV diazepam or lorazepam. Give fosphenytoin or phenytoin if the seizures persist. In severe cases, patients can be given pentobarbital. Remember to protect the airway and intubate if necessary.

For a list of commonly used **antiepileptic medications**, see Table 18-5.

IMPORTANT POINTS

1. Hypertension can cause seizures or convulsions, headache, confusion, or mental status changes.
2. All anticonvulsants are teratogenic, and women need counseling about the risks of pregnancy. Do a pregnancy test before starting an anticonvulsant. Valproic acid is a major contributor to the risk. Polypharmacy increases the risk. There is limited human information of the risks to fetuses with the newer antiepileptic medications.
3. Cysticercosis is caused by infection with the larval form of *Taenia solium*, the pork tapeworm, and most often is seen in AIDS patients and in immigrants. On CT scan with contrast, you may be able to see the viable cysts, which appear as non-enhancing, round, hypodense lesions. Old cysts that are no longer viable may calcify. Treat with albendazole or praziquantel.

TABLE 18-5 Commonly Used Antiepileptic Medications

NAME	USES	SIDE EFFECTS
Carbamazepine	Generalized tonic–clonic, partial seizures, trigeminal neuralgia	Nausea, vomiting, rash, pancytopenia
Ethosuximide	Absence seizures	Nausea, vomiting, drowsiness
Lamotrigine	Partial seizures, adjunct for generalized seizures	Rash (Stevens-Johnson syndrome), nausea
Levetiracetam	Adjunctive for partial, myoclonic, and generalized seizures	Fatigue, somnolence, dizziness, agitation
Phenobarbital	Generalized and partial seizures	Severe respiratory or CNS depression, drowsiness, osteoporosis with long-term use
Phenytoin	Generalized and partial seizures	Gingival hypertrophy, rash, increased body hair, ataxia
Topiramate	Partial seizures	Weight loss, fatigue, dizziness, paresthesias
Valproic acid	Generalized and partial seizures	Weight gain, insulin resistance, nausea vomiting, blood dyscrasias
Zonisamide	Generalized and partial seizures, myoclonic epilepsy	Somnolence, ataxia, fatigue, dizziness

CNS, central nervous system.

OTHER NEUROLOGIC DISORDERS

Multiple Sclerosis

Look for insidious onset of neurologic symptoms in women ages 20 to 40 years with exacerbations and remissions. Common presentations include paresthesias and numbness, weakness and clumsiness, visual disturbances (decreased vision and pain caused by *optic neuritis*, diplopia caused by CN involvement), gait disturbances, incontinence or urgency, and vertigo. Also look for emotional lability or other mental status changes. Internuclear ophthalmoplegia and scanning speech are classic; Babinski sign may be positive.

MRI, the most sensitive diagnostic tool, shows demyelination plaques (Fig. 18-3). Look for increased immunoglobulin G (IgG) or oligoclonal bands and possibly myelin basic protein in the CSF.

The disease course is variable, but long-term prognosis poor. Treatment is variably effective and includes interferon, glatiramer, mitoxantrone, natalizumab, cyclophosphamide, and methotrexate. Acute exacerbations are treated with corticosteroids.

Peripheral Neuropathies

Nerve conduction velocity is slowed with a peripheral neuropathy, which can be motor (lower motor neuron signs), sensory, or autonomic. Multiple causes include:

○ **Metabolic: Diabetes mellitus** (autonomic and sensory neuropathy), uremia, hypothyroidism
○ **Nutritional:** Deficiencies of vitamin B_{12}, B_6 (look for history of isoniazid use), thiamine (dry beriberi), or vitamin E
○ **Toxins and medications:** Lead (classic symptom is wristdrop or footdrop; look for coexisting CNS or abdominal symptoms) or other heavy metals, **isoniazid**, vincristine, ethambutol (especially optic neuritis), aminoglycosides (especially CN VIII)
○ **Postinfection, postimmunization, and autoimmune:** Guillain-Barré syndrome, systemic lupus erythematosus, polyarteritis nodosa, scleroderma, sarcoidosis, amyloidosis
○ **Trauma:** Carpal tunnel syndrome (median nerve entrapment at the wrist), pressure paralysis (radial nerve palsy in alcoholics), or fractures. Carpal tunnel syndrome usually is caused by repetitive physical activity but may be a manifestation of acromegaly or hypothyroidism. Look for positive Tinel and Phalen signs.
○ **Infectious:** Lyme disease, diphtheria, HIV, leprosy

Syncope

Syncope can be caused by any number of conditions. Vasovagal syncope, medications, and orthostatic hypotension are the most common causes.

○ **Cardiac:** Arrhythmias, ischemia, heart block, valvular disease. These are the most common life-threatening causes of syncope.
○ **Hemorrhage:** Ruptured abdominal aortic aneurysm, gastrointestinal bleeding, trauma, and so on

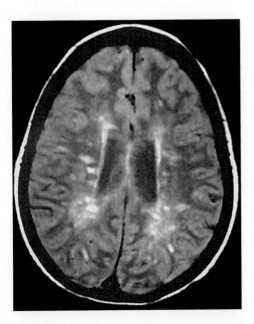

FIGURE 18-3 Multiple sclerosis on magnetic resonance image. The periventricular distribution and oval shape are typical of demyelination.

○ Pulmonary embolism
○ **Neurologic:** Subarachnoid hemorrhage, transient ischemic attack, stroke, seizure
○ **Vasovagal** (or neurocardiogenic syncope): Increased vagal tone from stress, fear, or a Valsalva maneuver such as with urination. Patients usually experience a prodrome of dizziness, lightheadedness, warmth, nausea, and diaphoresis before losing consciousness.
○ **Orthostatic hypotension:** Defined as a decrease in blood pressure of more than 20 mm Hg or a reflex tachycardia of greater than 20 beats/min upon standing or sitting up. Diagnosis is by checking orthostatic vital signs.
○ **Carotid sinus hypersensitivity:** Look for patients with a tight collar and patients who have syncope while shaving or turning their heads.
○ **Medication effect:** Look for antihypertensives, diuretics (decreased fluid status), and antipsychotics (increased QT interval).

The workup of syncope consists of first ruling out dangerous causes of syncope. You should always start with an electrocardiogram for all patients to evaluate for ischemia, arrhythmia, and heart block and then guide the rest of the workup by symptomatology. An example is getting a head CT for a patient who experienced syncope right after having the most severe headache of his life. For vasovagal syncope, look for precipitating symptoms in the question such as getting blood drawn or a patient with benign prostatic hyperplasia trying to urinate.

Vitamin Deficiencies

Vitamin deficiencies can present with neurologic signs and symptoms:
○ **Vitamin A:** Vision loss
○ **Thiamine (vitamin B$_1$):** Peripheral neuropathy, confusion, ophthalmoplegia, nystagmus, ataxia, confusion, delirium, dementia
○ **Vitamin B$_6$:** Peripheral sensory neuropathy. Watch for isoniazid as a cause and give prophylactic B$_6$ (pyridoxine) to patients taking isoniazid if given the choice on Step 2.
○ **Vitamin B$_{12}$:** Dementia, peripheral neuropathy, loss of vibration sense in lower extremities, loss of position sense, ataxia, spasticity, hyperactive reflexes, positive Babinski sign, and macrocytic anemia
○ **Vitamin E:** Loss of proprioception or vibratory sensation, areflexia, ataxia, and gaze palsy

QR CODE

The QR code includes three USMLE-style questions and answers. For more questions, redeem the PIN code on the inside cover for the Crush Step 2 question bank powered by USMLE Consult.
Please see the Introduction for instructions on how to access content using the QR codes.

Question

A 66-year-old man presents to the emergency department (ED) with a chief complaint of transient blindness in the right eye that lasted 2 minutes and subsequently resolved before he reached the ED. He describes the vision loss as "someone pulling a shade down in front of my eye." His medical history is significant for long-standing hypertension, diabetes, a myocardial infarction 6 months ago, and tobacco abuse. His medications include amlodipine, glipizide, and pioglitazone. Vital signs and physical examination are within normal limits other than obesity. Laboratory tests reveal the following:

Hemoglobin	16 g/dL
Mean corpuscular volume	90 μm/cell
Creatinine	1.3 mg/dL
BUN	15 mg/dL
Sodium	140 mEq/L
Potassium	4.1 mEq/L
Chloride	106 mEq/L
CO_2	27 mEq/L

Which of the following is FALSE?
(A) A carotid duplex scan (ultrasonography) should be ordered.
(B) The patient should have a fasting lipid profile analysis done.
(C) The patient should be put on an angiotensin-converting enzyme inhibitor, such as captopril.
(D) The patient should undergo urgent carotid endarterectomy for the best long-term prognosis.
(E) The patient likely would benefit from being put on a β-blocker, such as metoprolol.

19 NEUROSURGERY

CRANIUM AND SKULL

Whenever intracranial hemorrhage is suspected, order a computed tomography (CT) head scan without contrast. Blood shows up as white and can cause a midline shift.

Subdural Hematoma
Subdural hematoma (Fig. 19-1) is caused by bleeding from veins that bridge the cortex and dural sinuses. The hematoma is crescent shaped; it is common in people with alcoholism and after head trauma. Patients can present immediately after trauma or up to 1 to 2 months later. If the Step 2 question includes a history of head trauma, always consider the diagnosis of a subdural hematoma. Treat with surgical evacuation.

Epidural Hematoma
Epidural hematoma is caused by bleeding from meningeal arteries (classically, the middle meningeal artery). The hematoma is lenticular shaped (i.e., lens or biconvex shaped, Fig. 19-2). It is almost always associated with a skull fracture (classically, fracture of the temporal bone). More than 50% of patients have an ipsilateral blown pupil (dilated, fixed, nonreactive pupil). The classic history is a head trauma with loss of consciousness followed by a lucid interval of minutes to hours and then neurologic deterioration. Treat with surgical evacuation.

Subarachnoid Hemorrhage
Subarachnoid hemorrhage is caused by blood between the arachnoid and the pia mater. The most common cause is trauma followed by ruptured berry aneurysm. Blood is seen in ventricles and around (but not in) the brain or brainstem. Patients classically present with the "worst headache of my life," although many die before they reach the hospital or may be unconscious. Awake patients have signs of meningitis (positive Kernig and Brudzinski signs). Remember the association between polycystic kidney disease and berry aneurysms. Although CT without contrast is always the test of choice, a lumbar tap shows grossly bloody cerebrospinal fluid (CSF).

Treat with support, anticonvulsants, and observation. In the absence of a trauma history, do a cerebral angiogram or magnetic resonance angiogram to look for aneurysms and arteriovenous malformations, which can often be treated with open or endovascular surgery.

Intracerebral Hemorrhage
Intracerebral hemorrhage is bleeding into the brain parenchyma. The most common cause is hypertension; other causes include arteriovenous malformations, coagulopathies, tumor, and trauma. Two-thirds of hypertensive hemorrhages occur in the basal ganglia. Patients often present with coma; if awake, they have contralateral hemiplegia and hemisensory deficits. On CT, blood (white) is seen in brain parenchyma and sometimes extends into the ventricles. Surgery is reserved for large bleeds that are accessible (particularly cerebellar bleeds).

After a history of trauma, a dilated, unreactive (blown) pupil on only one side most likely represents impingement of the ipsilateral third cranial nerve and impending uncal herniation caused by increased intracranial pressure (ICP). Of the different intracranial bleeds, this is most commonly seen with epidural hematomas. Do not do a lumbar tap on any patient with a blown pupil; you might precipitate uncal herniation and death. First do a noncontrast CT (second choice is magnetic resonance imaging [MRI]).

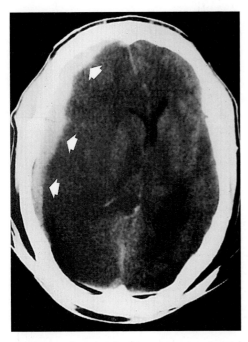

FIGURE 19-1 Subdural hematoma (*arrows*).

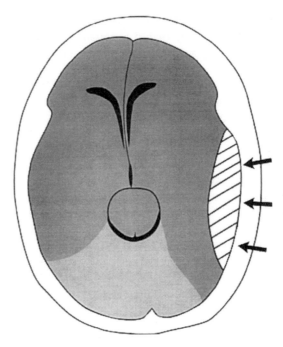

FIGURE 19-2 Biconvex epidural hematoma overlying the left temporal lobe (*arrows*).

Skull Fractures

Basilar skull fracture is diagnosed most confidently with CT of the head but is often suspected clinically based on one or more of four classic signs:

○ Battle sign: Postauricular ecchymosis
○ CSF otorrhea or rhinorrhea: Clear fluid from the ears or nose
○ Hemotympanum: Blood behind the eardrum
○ Raccoon eyes: Periorbital ecchymosis

IMPORTANT POINTS

1. Skull fractures of the calvarium are evaluated with noncontrast CT scan. Surgical indications are contamination (cleaning and debridement), impingement on brain parenchyma, or open fracture with CSF leak. Otherwise, fractures may be observed and generally heal on their own.
2. Head trauma may also cause cerebral contusion or shear injury of the brain parenchyma, which might or might not show up on a CT or MRI, but both can cause temporary or permanent neurologic deficits.

Increased Intracranial Pressure

Normal ICP is 5 to 15 mm Hg. Increased ICP (intracranial hypertension) is suggested by bilaterally dilated and fixed pupils. Other symptoms include headache, papilledema, nausea and vomiting, and mental status changes. Look also for the classic Cushing triad (increasing blood pressure, bradycardia, and respiratory irregularity).

The first step is to put the patient in the reverse Trendelenburg (head-up) position and intubate. After being intubated, the patient should be hyperventilated to rapidly lower the ICP. This approach decreases intracranial blood volume by causing cerebral vasoconstriction. If the decrease in ICP is not sufficient, mannitol diuresis can be tried to lessen cerebral edema. Furosemide is also used but is less effective. Barbiturate coma and decompressive craniotomy (burr holes) are last-ditch measures. Anticonvulsant therapy should be started if seizures are suspected; prophylactic anticonvulsants are controversial but may be warranted in some cases.

> *Cerebral perfusion pressure equals blood pressure minus ICP. In other words, do not treat hypertension initially in a patient with increased ICP; hypertension is the body's way of trying to increase cerebral perfusion.*

> *Never do a lumbar tap on any patient with signs of increased ICP until a CT scan is done first. If the CT findings are negative, you can proceed to a tap if one is needed or indicated.*

Venous Sinus Thromobosis

The risk factors for dural venous sinus thrombosis are similar to those for deep venous thrombosis in other areas, including hypercoagulable state, trauma, dehydration, pregnancy, oral contraceptive use, infections (e.g., extension of sinusitis or mastoiditis intracranially), nephrotic syndrome, and local tumor invasion. The diagnostic test of choice is MRI. Although hemorrhagic infarcts are common with dural venous thrombosis, treatment with anticoagulation improves outcomes.

Hydrocephalus

In children, look for increasing head circumference, increased ICP, bulging fontanelle, scalp vein engorgement, and paralysis of upward gaze. The most common causes include congenital malformations, tumors, and inflammation (hemorrhage, meningitis). Treat the underlying cause, if possible; otherwise, a surgical shunt is created to decompress the ventricles.

Neoplasms

Astrocytoma (Fig. 19-3) arises in the brain parenchyma (most commonly in the cerebral hemispheres) and typically affects those who are 30 to 50 years old. Patients may present with headache, focal neurologic deficits, or seizures. Astrocytomas are treated with radiation and resection if possible. The prognosis is better than that for glioblastoma multiforme.

Pilocytic astrocytoma is a slowly growing, well-demarcated tumor that generally is cystic. They occur predominantly in children and young adults and most frequently arise in the cerebellar hemispheres and around the third ventricle. Pilocytic astrocytomas enhance on CT and MRI. Surgical resection is the treatment of choice.

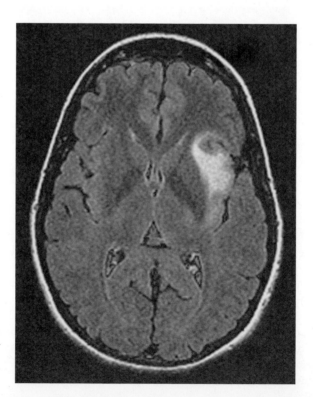

FIGURE 19-3 Astrocytoma. Fluid attenuated inversion recovery (FLAIR) magnetic resonance image showing a mass without ring enhancement. *(From Bope E, Kellerman R, Rakel R: Conn's Current Therapy 2010. Philadelphia, Saunders, 2010, p. 979.)*

Glioblastoma multiforme (grade IV astrocytoma) is a rapidly progressive tumor with a poor prognosis. Clinical manifestations depend on the location and size of the tumor. These include headache, seizures, memory loss, motor weakness, and visual symptoms. Endothelial proliferation or tumor necrosis leads to ring-enhancing lesions on MRI (Fig. 19-4). The initial treatment is surgical resection with postoperative adjuvant radiation and chemotherapy.

Acoustic neuroma is derived from Schwann cells and is thus also called schwannoma. The average age of diagnosis is 50 years. The most common symptoms are asymmetric hearing loss and tinnitus, although vertigo and symptoms of cranial nerve compression may occur as well (facial numbness or pain from trigeminal nerve compression; facial paresis or taste disturbance from facial nerve compression). MRI is the imaging procedure of choice (Fig. 19-5), and surgery is usually curative.

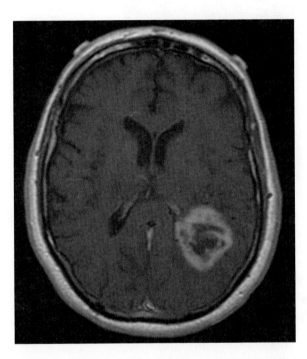

FIGURE 19-4 Glioblastoma multiforme. Magnetic resonance image with a ring-enhancing mass with central necrosis. *(From Bope E, Kellerman R, Rakel R: Conn's Current Therapy 2010. Philadelphia, Saunders, 2010, p. 980.)*

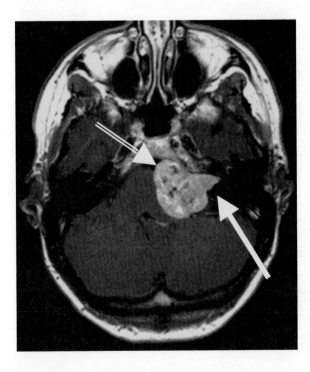

FIGURE 19-5 Acoustic neuroma. Magnetic resonance T1-weighted image showing a mass within the internal auditory canal. *(From Goldman L, Ausiello D: Cecil Medicine, 23rd edition. Philadelphia, Saunders, 2008.)*

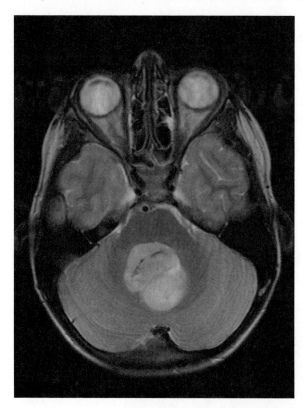

FIGURE 19-6 Medulloblastoma. Magnetic resonance T2-weighted image showing a heterogeneous mass typically in the posterior fossa or cerebellum. *(From Adam A, Dixon AK: Grainger & Allison's Diagnostic Radiology, 5th edition. London, Churchill Livingstone, 2008.)*

Ependymomas arise from the ependymal cells lining the ventricular system. These generally are low-grade tumors, are most common in children (average age at diagnosis, 5 years), and may result in obstructive hydrocephalus. Ependymomas are treated with surgical resection and radiation.

Medulloblastoma (Fig. 19-6) is an embryonal tumor typically arising in the roof of the fourth ventricle in children, resulting in increased ICP and obstructive hydrocephalus. Medulloblastoma is highly malignant and may seed the subarachnoid space. It is treated with surgical resection, radiation, and chemotherapy.

Meningioma (Fig. 19-7) may vary histologically from benign (the great majority) to malignant and originates from the dura mater or arachnoid. The presentation depends on the location, although meningioma is often an incidental finding. The incidence increases with age. Prognosis

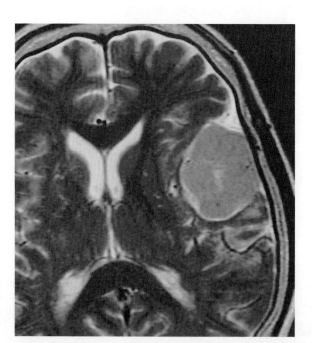

FIGURE 19-7 Meningioma. Magnetic resonance T2-weighted image showing an isointense mass arising from the meninges. *(From Adam A, Dixon AK: Grainger & Allison's Diagnostic Radiology, 5th edition. London, Churchill Livingstone, 2008.)*

generally is good. Active surveillance may be appropriate for a meningioma discovered incidentally. Surgical resection is indicated for larger or symptomatic meningiomas; radiation therapy is used if the meningioma is not in an accessible location.

SPINAL CORD

Trauma

Spinal cord trauma often manifests with spinal shock (loss of reflexes, loss of motor function, and hypotension). Get standard trauma radiographs (cervical spine, chest, pelvis) as well as additional spine x-rays and CT scans based on physical examination. MRI is the best noninvasive method to assess cord injury and compression. Give corticosteroids for spinal cord injuries (proven to improve outcome). Surgery is done for incomplete neurologic injury (some residual function is maintained) in the presence of correctable external compression (e.g., spine subluxation, bone chip).

Compression

Spinal cord compression usually is defined as acute or subacute. Most cases of acute spinal cord compression result from trauma. Look for the appropriate history. Subacute compression is often caused by metastatic cancer but also may result from a primary neoplasm, subdural or epidural abscess, or hematoma (especially after a lumbar tap or epidural or spinal anesthesia in a patient with a bleeding disorder or a patient taking anticoagulation). Patients present with local spinal pain (especially with bone metastases) and neurologic deficits below the lesion (hyperreflexia, positive Babinski sign, weakness, sensory loss).

The first steps in the emergency department are to get a confirmatory CT or MRI and then give high-dose corticosteroids. Radiotherapy can be used for metastases from a known primary tumor that is radiosensitive. Alternatively, surgical decompression may be done.

○ The prognosis is most closely related to pretreatment function; the longer you wait to treat, the worse the prognosis.

○ For hematoma or for subdural or epidural abscess (seen especially in patients with diabetes and usually caused by infection with Staphylococcus aureus), surgery is indicated for decompression and drainage.

Syringomyelia

Syringomyelia is a central pathologic cavitation of the spinal cord, usually in the cervical or upper thoracic region. Syringomyelia is sometimes idiopathic but classically occurs with Arnold-Chiari malformation or because of a tumor or past trauma. The classic presentation is a bilateral loss of pain and temperature sensation below the lesion in the distribution of a cape because of involvement of the lateral spinothalamic tracts. The cavitation in the spinal cord gradually widens to involve other tracts, causing motor and sensory deficits. MRI is the imaging study of choice to confirm the diagnosis and exclude underlying Chiari malformation and tumor, and treatment is surgical (e.g., creation of a shunt, decompression of the skull base with a Chiari malformation, treatment of any causative tumor).

Neural Tube Defects

A triangular patch of hair over the lumbar spine indicates spina bifida occulta. Serious defects are obvious and occur most commonly in the lumbosacral region. Meningocele is defined as meninges outside the spinal canal; myelomeningocele is defined as central nervous system tissue plus meninges outside the spinal canal. Most importantly, giving folate to potential mothers reduces the incidence of neural tube defects. MRI is used to assess the extent of malformation if it is not obvious. No imaging or treatment is needed for spina bifida occulta, which occurs in up to 10% of the population.

QR CODE

The QR code includes three USMLE-style questions and answers. For more questions, redeem the PIN code on the inside cover for the Crush Step 2 question bank powered by USMLE Consult.

Please see the Introduction for instructions on how to access content using the QR codes.

Question

A 42-year-old man is brought to the emergency department (ED) after sustaining a closed head injury and being knocked unconscious. He is intubated when you see him in the ED. A computed tomography scan of the head is performed and is negative for intracranial bleed or fracture. A few hours later, the patient wakes up and extubates himself. His oxygen saturation remains stable after extubation, his disorientation clears, and the patient claims to be fine other than "one heckuva headache." A few hours later, the nurse calls you because the patient has developed high blood pressure. When you go to see the patient, you look over the vital signs from admission and compare them with the current values:

	INITIAL	CURRENT
Temperature	98.6°F	99.1°F
Blood pressure	124/80 mm Hg	198/118 mm Hg
Pulse rate	110 beats/min	50 beats/min
Respirations	16 breaths/min	6 breaths/min

The patient's respirations are irregular, with rapid respirations interspersed with random cessation of respirations for several seconds and slow respirations at other times. The patient is disoriented. What is the most likely underlying pathophysiologic abnormality?
(A) Infection
(B) Hypoxia
(C) Increased intracranial pressure
(D) Acute cocaine withdrawal with delirium
(E) Intensive care unit–induced delirium

20 OBSTETRICS

GENERAL PREGNANCY

Terms and Definitions

Previable	<24 weeks' gestational age
Preterm	24–36 weeks, 6 days' gestational age
Term	37–42 weeks' gestational age
Postdates	40–41 weeks, 6 days' gestational age
Postterm	>42 weeks' gestational age

IMPORTANT POINTS

1. The most common cause of secondary amenorrhea is pregnancy. Always do a pregnancy test first when a patient presents with amenorrhea. Pregnancy also must be ruled out as a cause of primary amenorrhea.
2. A woman may be (or say that she is) taking oral contraceptives and still be pregnant. No contraception is 100% effective, especially when you factor in adherence.
3. Signs and symptoms of pregnancy: Amenorrhea, morning sickness, visualization of gestational sac or fetus on ultrasonography, Chadwick sign (dark discoloration of the vulva and vaginal walls), auscultation of fetal heart toes, Hegar sign (softening and compressibility of the lower uterine segment), linea nigra, chloasma, weight gain, uterine contractions, and palpation or ballottement of fetus.
4. Give all pregnant patients folate (0.4 mg/day) to prevent neural tube defects. Ideally, all women of reproductive age should take folate because it is most effective in the first trimester when most women do not know they are pregnant. Iron is often given routinely during pregnancy to prevent anemia.
5. Macrosomia (or positive history in previous children) is caused by maternal diabetes mellitus until proven otherwise.
6. It is important to determine accurate dating of the pregnancy. In women with regular menstrual cycles, calculate the estimated date of delivery using Naegele's rule (using the last menstrual period, subtract 3 months and add 7 days).

Routine laboratory tests in pregnant patients:
- **Blood type, Rh type, and antibody screen:** At first visit (for identification of possible isoimmunization or Rh incompatibility). Perform sickle prep or hemoglobin electrophoresis in appropriate populations.
- **Chlamydia screening:** The Centers for Disease Control and Prevention advocates testing all pregnant women, but the American Congress of Obstetricians and Gynecologists (ACOG) recommends screening women at higher risk (e.g., age younger than 25 years, new sexual partner or more than one sexual partner, history of sexually transmitted disease [STD], drug use).

- ⚪ **Complete blood count:** At first visit to see if the patient is anemic (pregnancy can aggravate anemia)
- ⚪ **Down syndrome screening:** Should be offered to all pregnant patients. There are multiple ways to screen. Discussed in more detail later.
- ⚪ **First trimester screen:** See discussion below.
- ⚪ **Group B beta-hemolytic streptococcus (GBS) screen:** Screen at 35 to 37 weeks' gestation with a swab of the lower vagina and rectum.
- ⚪ **Glucose screen:** At first visit if the patient has risk factors for diabetes mellitus (obesity, family history, age older than 30 years); otherwise, do at 24 to 28 weeks. Screen with fasting serum glucose *and* serum glucose 1 hour after an oral glucose load. If the 1 hour glucose is greater than 140 mg/dL, perform a 3-hour glucose tolerance test (GTT).
- ⚪ **Hepatitis B antigen testing:** To prevent perinatal transmission
- ⚪ **HIV test:** The ACOG advocates an "opt-out" approach to screening rather than an "opt-in" approach to increase screening.
- ⚪ **Pap smear:** Give to every patient at first visit if she is due. Pregnancy does not change the frequency of screening.
- ⚪ **Rubella antibody screen:** If the patient is found to be nonimmune, counsel her to get postpartum immunization.
- ⚪ **Serum alpha fetoprotein (AFP):** Performed at 15 to 20 weeks' gestation, primarily to detect open spina bifida and anencephaly
- ⚪ **Syphilis test:** At first visit (mandated in most states) and subsequent visits if the patient is at high risk
- ⚪ **Thyroid function:** Maternal hypothyroidism may affect fetal neurologic development. Maternal hyperthyroidism can lead to fetal and maternal complications.
- ⚪ **Urinalysis:** At first visit and every visit (screen for preeclampsia and bacteriuria; not a good screen for diabetes mellitus)
- ⚪ **Urine culture:** Obtained at 12 to 16 weeks' gestation to screen for asymptomatic bacteriuria.
- ⚪ **Varicella:** All pregnant women should be tested for immunity to varicella.
- ⚪ **Tuberculosis skin test:** For women at higher risk.

Testing for gonorrhea for women at higher risk of infection. Testing for toxoplasmosis is controversial. If asked, you should do chlamydia and gonorrhea cultures for any pregnant teenager. Testing for STDs should be repeated in the third trimester for women who continue to be at risk or for women who acquire a risk factor during pregnancy.

Common pregnancy changes, signs, and complaints include nausea and vomiting (morning sickness), amenorrhea, heavy (possibly even painful) feeling of the breasts, increased pigmentation of the nipples and areolae (and Montgomery tubercles), backache, linea nigra, chloasma, striae gravidarum, *mild* ankle edema, heartburn, and increased frequency of urination.

Normal physiologic changes in pregnancy:

- ⚪ **Laboratory tests:** Erythrocyte sedimentation rate is markedly elevated (*worthless* test in pregnancy). Thyroxine and thyroxine-binding globulin increase, but free thyroxine is normal. Hemoglobin increases, but plasma volume increases more, so the net result is a decreased hematocrit and hemoglobin; blood urea nitrogen (BUN) and creatinine decrease because glomerular filtration rate (GFR) increases (high end of normal range for BUN and creatinine indicate renal disease in pregnancy); white blood cell count increases; and alkaline phosphatase increases markedly. Mild proteinuria and glycosuria are *normal* in pregnancy. Electrolytes and liver function tests remain normal.
- ⚪ **Cardiovascular changes:** Blood pressure decreases slightly because of decreased systemic vascular resistance, heart rate increases (by up to 50%), stroke volume increases, and cardiac output increases (≤50%). A systolic ejection murmur and audible S3 are normal.
- ⚪ **Endocrinologic changes:** The placenta produces human placental lactogen (HPL), which acts as an insulin antagonist, leading to postprandial hyperglycemia. This can lead to or worsen gestational diabetes. Total and free cortisol levels increase because of production from the fetal adrenal glands and the placenta.
- ⚪ **Pulmonary changes:** Minute ventilation increases because of increased tidal volume with the same or only slightly increased respiratory rate. Residual volume and carbon dioxide decrease (together, these changes result in physiologic hyperventilation and respiratory alkalosis of pregnancy).
- ⚪ **The average weight gain** in pregnancy is 28 lb (12.5 kg). With a greater weight gain, think of diabetes mellitus. With a smaller weight gain, think of hyperemesis gravidarum or psychological or major systemic disease.

PRENATAL CARE

At every prenatal visit, listen for fetal heart tones, evaluate uterine size for any **size–date discrepancy,** and perform urinalysis. Uterine size is evaluated by measuring the distance from the symphysis pubis to the top of the fundus in centimeters. Between roughly 20 and 35 weeks, the measurement in centimeters should equal the number of weeks of gestation. A discrepancy greater than 2 to 3 cm is called a size–date discrepancy, and ultrasonography should be done to evaluate further. Possible explanations include inaccurate dates, intrauterine growth retardation, and multiple gestation.

IMPORTANT POINTS

1. At 12 weeks' gestation, the uterus enters the abdomen and may be palpable at the pubic symphysis; at roughly 20 weeks, it reaches the umbilicus.
2. Fetal heart tones and cardiac activity can be detected with transvaginal ultrasound at 5.5 to 7 weeks, heard with Doppler at 10 to 12 weeks, and heard with a stethoscope at 16 to 20 weeks.
3. Ultrasonography is most accurate at estimating fetal age at 5 to 12 weeks using the fetal crown–rump length.
4. Quickening (when the mother first detects fetal movements) usually occurs at 18 to 20 weeks in a primigravida and 16 to 18 weeks in a multigravida.

Treat asymptomatic bacteriuria in pregnancy (but not in other patients) because 20% of patients develop cystitis or pyelonephritis if untreated. This is thought to be caused by progesterone decreasing the tone of the ureters and the uterus compressing the ureters. Give penicillin, cephalosporin, or nitrofurantoin.

Human chorionic gonadotropin (hCG) roughly doubles every 2 days in the first trimester of pregnancy. An hCG that stays the same or increases only slowly with serial testing indicates a fetus in trouble or fetal demise. A rapidly increasing hCG or one that does not decrease after delivery can indicate a hydatiform mole or choriocarcinoma. The standard hCG home pregnancy test becomes positive roughly 2 weeks after conception (about the time when the woman realizes that her period is late).

PREPARTUM PREGNANCY ISSUES

Abortion

Abortion is defined as termination of a pregnancy at less than 20 weeks (fetus <500 g). The following specific terms also imply that the event occurs at earlier than 20 weeks' gestation:
- **Threatened abortion:** Uterine bleeding without cervical dilation and no expulsion of tissue. Treat with intravenous (IV) fluids (or blood, if needed), bedrest, pelvic rest, and RhoGAM (Rh immune globulin) if the patient is Rh negative. Do dilation and curettage (D&C) if the fetus dies and is not promptly expelled.
- **Inevitable abortion:** Uterine bleeding with cervical dilation and crampy abdominal pain and no tissue expulsion. Treat with IV fluids, RhoGAM if the patient is Rh negative, and D&C.
- **Incomplete abortion:** Passage of some products of conception through the cervix. Treat with IV fluids, RhoGAM if the patient is Rh negative, and D&C.
- **Complete abortion:** Expulsion of all products of conception from the uterus. Treat with serial hCG testing to make sure that hCG drops to zero, consider D&C, and give RhoGAM if the patient is Rh negative.
- **Missed abortion:** Fetal death with no expulsion of tissue (often for several weeks). Treat with D&C if less than 14 weeks or attempted delivery if greater than 14 weeks. Give RhoGAM if the patient is Rh negative.
- **Induced abortion:** Intentional termination of pregnancy before 20 weeks' gestation; may be elective (requested by patient) or therapeutic (to maintain the health of the mother).

○ **Recurrent abortion:** Two or three successive unplanned abortions. History and physical exam may show:
  ○ Infectious etiology (*Listeria, Mycoplasma,* or *Toxoplasma* spp.; syphilis)
  ○ Inherited thrombophilia (factor V Leiden, G20210A gene mutation, antithrombin deficiency, deficiency of protein C or protein S)
  ○ Environmental influences (alcohol, tobacco, drugs)
  ○ Diabetes mellitus
  ○ Hypothyroidism
  ○ Systemic lupus erythematosus (especially with positive antiphospholipid or lupus anticoagulant antibodies)
  ○ Cervical incompetence (watch for history of patient's mother taking diethylstilbestrol [DES] during pregnancy and patient with recurrent second trimester abortions; treat future pregnancies with a cervical cerclage at 14–16 weeks)
  ○ Congenital female tract abnormalities (correct if possible to restore fertility)
  ○ Fibroids (remove them)
  ○ Chromosomal abnormalities (e.g., maternal or paternal translocations)

 In women with antiphospholipid antibodies and previous problem pregnancies, low-dose aspirin may help in subsequent pregnancies. Normally, aspirin and other nonsteroidal antiinflammatory drugs (NSAIDs) should be avoided in pregnancy; use acetaminophen instead. Subcutaneous unfractionated heparin or low-molecular-weight heparin also can be used to treat antiphospholipid syndrome in pregnancy.

Testing

Alpha Fetoprotein Levels

Maternal alpha fetoprotein (AFP) is used to screen for neural tube defects and is most accurate when measured between 15 and 20 weeks' gestation. A low AFP may represent Down syndrome, fetal demise, or inaccurate dates. A high AFP may a represent neural tube defect (e.g., anencephaly, spina bifida), ventral wall defect (e.g., omphalocele, gastroschisis), multiple gestation, or inaccurate dates.

If the AFP is elevated, repeat the test. As many as 30% of elevated maternal serum AFP test results may be elevated but are normal upon repeat testing. The initial elevation is not associated with an increased risk of neural tube defects. If the AFP remains elevated, the patient is advised first to undergo ultrasonography to determine whether a neural tube defect or other anomaly is present. Ultrasonography is also used to confirm gestational age, number of fetuses, and fetal viability. Further evaluation with amniocentesis may be required if the ultrasound findings are uncertain or there is a concern for nonvisualized neural tube defects (via elevated AFP level in amniotic fluid [AF] or detection of acetylcholinesterase in AF). There is a small risk of miscarriage after amniocentesis.

Down Syndrome Screening

Several tests are available to screen for Down syndrome, including the first trimester combined test, integrated tests, and the quadruple test. The American College of Obstetricians and Gynecologists recommends that all women be offered screening before 20 weeks' gestation.

The **first trimester combined test** is performed at 10.5 to 13 weeks' gestation. The test involves determination of nuchal translucency (NT) by ultrasonography combined with serum pregnancy-associated plasma protein-A (PAPP-A) and serum human chorionic gonadotropin (hCG). Chorionic villus sampling (CVS) is used for women who have this first trimester screening and test positive.

Integrated tests:
○ The **full integrated test** includes an ultrasound measurement of nuchal translucency at 10 to 13 weeks' gestation; PAPP-A at 10 to 13 weeks' gestation; and AFP, unconjugated estradiol (uE3), hCG, and inhibin A at 15 to 18 weeks' gestation. Results of the full integrated test are not available until the second trimester.
○ The **serum integrated test** is the same as the full integrated test but without the ultrasound evaluation of nuchal translucency. This test is used in areas where expertise in the ultrasound measurement of nuchal translucency is not available. Results of the serum integrated test are not available until the second trimester.

○ **Stepwise sequential testing** has been developed to provide a risk estimate during the first trimester. The first trimester portion of the integrated screen is performed. If the tests indicate a very high risk of having an affected fetus, CVS is offered. Women whose results do not place them at very high risk of having an affected fetus go on to have the second trimester portion of the screening.

○ **Contingent testing** is being evaluated in clinical trials, and concerns exist about the performance of this screening modality. You are not likely to be asked about it on the USMLE.

The **quadruple test** includes the serum markers AFP, uE3, hCG, and inhibin A. The quadruple test is the best available test for women who present for prenatal care in the second trimester but can be used for women who receive earlier prenatal care. It is performed at 15 to 18 weeks' gestation.

Quadruple Test Interpretation

	Trisomy 21	Trisomy 18	Trisomy 13
Alpha-fetoprotein	Decreased	Decreased	Depends on defects
Estriol	Decreased	Decreased	Depends on defects
HCG	Elevated	Decreased	Depends on defects
Inhibin A	Elevated	Decreased	N/A

N/A, not applicable.

If a woman has a positive screening test result for Down syndrome, the next step is to offer fetal karyotype determination. This is done by CVS in the first trimester and by amniocentesis in the second trimester. CVS can be done at 9 to 12 weeks' gestation (earlier than amniocentesis) and generally is reserved for women with previously affected offspring or a known genetic disease. It offers the advantage of a first trimester abortion if the fetus is affected. CVS is associated with a slightly higher miscarriage rate than amniocentesis.

 Chorionic villus sampling can detect genetic or chromosomal disorders but not neural tube defects.

Diabetes Mellitus

○ **Problems in pregnant diabetic mothers:** Polyhydramnios, preeclampsia, and complications of diabetes

○ **Problems in infants born to diabetic mothers:** Macrosomia or intrauterine growth retardation (IUGR); respiratory distress syndrome; cardiovascular, colon (e.g., left colon hypoplasia), craniofacial (e.g., cleft lip or palate), and neural tube defects; caudal regression syndrome (lower half of the body incompletely formed), and **postdelivery hypoglycemia** in the fetus (from fetal islet-cell hypertrophy caused by maternal and thus fetal hyperglycemia). After birth, the infant is cut off from the mother's glucose, and the hyperglycemia goes away, but islet cells still overproduce insulin and cause hypoglycemia. Treat with IV glucose.

○ **Treat diabetes mellitus** with a combination of diet, exercise, and insulin (oral hypoglycemic agents should be used with caution). Tighter control results in better outcomes for the mother and infant. Check hemoglobin A1c (HbA1c) to determine compliance and glucose fluctuations.

○ **In evaluating amniotic fluid (AF).** to determine fetal lung maturity, phosphatidylglycerol concentration is better than the lecithin-to-sphingomyelin ratio when the mother has diabetes.

Ectopic Pregnancy

A major risk factor is a history of pelvic inflammatory disease (10-fold increase in ectopic pregnancies). Other risk factors include previous ectopic pregnancy, history of tubal sterilization or tuboplasty, pregnancy that occurs with an intrauterine device in place, and DES exposure (which can cause tubal abnormalities in women exposed in utero).

Classic symptoms of ectopic pregnancy are amenorrhea, vaginal bleeding, and abdominal pain. Patients also have positive hCG test result. If you palpate an adnexal mass, you may be palpating an ectopic pregnancy or a corpus luteum cyst, which can coexist with a tubal pregnancy or a threatened abortion (both can have similar symptoms). Order an ultrasonography scan to look for a gestational sac or fetus. When in doubt and the patient is doing poorly (hypovolemia, shock, severe abdominal pain, or rebound tenderness), do urgent ultrasonography while stabilizing the patient and prepare for laparoscopy for definitive diagnosis and treatment if necessary.

Tubal Pregnancy

If the patient is stable and the conceptus is less than 3 cm in greatest diameter, tubal pregnancy can be treated with salpingostomy and removal, leaving the tube open to heal on its own. In reliable patients who desire to avoid surgery, methotrexate can be given to cause medical abortion. If the patient is unstable or the ectopic pregnancy has ruptured or is larger than 3 cm, salpingectomy is required. Give RhoGAM after treatment for Rh-negative patients.

Hyperemesis Gravidarum

Hyperemesis gravidarum is intractable nausea and vomiting beyond 14 to 16 weeks' gestation that can lead to dehydration, electrolyte disturbances, and poor weight gain or weight loss (5% of prepregnancy weight). It is more common in younger patients with their first pregnancies, molar pregnancies, and underlying social stressors or psychological problems. Treat with supportive care, including small, frequent meals and antiemetics (fairly safe in pregnancy). Outpatient treatment sometimes is acceptable unless the patient has severe dehydration or electrolyte disturbances, in which case, admit for treatment.

Pharmacology

Drugs that are not safe in pregnancy are shown in Table 20-1.

Drugs that are generally **safe in pregnancy** include acetaminophen (*not* NSAIDs or aspirin), penicillin, cephalosporins, erythromycin, nitrofurantoin, H_2 blockers, antacids, heparin, hydralazine, methyldopa, labetalol, insulin, and docusate.

Transvaginal Ultrasonography

Transvaginal ultrasonography detects an intrauterine gestational sac at roughly 5 weeks and a fetus at 5.5 to 7 weeks. Use this information in trying to determine the possibility of an ectopic pregnancy. If the patient's last menstrual period (LMP) was 4 weeks ago and the pregnancy test result is positive, you cannot rule out an ectopic pregnancy with ultrasonography. If, however, the patient's LMP was 10 weeks ago, there is a positive pregnancy test result, and ultrasonography of the uterus shows no gestational sac, think of ectopic pregnancy. If hCG is greater than 2000 mIU, you should be able to visualize a gestational sac with transvaginal ultrasonography.

MATERNAL-TO-FETAL INFECTIONS

Torch Infections

Most intrauterine fetal infections can cause mental retardation, microcephaly, hydrocephalus, hepatosplenomegaly, jaundice, anemia, low birth weight, or IUGR.

○ *Toxoplasma gondii:* Look for exposure to cats; specific defects include intracranial calcifications and chorioretinitis.

○ **Other:** Varicella zoster (limb hypoplasia and scarring of the skin) and syphilis (rhinitis, saber shins, Hutchinson teeth, interstitial keratitis, skin lesions)

○ *Rubella:* Worst in first trimester (some authorities recommend abortion if the mother contracts rubella in the first trimester). Always check antibody status on first visit if the patient has a poor immunization history. Look for cardiovascular defects (patent ductus arteriosus, ventral septal defect), deafness, cataracts, and microphthalmia.

○ *Cytomegalovirus:* Most common; look for deafness, cerebral calcifications, and microphthalmia.

○ *Herpes:* Look for vesicular skin lesions (with positive Tzanck smears) and a history of maternal herpes lesions.

TABLE 20-1 Teratogenic Agents*

AGENT	DEFECT(S) CAUSED
Alcohol	Fetal alcohol syndrome
ACE inhibitors	Fetal renal damage, oligohydramnios
Aminoglycosides	Deafness
Aminopterin	IUGR, CNS defects, cleft lip, cleft palate
Angiotensin receptor blockers	Fetal renal damage, oligohydramnios
Antineoplastics	Many
Birth control pills	VACTERL syndrome
Carbamazepine	Fingernail hypoplasia, craniofacial defects
Cigarettes	IUGR, low birth weight, prematurity
Cocaine	Cerebral infarcts, mental retardation
Diazepam	Cleft lip, cleft palate
Diethylstilbestrol	Clear cell vaginal cancer, adenosis, cervical incompetence
Fluoroquinolones	Cartilage damage
Sulfonamides	Kernicterus
Iodine	Goiter, congenital hypothyroidism
Isotretinoin†	CNS, craniofacial, ear, and cardiovascular defects
Lithium	Cardiac (Ebstein) anomalies
Phenytoin (diphenylhydantoin)	Craniofacial and limb defects, mental retardation, cardiovascular defects
Progesterone	Masculinization of female fetus
Radiation	IUGR, CNS and face defects, leukemia
Tetracycline	Yellow or brown teeth
Thalidomide	Phocomelia (absence of long bones and flipperlike appearance of the hands)
Trimethadione	Craniofacial and cardiovascular defects, mental retardation
Valproic acid	Spina bifida, hypospadias
Warfarin	Craniofacial and CNS defects, IUGR, stillbirth

*Note: Marijuana and LSD (lysergic acid diethylamide) have not been confirmed as teratogens.
†Vitamin A in general is considered teratogenic when recommended intake levels are exceeded.
ACE, angiotensin-converting enzyme; CNS, central nervous system; IUGR, Intrauterine growth retardation VACTERL, vertebral, anal, cardiac, tracheoesophageal, renal, and limb malformations.

With all in utero infections that can cause problems with the fetus, the mother may be asymptomatic (subclinical infection), and the infant may even be asymptomatic at birth, only to develop symptoms later (e.g., learning disability, mental retardation).

Human Immunodeficiency Virus

In untreated HIV-positive patients, transmission to the fetus occurs in roughly 25% of cases. With prenatal zidovudine (AZT) treatment of the mother and administration of AZT (or other antiretroviral) to the infant for 6 weeks after birth, HIV transmission is reduced to less than 10%. A noninfected infant might still be HIV positive on enzyme-linked immunosorbent assay testing because maternal antibodies can cross the placenta. Within 6 months, the test result reverts to negative. Children are thus tested with a DNA polymerase chain reaction test after birth to directly detect the HIV virus. HIV-positive mothers should *not* breastfeed because milk can transmit HIV to the infant.

Herpes

When the mother has genital herpes simplex virus (HSV) infection, delay the decision of whether to do a cesarean section until the mother goes into labor. If at the time of true labor she has lesions of HSV, do a cesarean section to prevent transmission to the fetus. If at the time of true labor the mother has no HSV lesions, deliver the infant vaginally.

Hepatitis B

If the mother has hepatitis B, give the infant the first hepatitis B vaccine shot and hepatitis B immunoglobulin at birth.

Varicella

If the mother gets chickenpox in the last 5 days of pregnancy or first 2 days after delivery, give the infant varicella zoster immunoglobulin.

Chlamydia

In pregnancy, treat chlamydial infection with azithromycin, amoxicillin, or erythromycin base (not doxycycline). Remember the association with neonatal conjunctivitis and pneumonia.

Group B Streptococcus

Routine screening is usually performed at 36 weeks' gestation. If the result is positive, the patient is treated with penicillin or ampicillin at delivery. Patients also should be treated with penicillin if they have had a previous GBS-infected neonate, preterm labor, membrane rupture longer than 18 hours, or GBS-positive urine culture. The goal of treatment is to prevent neonatal sepsis and maternal endometritis.

IMPORTANT POINTS

1. Immunoglobulin G (IgG) is the only maternal antibody that crosses the placenta. An elevated neonatal IgM concentration is never normal, but an elevated neonatal IgG often represents maternal antibodies.
2. If a woman has tuberculosis in pregnancy (positive purified protein derivative [PPD] test and suspicious chest radiograph plus a positive sputum culture), treat as you would any other patient. If the patient is a known recent PPD converter but has a negative chest radiograph, she has latent tuberculosis. Treat with isoniazid as in a nonpregnant patient. Make sure to give the mother vitamin B_6 with isoniazid to prevent nutritional defects in her and the fetus. Avoid streptomycin, which can cause deafness and nephrotoxicity in fetuses.

OTHER CONDITIONS IN PREGNANCY

Cholestasis of Pregnancy

Cholestasis of pregnancy presents with itching (palms and soles), abnormal liver function tests, or jaundice during pregnancy. Cholestasis increases the risk of premature birth, meconium aspiration, and intrauterine demise. The only treatment is delivery, but ursodeoxycholic acid or cholestyramine can help with symptoms.

Acute fatty liver of pregnancy is a more serious disorder that occurs in the third trimester or after delivery and usually progresses to hepatic coma. Treatment includes IV fluids, IV glucose, and fresh-frozen plasma. Vitamin K does not work because the liver is in temporary failure.

Gestational Trophoblastic Disease

In a sense, the products of conception become a tumor that can be malignant (e.g., choriocarcinoma) or benign (e.g., hydatidiform mole). Look for preeclampsia before the third trimester, an hCG that does not return to zero after delivery (or abortion) or that rapidly rises during pregnancy, first- or second-trimester bleeding with possible expulsion of "grapes", uterine size or date discrepancy, and a "snowstorm" pattern on ultrasonography. Hydatidiform moles can be characterized as complete or incomplete (partial) moles. **Complete moles** are 46 XX (all chromosomes from the father) and have no fetal tissue; **incomplete moles** are usually 69 XXY and contain fetal tissue. Gross appearance suggests a *bunch of grapes*.

Treat with uterine D&C and then follow hCG until it falls to zero. If hCG does not fall to zero or rises, the patient has either an invasive mole or choriocarcinoma; in either case, the patient needs chemotherapy (usually *methotrexate* or actinomycin D).

Intrauterine Growth Retardation

Intrauterine growth retardation is defined as size below the tenth percentile for age. The causes are many and are best understood in broad terms as caused by one of three factors: maternal (e.g., smoking, alcohol or drugs, lupus erythematosus), fetal (e.g., TORCH infections, congenital anomalies), or placental (e.g., hypertension, preeclampsia). Ultrasonography should be done on all patients who have a size–date discrepancy greater than 2 to 3 cm or risk factors for pregnancy problems (e.g., hypertension; diabetes mellitus; renal disease; lupus erythematosus; cigarette, alcohol, or drug use; history of previous problems). IUGR is usually classified as symmetric or asymmetric based on how many ultrasound parameters are smaller than expected. Ultrasound parameters measured for IUGR determination include biparietal diameter, head circumference, abdominal circumference, and femur length. Symmetric IUGR occurs when all parameters are "symmetrically" decreased and generally is caused by an insult that occurred early in pregnancy. Asymmetric IUGR occurs when only one parameter is decreased (usually abdominal circumference) and results from an insult late in pregnancy.

Multiple Gestations

If sex or blood type is different, twins are dizygotic. If the placentas are monochorionic, the twins are monozygotic. These three simple factors differentiate monozygotic from dizygotic twins in 80% of cases. The remaining 20% require HLA-typing studies. Complications of multiple gestations (the higher the number of fetuses, the higher the risk of most of these conditions) include the following:

○ **Maternal:** Anemia, hypertension, premature labor, postpartum uterine atony, postpartum hemorrhage, preeclampsia, gestational diabetes
○ **Fetal:** Polyhydramnios, malpresentation, placenta previa, abruptio placentae, velamentous cord insertion or vasa previa, premature rupture of membranes (PROM), prematurity, umbilical cord prolapse, IUGR, congenital anomalies, increased perinatal morbidity and mortality

With vertex–vertex presentations, you can try vaginal delivery for both infants; with any other combination of presentations, do a cesarean section.

Oligohydramnios

Oligohydramnios is defined as AF below 500 mL or an AF index below 5. Causes include rupture of membranes, postmaturity, genitourinary tract abnormalities (renal agenesis, polycystic kidney disease, genitourinary obstruction), or chronic uteroplacental insufficiency (associated with a fetus that is small for gestational age). Oligohydramnios can cause fetal problems such as pulmonary hypoplasia, cutaneous and skeletal abnormalities caused by compression, and hypoxia caused by umbilical cord compression.

Polyhydramnios

Polyhydramnios is defined as AF greater than 2000 to 2500 mL or an AF index greater than 25. Causes include maternal diabetes mellitus, multiple gestation, neural tube defects (anencephaly, spina bifida), gastrointestinal anomalies (omphalocele, esophageal atresia), and hydrops fetalis. Polyhydramnios can cause maternal dyspnea (overdistended uterus compromising pulmonary function), postpartum uterine atony with resultant postpartum hemorrhage, preterm labor, fetal malpresentation, and umbilical cord prolapse.

Postterm Pregnancy

Postterm pregnancy is defined as pregnancy after 42 weeks of gestation. Generally, if gestational age is known to be accurate, labor is induced (e.g., by oxytocin) if the cervix is favorable. If the cervix is not favorable or the dates are uncertain, do twice-weekly nonstress test (NST) and biophysical profile (BPP) (see later discussion). At 41 weeks' gestation, most authorities advise induction of labor or cesarean section. Both prematurity and postmaturity increase perinatal morbidity and mortality. Prolonged gestation is common in association with anencephaly and placental sulfatase deficiency.

Preeclampsia

Preeclampsia is defined as new-onset hypertension plus proteinuria occurring after 20 weeks gestation. To make the diagnosis, the patient must have blood pressure above 140/90 mm Hg on two separate occasions more than 6 hours apart and greater than 2+ protein on urinalysis or greater than 300 mg protein on 24-hour urine collection. Nondependent edema is usually noted. A patient is classified as having severe preeclampsia if she has blood pressure above 160/110 mm Hg and greater than 2 to 4+ protein on urinalysis or greater than 5 g of protein on 24-hour urine collection. Severe preeclampsia often is associated with headache, visual disturbance, HELLP (**h**emolysis, **e**levated **l**iver enzymes, **l**ow **p**latelets) syndrome, and right upper quadrant or epigastric pain.

The main **risk factors** for preeclampsia (in order of importance) are chronic renal disease, chronic hypertension, family history, multiple gestation, primiparity, age older than 40 years (although the classic case is a young woman with her first child), diabetes mellitus, and black race. **Treatment** is delivery if the patient is at term. If the patient is premature and has mild disease, treat hypertension with labetalol or hydralazine and bedrest. Observe the patient carefully. If the patient has severe disease (oliguria, mental status changes, headache, blurred vision, pulmonary edema, cyanosis, HELLP syndrome, blood pressure above 160/110 mm Hg, or progression to eclampsia [seizures]), deliver regardless of gestational age because both the mother and infant might die.

Of note, preeclampsia is not synonymous with gestational hypertension because gestational hypertension does not involve significant proteinuria (<2+ protein on urinalysis). Gestational hypertension occurs after 20 weeks of gestation and resolves by 12 weeks postpartum. If a patient is hypertensive before 20 weeks of gestation, consider molar pregnancy or chronic hypertension.

IMPORTANT POINTS

1. Mild ankle edema is normal in pregnancy, but severe ankle edema or hand edema is likely to be preeclampsia.
2. If preeclampsia symptoms develop before the third trimester, think of hydatiform mole or choriocarcinoma.
3. Hypertension plus proteinuria in a pregnant patient is preeclampsia until proven otherwise.
4. Preeclampsia plus seizures =eclampsia. Eclampsia can be prevented by regular prenatal care. Catch it in preeclamptic stage and treat appropriately.
5. Use magnesium sulfate for eclamptic seizures (also lowers blood pressure). Toxic magnesium effects include hyporeflexia (first sign of toxicity), respiratory depression, central nervous system depression, coma, and death. If toxicity occurs, the first step is to stop the magnesium infusion.
6. Do not wait to follow up and remeasure very high blood pressure in a pregnant patient (likely you would in nonpregnant patients with nonemergent elevated blood pressure levels). Err on the safe side; assume that it represents preeclampsia and start treatment.
7. Do not try to deliver the infant until the mother is stable (do not do a cesarean section while the mother is having a seizure!).
8. Preeclampsia and eclampsia cause uteroplacental insufficiency, IUGR, fetal demise, and increased maternal morbidity and mortality.
9. Preeclampsia and eclampsia are not risk factors for future development of hypertension or end-organ effects of hypertension.

Premature Rupture of Membranes

Premature rupture of membranes is rupture of the amniotic sac before the onset of labor. Diagnosis of rupture of the membranes (whether premature or not) is based on history and sterile speculum examination, which will show pooling of AF, ferning pattern when the fluid is placed on a microscopic slide and allowed to dry, or a positive nitrazine test result (nitrazine paper turns blue in the presence of AF). Ultrasonography also should be done to assess AF volume (as well as gestational age and any anomalies that may be present). Spontaneous labor often follows membrane rupture. If labor does not occur within 6 to 8 hours and the patient is at term, labor should be induced. If the cervix is highly unfavorable, you can wait 24 hours to attempt induction. PROM should be distinguished from prolonged rupture of membranes, which is rupture of membranes longer than 18 hours. Prolonged rupture of membranes carries an increased risk of infection, both to the mother (chorioamnionitis) and infant (neonatal sepsis, pneumonia, meningitis), usually from GBS, *Escherichia coli,* or *Listeria* spp.

Preterm premature rupture of membranes (PPROM) is PROM that occurs before 36 to 37 weeks' gestation. Risk of infection increases with the duration of ruptured membranes. Do a culture and Gram stain of AF. If the results are negative, treat with pelvic rest and bedrest and frequent follow-up. If positive for GBS, treat the mother with penicillin or ampicillin even if she is asymptomatic.

Preterm Labor

Preterm labor is defined as labor between 20 and 37 weeks' gestation. It is the primary cause of neonatal morbidity and mortality. Risk factors include multiple gestation, infection, PROM, uterine anomalies, previous preterm labor or delivery, polyhydramnios, placental abruption, poor maternal nutrition, and low socioeconomic status. Treat with lateral decubitus position, bed and pelvic rest, oral or IV fluids, and oxygen administration (all might stop the contractions). Then give a tocolytic (β_2 agonist or magnesium sulfate) if no contraindications are present (heart disease, hypertension, diabetes mellitus, hemorrhage, ruptured membranes, cervix dilated >4 cm). After the patient is stable, she may be discharged on an oral tocolytic. *Do not* tocolyze the mother if it is dangerous to do so (preeclampsia, severe hemorrhage, chorioamnionitis, IUGR, fetal demise, or fetal anomalies incompatible with survival). Often steroids are given with tocolysis (if the infant is 24–34 weeks old) to hasten fetal lung maturity.

Fetal fibronectin may be detected in vaginal secretions of women presenting with signs and symptoms of preterm labor. The test is most helpful when the result is negative between 22 and 34 weeks because it indicates a very low likelihood of delivery in the next 2 weeks. Thus, a more conservative, observational approach can be used. When fetal fibronectin is positive in this setting, the woman remains at a higher risk for delivery in the next 2 weeks, and a more aggressive approach to tocolysis and fetal lung maturity hastening is typically used.

Rh Incompatibility and Hemolytic Disease of The Newborn

Rh incompatibility and hemolytic disease of the newborn occur when the mother is Rh negative and the infant is Rh positive. If both mother and father are Rh negative, there is nothing to worry about—the infant will be Rh negative. If the father is Rh positive, the infant has a 50% chance of being Rh positive. If the potential for hemolytic disease exists, check maternal Rh antibody titers every month, starting in the seventh month of gestation. Give RhoGAM automatically at 28 weeks and within 72 hours after delivery as well as after any procedures that can cause transplacental hemorrhage (e.g., amniocentesis).

The development of disease requires previous **sensitization.** In other words, if a nulliparous mother has never received blood products, her first Rh-positive infant will often not be affected by hemolytic disease (except in the rare case of sensitization during the first pregnancy from undetected fetomaternal bleeding, which usually occurs later in the pregnancy and can be prevented by RhoGAM administration at 28 weeks in most instances). The second Rh-positive infant, however, will be affected—unless you, the astute board taker/physician, administer RhoGAM appropriately. Any history of blood transfusion, abortion, ectopic pregnancy, stillbirth, or delivery can cause sensitization. If you check maternal Rh antibodies and they are strongly positive, RhoGAM is worthless because sensitization has already occurred. RhoGAM administration is a good example of **primary prevention**.

RhoGAM Summary

Give RhoGAM only when the mother is Rh negative and the father's blood type is unknown or Rh positive. During routine prenatal care, check for Rh antibodies at the first visit. If the test is positive, *do not* give RhoGAM—you are too late. Otherwise, give RhoGAM routinely at 28 weeks and immediately after delivery. Also give RhoGAM after an abortion, stillbirth, ectopic pregnancy, amniocentesis, CVS, and any other invasive procedure during pregnancy that can cause transplacental bleeding.

If fetal lungs are immature (lecithin-to-sphingomyelin ratio <2:1 or prostaglandin negative) and the fetus is between 24 and 34 weeks' gestational age, corticosteroid administration can hasten lung maturity and thus reduce the risk of respiratory distress syndrome.

IMPORTANT POINTS

1. If not detected and prevented, Rh incompatibility can lead to fetal hydrops (edema, ascites, pleural and pericardial effusions) and death.

2. AF spectrophotometry gauges the severity of fetal hemolysis.

3. Treatment of hemolytic disease involves delivery if the fetus is mature. Check lung maturity with the lecithin-to-sphingomyelin ratio. Intrauterine transfusion is invasive but can be performed if needed; phenobarbital helps the fetal liver break down bilirubin by inducing enzymes.

4. ABO blood group incompatibility also can cause hemolytic disease of the newborn when the mother has type O blood and the infant has type A, B, or AB blood. Previous sensitization is not required because IgG antibodies, which can cross the placenta, occur naturally in patients with blood type O (but not in mothers with other blood types). Usually the disease is less severe than with Rh incompatibility, but treatment is the same. Other minor blood antigens also cause a reaction in rare cases.

Surgical Conditions

Pregnant women can have the same surgical conditions as nonpregnant women. In general, treat the disease regardless of pregnancy. This general rule always works with acute surgical conditions (e.g., appendicitis, cholecystitis). With semi-urgent conditions (e.g., ovarian neoplasm), it is best to wait until the second trimester when the patient is most stable. Purely elective cases are avoided. Appendicitis can manifest with right upper quadrant pain or tenderness because of displacement of the appendix by the uterus. Consider exploratory laparotomy if you are unsure and if the patient has peritoneal signs.

Third Trimester Bleeding

For third trimester bleeding (very high yield), *always* have ultrasonography done before pelvic examination. Repeat: *Always* do an ultrasonography before pelvic examination. The differential diagnosis includes:

○ **Abruptio placentae:** This is premature detachment of a normally situated placenta. Predisposing factors include hypertension (with or without preeclampsia), trauma, polyhydramnios with rapid decompression after membrane rupture, cocaine or tobacco use, and PPROM. *Do not* forget that the patient can have this condition without visible bleeding (blood may be contained behind the placenta). Patients have pain, uterine tenderness, and increased uterine tone with a hyperactive contraction pattern. Fetal distress also is present. Abruptio placentae can cause disseminated intravascular coagulation if fetal products enter the maternal circulation. Ultrasonography detects less than 5% of cases. Treat with IV fluids (and blood if needed) and rapid delivery (vaginal preferred).

○ **Bleeding disorder:** Rarely manifests before delivery (more common after delivery)

○ **"Bloody show":** With cervical effacement, a blood-tinged mucus plug may be released from the cervical canal and heralds the onset of labor. This event is *normal* and is a diagnosis of exclusion in the evaluation of third trimester bleeding.

○ **Cervical cancer:** Can occur in pregnant patients, too!

○ **Cervical or vaginal lesions:** Examples include herpes simplex virus, gonorrhea, chlamydial, or candidal infection.

○ **Cervical or vaginal trauma:** Usually from intercourse

○ **Fetal bleeding:** Usually from vasa previa or velamentous insertion of the cord. The major risk factor is multiple gestation (the higher the number of fetuses, the higher the risk). Bleeding is *painless,* and the mother is completely stable while the fetus shows worsening distress (tachycardia initially and then bradycardia as the fetus decompensates). The Apt test is positive on uterine blood and differentiates fetal from maternal blood. Treat with immediate cesarean section.

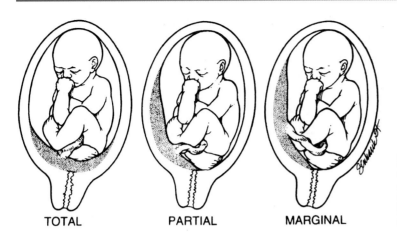

TOTAL   PARTIAL   MARGINAL

FIGURE **20-1** Three variations of placenta previa. *(From Gabbe SG, Niebyl JR, Simpson JL (eds): Obstetrics: Normal & Problem Pregnancies. New York, Churchill Livingstone, 1986, p 495.)*

○ **Placenta previa** (Fig. 20-1): True placenta previa occurs when the placenta implants in an area where it covers the cervical os. Predisposing factors include multiparity, increasing age, multiple gestation, and prior previa. This condition is why you *always* do ultrasonography before pelvic examination. Bleeding is painless and may be profuse. Ultrasonography is 95% to 100% accurate in diagnosis. Cesarean section is mandatory for delivery, but you may try to admit the patient with bedrest and pelvic rest and tocolysis if the patient is preterm and stable and the bleeding stops.

○ **Uterine rupture:** Predisposing factors include previous uterine surgery, trauma, oxytocin, grand multiparity (several previous deliveries), excessive uterine distension (e.g., multiple gestation, polyhydramnios), abnormal fetal lie, cephalopelvic disproportion, and shoulder dystocia. Uterine rupture is characterized by *extreme pain* of sudden onset and is often associated with maternal hypotension or shock. Fetal parts may be felt in the abdomen, or the abdominal contour might change. Treat with immediate laparotomy and usually hysterectomy after delivery.

In all patients with third trimester bleeding, initiate **treatment** with IV fluids and give blood if needed. Give oxygen and get a complete blood count, coagulation profiles, and ultrasound scan. Set up fetal and maternal monitoring. Do a drug screen if you are suspicious (cocaine causes placental abruption). Give RhoGAM if the mother is Rh negative. The Kleihauer-Betke test quantifies fetal blood in maternal circulation and is sometimes used to calculate the dose of RhoGAM.

EVALUATION OF FETAL WELL-BEING

Nonstress Test

With the mother resting, fetal heart rate tracing is obtained for 20 minutes. A normal strip has at least two accelerations of the heart rate, each of which is at least 15 beats/min above baseline and lasts at least 15 seconds. This is the first screening test to evaluate fetal well-being; it is often done in the context of a biophysical profile.

Biophysical Profile

The BPP includes four measurements:

○ **NST:** See above.

○ **AF index:** Measures vertical pockets of AF (in centimeters) in each of the four quadrants. The sum of the highest vertical pocket in each quadrant is used to determine whether oligohydramnios or polyhydramnios is present (AF index <5 cm = oligohydramnios; AF index >25 cm = polyhydramnios).

○ **Fetal breathing movements:** Fetuses should have at least 30 breathing movements in 10 minutes.

○ **Fetal movements:** Fetuses should have at least three body movements (e.g., flexion, extension, rotation) in 10 minutes.

If the fetus scores low on the BPP, the next test is the contraction stress test. With high-risk pregnancies (e.g., IUGR, diabetes mellitus, hypertension, alcohol or drug use, postterm pregnancy, history of problem pregnancies, maternal or physician concern), the BPP often is done once or even twice a week in the third trimester until delivery.

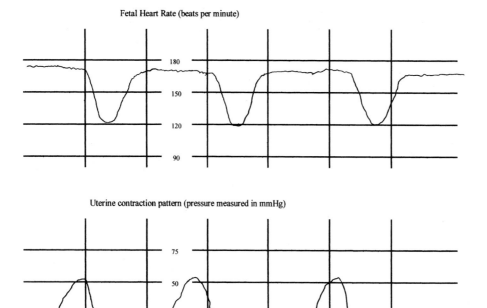

Fetal Heart Rate (beats per minute)

Uterine contraction pattern (pressure measured in mmHg)

Figure 20-2 Positive contraction stress test with late decelerations. The nadir (i.e., valley or low point) of the fetal heart rate occurs just after the peak of each uterine contraction. This is a worrisome pattern and generally indicates uteroplacental insufficiency.

The **contraction stress test** (Fig. 20-2) is a test for uteroplacental dysfunction. Contractions can be spontaneous or stimulated (oxytocin or nipple stimulation), and the fetal heart strip is monitored. Contractions need to be adequate (three contractions in 10 minutes) for an accurate test result. If late decelerations are seen on the fetal heart strip with each contraction, the test result is positive, and a cesarean section is usually done if feasible.

LABOR AND DELIVERY

True Labor
Normal contractions occur at least every 3 minutes, are fairly regular, and are associated with cervical changes (effacement and dilation). **False labor** (Braxton-Hicks contractions) is characterized by irregular contractions with no cervical changes.

Normal Labor
Characteristics of normal labor are shown in Table 20-2.

 Signs of placental separation: fresh show of blood from vagina, the umbilical cord lengthens, and the fundus rises and becomes firm and globular

 Cardinal movements of labor: engagement, flexion, descent, internal rotation, extension, external rotation (restitution), and expulsion

Protraction and Arrest
Protraction disorder occurs when true labor has begun if the mother takes longer than she should (see Table 20-2), although labor is still progressing slowly. **Arrest disorder** (failure to progress) occurs when true labor has begun if no change in dilation (as opposed to the slow change of protraction disorder) occurs over 2 hours *or* if no change occurs in descent over 1 hour. First rule out abnormal lie or cephalopelvic disproportion. If everything is okay, treat with labor augmentation (oxytocin, prostaglandin gel, amniotomy). If this approach does not work, manage expectantly and do a cesarean section at the first sign of trouble.

TABLE 20-2 Characteristics of Normal Labor

STAGE	CHARACTERISTICS	PRIMIGRAVIDA	MULTIGRAVIDA
First	Onset of true labor to full cervical dilation	<20 h	<14 h
Latent phase	From 0 to 3–4 cm dilation (slow, irregular)	Highly variable	Highly variable
Active phase	From 3–4 cm to full dilation (rapid, regular)	>1 cm/h dilation	>1.2 cm/h dilation
Second	From full dilation to birth of infant	30 min–3 h	5–30 min
Third	From delivery of infant to delivery of placenta	0–30 min	0–30 min
Fourth	From placental delivery to maternal stabilization	≤48 h	≤48 h

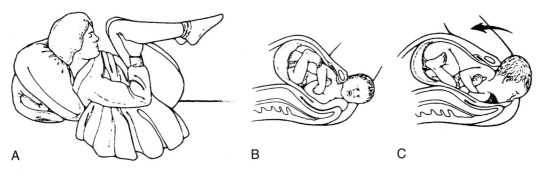

FIGURE 20-3 A, The McRobert maneuver with the legs flexed on the maternal abdomen and chest. Compared with the angle with the legs extended in lithotomy **(B),** the angle of inclination of the pelvic area is increased when the legs are flexed **(C);** thus, the shoulder of the infant might become disengaged. *(From Ratcliffe SD, Byrd JE, Sakornbut EL: Handbook of Pregnancy and Perinatal Care in Family Practice. Philadelphia, Hanley & Belfus, 1996.)*

The most common cause of failure to progress (protraction or arrest disorder), also known as dystocia (difficult birth), is cephalopelvic disproportion, defined as disparity between the size of the infant's head and the mother's pelvis. Labor augmentation is *contraindicated* in this setting.

When **shoulder dystocia** occurs, the first step is the McRobert maneuver (Fig. 20-3). Ask the mother to flex her thighs sharply against her abdomen. This maneuver might free the impacted anterior shoulder. Other maneuvers include applying suprapubic pressure, Woods screw maneuver (rotates the fetus so the anterior shoulder emerges from behind the maternal symphysis), delivery of the posterior arm, and fracture of the clavicle (risky). If these maneuvers to not work, options are limited. A cesarean section is usually the procedure of choice (after pushing the infant's head back up into the birth canal).

Hastening Labor

Contraindications to labor induction and augmentation (similar to contraindications to vaginal delivery) are:

○ Placenta or vasa previa
○ Umbilical cord prolapse or presentation
○ Transverse fetal lie
○ Active genital herpes
○ Known cervical cancer
○ Known cephalopelvic disproportion
○ Prior classic (vertical) uterine cesarean section incision (increased rate of uterine rupture). After a cesarean section with a lower (horizontal) uterine incision, the patient may deliver future pregnancies vaginally (but with a slightly increased risk).

You may try oxytocin to augment ineffective uterine contractions. Watch out for uterine hyperstimulation (painful, overly frequent, and poorly coordinated uterine contractions), uterine rupture, fetal heart rate decelerations, and water intoxication (from the antidiuretic hormone–like effect of oxytocin). Treat all of these symptoms by first discontinuing oxytocin infusion (half-life is <10 min). Prostaglandin E_2 (dinoprostone) or misoprostol also may be used locally to induce (ripen) the cervix and is highly effective in combination with (often before) oxytocin.

Prostaglandin E_2 also can cause uterine hyperstimulation. Amniotomy hastens labor but exposes the fetus and uterine cavity to possible infection if labor does not occur.

Fetal Heart Monitoring

Fetal heart monitoring is routinely done during labor and delivery, but its benefit is controversial. At term, the normal heart rate is 120 to 160 beats/min. Any value outside this range is worrisome. Know what a basic fetal heart strip with uterine contraction patterns looks like and know the following abnormalities:

○ **Early deceleration:** Peaks match up (fetal heart deceleration nadir and uterine contraction peak). **Early deceleration** signifies **head compression** (probable vagal response) and is *normal.*
○ **Variable deceleration:** Variable with relation to uterine contractions. The most commonly encountered abnormality, **variable deceleration** signifies **umbilical cord compression**. Place the mother in a lateral decubitus position, administer oxygen by face mask, and stop any oxytocin infusion. If bradycardia is severe (<80–90 beats/min) or does not resolve, measure fetal scalp pH.
○ **Late deceleration:** Fetal heart deceleration comes after uterine contraction. **Late deceleration** signifies **uteroplacental insufficiency** and is the most worrisome pattern. Place the mother in a lateral decubitus position, give oxygen by face mask, and stop oxytocin if it is being given. Then give IV fluids if the mother is hypotensive (especially with epidural anesthesia). If late decelerations persist, measure fetal scalp pH. Consider preparing for operative delivery.
○ **Short-term variability (beat-to-beat variability):** Reflects the interval between successive heart beats. The normal value is 5 to 25 beats/min. Variability consistently less than 5 beats/min is worrisome, especially when combined with decelerations. Measure fetal scalp pH.
○ **Long-term variability:** A 1-minute strip normally shows changes in the baseline heart rate. Fewer than three cycles per minute is worrisome, especially when combined with decelerations. Measure fetal scalp pH. *Special warning:* Long-term variability is decreased normally during fetal sleep.
○ **Fetal tachycardia:** Heart rate greater than 160 beats/min. Poor indicator of fetal distress unless prolonged or marked. Often associated with oxytocin administration, maternal fever, or intrauterine infection.

 Any fetal scalp pH below 7.2 is an indication for immediate cesarean delivery. If pH is greater than 7.2, in general, continue to observe.

Fetal Malpresentations

Although under specific guidelines, babies in some frank and complete breeches may be delivered vaginally, it is acceptable to do a cesarean section for *any* breech presentation. With shoulder presentation or incomplete or footling breech, cesarean section is mandatory. For face and brow presentations, watchful waiting is best because most convert to vertex presentations; if they do not convert, do a cesarean section. Breech presentations are shown in Figure 20-4.

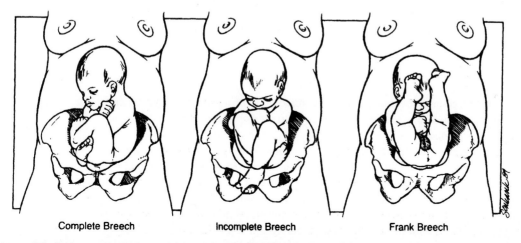

Complete Breech   Incomplete Breech   Frank Breech

Figure 20-4 Three possible breech presentations. *(From Gabbe SG, Niebyl JR, Simpson JL (eds): Obstetrics: Normal & Problem Pregnancies.* New York, Churchill Livingstone, 1986, p 465.)

Anesthesia

Epidural anesthesia is preferred in obstetric patients. General anesthesia involves a higher risk of aspiration and resulting pneumonia because the gastroesophageal sphincter is relaxed in pregnancy, and most patients have not been NPO (nothing by mouth). There are also concerns regarding the fetal effects of anesthesia. Spinal anesthesia can interfere with the mother's ability to push and has a higher incidence of hypotension than epidural anesthesia.

POSTPARTUM

IMPORTANT POINTS

1. The top causes of maternal mortality are pulmonary embolism, pregnancy-induced hypertension, and hemorrhage (most texts say in that order).
2. When a postpartum mother develops shortness of breath, tachypnea, chest pain, hypotension, or disseminated intravascular coagulation, think of AF pulmonary embolism.
3. If a postpartum patient goes into shock and you see no bleeding, think of AF embolism, uterine inversion, or concealed hemorrhage (e.g., uterine rupture with bleeding into the peritoneal cavity)

Breastfeeding

If a woman does not want to breastfeed, prescribe tight-fitting bras, ice packs, and analgesia. Medications for the suppression of lactation (e.g., bromocriptine and estrogens or oral contraceptive pills) are generally no longer recommended because of risks of thromboembolism and stroke.

If a woman does breastfeed, watch for **mastitis**, which usually develops in the first 2 months postpartum. The patient's breasts are red, indurated, and painful, and nipple cracks or fissuring may be seen. *Staphylococcus aureus* is the usual cause. Treat with analgesics (e.g., acetaminophen, ibuprofen), warm or cold compresses, and continued breastfeeding with the affected breast(s) even though it is painful (use a breast pump to empty the breast if needed) to prevent further milk duct blockage and abscess formation. An antistaphylococcal antibiotic (e.g., cephalexin, dicloxacillin) is usually given for more than mild symptoms. If a fluctuant mass develops or there is no response to antibiotics within a few days, an abscess is likely present and must be drained.

Breastfeeding is *contraindicated* in patients with HIV and in patients who use benzodiazepines, barbiturates, opiates, alcohol, caffeine or tobacco (in large amounts), antithyroid medications, lithium, chloramphenicol, anticancer agents, or ergot and its derivatives (e.g., methysergide).

Chorioamnionitis

Chorioamnionitis manifests with fever and a tender, irritable uterus (usually postpartum but may be antepartum in patients with PROM or PPROM). Do a culture and Gram stain of the cervix and AF and treat with antibiotics such as ampicillin plus gentamicin while awaiting culture results.

Postpartum Fever

Postpartum fever is defined as temperature above 100.4°F (38°C) for at least 2 consecutive days. Remember the seven Ws of postpartum fever: **w**omb (endometritis), **w**ind (atelectasis or pneumonia), **w**alk (deep venous thrombosis or pulmonary embolism), **w**ater (urinary tract infection), **w**ound (incision or episiotomy infection), **w**eaning (mastitis or engorgement), and **w**onder drug (drug fever).

Postpartum fever most commonly is caused by endometritis. Important predisposing factors are PROM or PPROM, prolonged labor, frequent vaginal examinations during labor, and manual removal of the placenta or retained placental fragments (good culture medium). Patients with endometritis have a tender uterus in addition to fever. Anaerobes usually are involved.

Clindamycin plus gentamicin is a good choice for endometritis; add extended coverage if the patient is doing poorly. Before antibiotics, do cultures of the endometrium, vagina, blood, and urine. Do not forget the easy causes of postpartum fever, such as urinary tract infection or atelectasis and pneumonia, especially after cesarean section.

If a postpartum fever does not resolve with broad-spectrum antibiotics, there are two main possibilities: progression to pelvic abscess or **pelvic thrombophlebitis**. Get a computed tomography (CT) scan, which will show an abscess. If an abscess is present, it needs to be drained. If no abscess is seen on CT, think of pelvic thrombophlebitis, which manifests with persistent spiking fevers and lack of response to antibiotics. Give heparin or low-molecular-weight-heparin for an easy cure (and retrospective diagnosis).

Postpartum Hemorrhage

Postpartum hemorrhage is defined as estimated blood loss of more than 500 mL during a vaginal delivery (>1000 mL during cesarean section). The most common cause is uterine atony (75%–80% of cases). Hemorrhage also may be caused by lacerations, retained placental tissue (placenta accreta, increta, or percreta), coagulation disorders (e.g., disseminated intravascular coagulation, von Willebrand disease), low placental implantation, and uterine inversion. The major risk factor for retained placental tissue is previous uterine surgery or cesarean section. Treatment might require a hysterectomy if conservative measures fail.

Retained Products of Conception

Retained products of conception is probably the most common cause of *delayed* postpartum hemorrhage. Remove the placenta manually to stop bleeding; then do curettage in the operating room under anesthesia. If placenta accreta, increta, or percreta is present (i.e., placental tissue grows abnormally into or through the myometrium), a hysterectomy is usually necessary to stop the bleeding.

Uterine Atony

Uterine atony is caused by overdistension of the uterus (multiple gestation, polyhydramnios, macrosomia), prolonged labor, oxytocin use, grand multiparity (history of five or more deliveries), and precipitous labor (<3 h). Treat with dilute oxytocin infusion and use bimanual compression and massage of the uterus while the infusion is running. If this approach fails, try ergonovine or another ergot drug (contraindicated with maternal hypertension) or prostaglandin F_{2a} or misoprostol. If this approach also fails, do a hysterectomy (can try ligating the uterine vessels if the patient strongly desires future fertility).

Uterine Inversion

The uterus inverts and can be seen outside the vagina, *usually as a result of pulling too hard on the umbilical cord.* Put the uterus back in place manually (anesthesia may be needed) and give IV fluids and oxytocin.

For the first several days after delivery, it is normal to have some vaginal discharge (lochia), which is red on the first few days and gradually turns to a white or yellowish-white color by day 10. If the lochia is foul smelling or if there is associated uterine tenderness or fever, suspect endometritis.

QR CODE

The QR code includes three USMLE-style questions and answers. For more questions, redeem the PIN code on the inside cover for the Crush Step 2 question bank powered by USMLE Consult.

Please see the Introduction for instructions on how to access content using the QR codes.

Question

Which of the following is a cause for a high maternal serum alpha-fetoprotein level performed at 17 weeks' gestation?
(A) Trisomy 18
(B) Down syndrome
(C) Intrauterine growth retardation
(D) Anencephaly
(E) Inaccurate dates with an actual gestation of only 14 weeks

21 ONCOLOGY

GENERAL

Blood dyscrasias are listed in Table 21-1. Types of cancer are ranked by incidence and mortality in Table 21-2.

IMPORTANT POINTS

1. In children and younger adults, leukemia is the most common cancer. Remember, however, that age has the most significant impact on the incidence and mortality rate of cancer. The incidence of cancer in the United States roughly doubles every 5 years after age 25 years; therefore, cancer most commonly affects older adults.
2. In most organs, the most common malignancy is metastatic. On Step 2, don't be fooled into saying that hepatocellular cancer is the most common malignancy of the liver if metastatic cancer is a choice. Some cancers, such as breast and colon, do not fit this rule of thumb.
3. Metastases to the spine can cause spinal cord compression (local spinal pain, reflex changes, weakness, sensory loss, paralysis). Spinal cord compression is an emergency, and the first step is to start high-dose corticosteroids. Magnetic resonance imaging (MRI) confirms the diagnosis. The next step is to treat with radiation. Surgical decompression is used if radiation fails or the tumor is known not to be radiosensitive. Prompt treatment is essential because outcome is closely linked to pretreatment function.

Table 21-3 lists genetic predispositions to cancer. Other diseases with an increased incidence of cancer include dermatomyositis, polymyositis, immunodeficiency syndromes, Bloom syndrome, and Fanconi anemia. Breast, ovarian, and colon cancer have well-known familial tendencies (along with some other types of cancer), but only rarely can a Mendelian inheritance pattern be demonstrated (e.g., *BRCA1* gene for breast cancer). Table 21-4 lists avoidable risk factors for cancer. Table 21-5 lists tumor markers for various kinds of cancer.

LUNG CANCER

Lung cancer is the number one cause of overall cancer mortality in the United States. The incidence is rising in women (because of increased smoking). Look for change in a chronic cough in a smoker. The more pack-years of tobacco use, the more suspicious you should be. Patients also can present with hemoptysis, pneumonia, or weight loss. Chest radiography might show mass (Fig. 21-4) or pleural effusion; with an effusion, perform thoracentesis and examine the fluid for malignant cells. After chest radiography, get a computed tomography (CT) scan and then a positron emission tomography (PET) scan in indeterminate cases. Tissue biopsy (e.g., via bronchoscopy, CT-guided biopsy, open lung biopsy) is needed to confirm malignancy and to define the histologic type. Non–small cell lung cancer may be treated with surgery if the cancer remains within the lung parenchyma (i.e., without

TABLE 21-1 Blood Dyscrasias

TYPE	AGE	WHAT TO LOOK FOR IN CASE DESCRIPTION; BUZZ WORDS
Acute lymphoblastic leukemia (ALL)	Children (peak at 3–5 y)	Pancytopenia (bleeding, fever, anemia), radiation therapy, Down syndrome
Acute myelogenous leukemia (AML)	>30 y	Pancytopenia (bleeding, fever, anemia), Auer rods, DIC
Chronic myelogenous leukemia (CML)	30–50 y	WBC count >50,000, Philadelphia chromosome, blast crisis, splenomegaly
Chronic lymphocytic leukemia (CLL)	>50 y	Male gender, lymphadenopathy, lymphocytosis, infections, smudge cells, splenomegaly
Hairy cell leukemia	Adults	Blood smear with hairlike projections (Fig. 21-1), splenomegaly
Mycosis fungoides, Sézary syndrome	>50 y	Plaque-like, itchy skin rash that does not improve with treatment, blood smear with cerebriform nuclei ("butt cells"), Pautrier abscesses in the epidermis
Burkitt lymphoma	Children	Associated with Epstein-Barr virus (in Africa)
CNS B-cell lymphoma	Adults	HIV/AIDS
T-cell leukemia	Adults	HTLV-1 is one cause
Hodgkin disease	15–34 y	Reed-Sternberg cells (Fig. 21-2), cervical lymphadenopathy, night sweats
Non-Hodgkin lymphoma	Any age	Small follicular type has best prognosis, large diffuse type has worst; primary tumor may be located in the GI tract
Myelodysplasia, myelofibrosis	>50 y	Anemia, teardrop cells, dry tap on bone marrow biopsy, high MCV and RBC distribution width index; associated with CML
Multiple myeloma	>40 y	Bence Jones protein (IgG, 50%; IgA, 25%), osteolytic lesions, high calcium level
Waldenstrom disease	>40 y	Hyperviscosity, IgM spike, cold agglutinins (Raynaud phenomenon with cold sensitivity)
Polycythemia vera	>40 y	High hemoglobin, pruritus (after hot bath or shower); treat with phlebotomy
Primary thrombocythemia	>50 y	Platelet count usually >1,000,000 mcL; patients might have bleeding or thrombosis

CNS, central nervous system; DIC, disseminated intravascular coagulation; GI, gastrointestinal; HTLV, human T-cell lymphotrophic virus; Ig, immunoglobulin; MCV, mean corpuscular volume; RBC, red blood cell; WBC, white blood cell.

TABLE 21-2 Cancer Statistics

RANK	OVERALL HIGHEST INCIDENCE		OVERALL HIGHEST MORTALITY RATE	
	Male	Female	Male	Female
First	Prostate	Breast	Lung	Lung
Second	Lung	Lung	Prostate	Breast
Third	Colon	Colon	Colon	Colon

involvement of the opposite lung, pleura, chest wall, spine, or mediastinal structures). Early metastases of small cell lung cancer make surgery inappropriate. Patients with small cell lung cancer and extensive non–small cell lung cancer are treated with chemotherapy with or without radiation. Usually a platinum-containing chemotherapy regimen (e.g., cisplatin) is used.

Weird, classic, and frequently tested consequences of lung cancer:

○ **Horner syndrome:** From invasion of cervical sympathetic chain by an apical (Pancoast) tumor. Look for *unilateral* ptosis, miosis, and anhidrosis (no sweating).
○ **Diaphragm paralysis:** From phrenic nerve involvement; results in elevated hemidiaphragm on chest radiography
○ **Hoarseness:** From recurrent laryngeal nerve involvement

TABLE 21-3 Genetic Predisposition to Cancer

DISEASE OR SYNDROME	INHERITANCE	TYPE OF CANCER (IN ORDER OF MOST LIKELY) AND OTHER INFORMATION
Retinoblastoma	Autosomal dominant	Retinoblastoma, osteogenic sarcoma (later in life)
MEN type I	Autosomal dominant	Parathyroid, pituitary, pancreas (islet cell tumors)
MEN type IIA	Autosomal dominant	Thyroid (medullary cancer), parathyroid, pheochromocytoma
MEN type IIB	Autosomal dominant	Thyroid (medullary cancer), pheochromocytoma, mucosal neuromas
Familial polyposis coli	Autosomal dominant	Hundreds of colon polyps that always become colon cancer
Gardner syndrome	Autosomal dominant	Familial polyposis plus osteomas and soft tissue tumors
Turcot syndrome	Autosomal dominant	Familial polyposis plus CNS tumors
Peutz-Jeghers syndrome	Autosomal dominant	Look for perioral freckles and multiple noncancerous GI polyps; increased incidence of noncolon cancer (stomach, breast, ovaries)
Neurofibromatosis, type 1	Autosomal dominant	Multiple neurofibromas (Fig. 21-3), café-au-lait spots; increased number of pheochromocytomas, bone cysts, Wilms tumor, leukemia
Neurofibromatosis, type 2	Autosomal dominant	Bilateral acoustic schwannomas
Tuberous sclerosis	Autosomal dominant	Adenoma sebaceum, seizures, mental retardation, glial nodules in brain; increased renal angiomyolipomas and cardiac rhabdomyomas
Von Hippel-Lindau disease	Autosomal dominant	Hemangiomas in cerebellum, renal cell cancer; cysts in liver or kidney
Xeroderma pigmentosum	Autosomal recessive	Skin cancer
Albinism	Autosomal recessive	Skin cancer
Down syndrome	Trisomy 21	Leukemia

GI, gastrointestinal; MEN, multiple endocrine neoplasia.

TABLE 21-4 Avoidable Risk Factors for Cancer Development

CANCER TYPE	RISK FACTOR (GREATEST IMPACT LISTED FIRST)
All cancer overall	Smoking (second is alcohol)
Bladder	Smoking, aniline dyes (rubber and dye industry), schistosomiasis (in immigrants)
Breast*	Combined estrogen and progesterone hormone replacement therapy, nulliparity, obesity, alcohol, high-fat diet (controversial), lack of exercise
Cervical	Smoking, sex (HPV infection), high parity
Clear cell cancer	DES exposure during pregnancy
Colorectal	High-fat and low-fiber diet, smoking, alcohol, obesity
Endometrial	Unopposed estrogen stimulation, obesity, tamoxifen
Esophagus	Smoking, alcohol
Leukemia	Chemotherapy, radiotherapy, other immunosuppressive drugs, benzene
Liver	Alcohol, vinyl chloride (liver angiosarcomas), aflatoxins
Lung	Smoking, asbestos (also nickel, radon, coal, arsenic, chromium, uranium)
Mesothelioma	Asbestos and smoking
Oral cavity	Smoking, alcohol
Pancreas	Smoking
Pharynx, larynx	Smoking, alcohol
Skin	Ultraviolet light exposure (e.g., sun), coal tar, arsenic
Renal cell	Smoking
Stomach	Alcohol, nitrosamines, nitrites (from smoked meats and fish)
Thyroid	Childhood head, neck, or chest irradiation

*Order of importance for avoidable breast cancer risk factors is uncertain and remains controversial. This list is presented in a random order.
DES, diethylstilbestrol; HPV, human papillomavirus.

TABLE 21-5 Tumor Markers

MARKER	CANCER(S)
Alpha fetoprotein	Liver, testicular (yolk sac)
Bladder tumor antigen, NMP 22	Bladder
CA 15-3, CA 27.29	Breast
CA 19-9	Pancreas, lung
CA-125	Ovarian
CEA	Colon, pancreas, other GI tumors
Chromogranin A	Carcinoid tumors, neuroblastoma
Human chorionic gonadotropin	Hydatiform moles, choriocarcinoma
β2-Microglobulin	Multiple myeloma, chronic lymphocytic leukemia
Prostate-specific antigen	Prostate (early)
S-100	Melanoma, CNS tumors, nerve tumors
Thyroglobulin	Thyroid

CEA, carcinoembryonic antigen; CNS, central nervous system; GI, gastrointestinal; NMP, nuclear matrix protein.

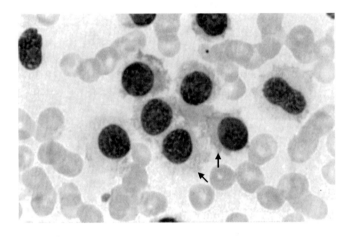

FIGURE 21-1 Peripheral blood film from a patient with hairy cell leukemia (HCL). The malignant cells show characteristic nuclear morphology and "hairy" cytoplasmic projections (*arrows*). This illustration is not typical of HCL because it is extremely unusual to find such large numbers of hairy cells circulating in the peripheral blood. *(From Wood ME: Hematology/Oncology Secrets, 2nd ed. Philadelphia, Hanley & Belfus, 1999.)*

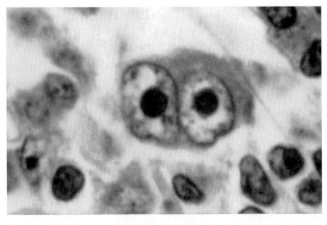

FIGURE 21-2 Lymph node from a patient with Hodgkin disease. A Reed-Sternberg cell shows the typical "owl eye" nuclear appearance. *(From Wood ME: Hematology/Oncology Secrets, 2nd ed. Philadelphia, Hanley & Belfus, 1999.)*

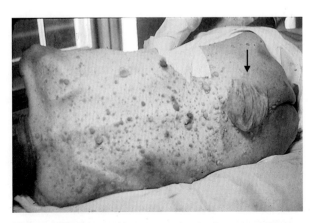

FIGURE 21-3 Neurofibromas and plexiform neurofibroma (*arrow*). *(From Fitzpatrick JE, Aeling JL: Dermatology Secrets. Philadelphia, Hanley & Belfus, 1996.)*

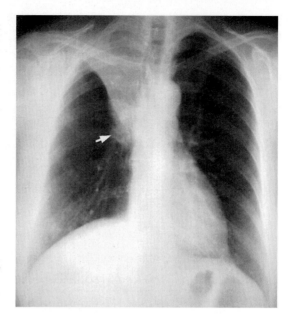

Figure 21-4 Convexity of the medial aspect of the minor fissure (*arrow*) is caused by a large central mass, with resulting right upper lobe atelectasis. This is known as the reverse S sign of Golden.

○ **Superior vena cava syndrome:** Look for edema and plethora (redness) of the neck and face and central nervous system symptoms (headache, visual symptoms, altered mental status). These are caused by compression of the superior vena cava with impaired venous drainage.

○ **Cushing syndrome:** From adrenocorticotropic hormone (ACTH) production by a small cell carcinoma

○ **Syndrome of inappropriate secretion of antidiuretic hormone (SIADH):** From antidiuretic hormone production by a small cell carcinoma

○ **Hypercalcemia:** From bone metastases or production of parathyroid hormone by a squamous cell carcinoma

○ **Eaton-Lambert syndrome:** Myasthenia gravis–like disease caused by lung cancer that spares the ocular muscles; the muscles become stronger with repetitive stimulation (opposite of myasthenia gravis)

○ **Hypertrophic pulmonary osteoarthropathy:** Clubbing and periostitis of the long bones of the upper and lower extremities most closely associated with adenocarcinoma of the lung.

Solitary pulmonary nodule on chest radiography: The first step is **comparison with previous chest radiographs.** If the nodule has remained the same size for more than 2 years, it is very unlikely to be cancer. If no old radiographs are available and the patient is older than 35 years or has more than a 5-year history of smoking, get a CT scan (and possibly a PET scan). If these are not definitely benign, get a biopsy of the nodule (via bronchoscopy or transthoracic needle biopsy if possible) for tissue diagnosis.

If the patient is younger than 35 years or has no smoking history, the cause is most likely infection (tuberculosis or fungi), hamartoma, or collagen vascular disease. The patient should undergo CT scan and careful observation with follow-up imaging in 3 to 6 months. Investigate for infection if the history is suspicious.

 Bronchoalveolar carcinoma is a subtype of lung cancer known to affect nonsmokers, Asians, and women.

BREAST CANCER

Incidence: Roughly one in eight women will develop breast cancer in her lifetime. Risk factors for breast cancer:

○ Personal history of breast cancer (biggest risk factor)

○ Family history in first-degree relatives

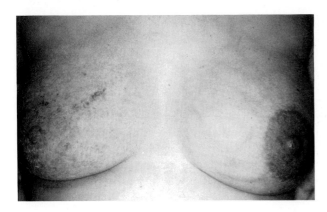

FIGURE 21-5 Paget disease of the nipple (*left side of figure*, right breast).

○ Age (breast cancer is rare before age 30 years; the incidence increases with age). Greatest risk in women older than 70 years.
○ Early menarche, late menopause, and late first pregnancy or nulliparity (more menstrual cycles = more risk)
○ Obesity
○ Atypical hyperplasia of the breast
○ Radiation exposure before age 30 years
○ Inherited gene mutations (e.g., *BRCA1*)
○ Excessive alcohol intake
○ The effect of hormonal stimulation (e.g., oral contraceptive pills, estrogen therapy) on the risk of developing breast cancer is controversial, but women with active or past breast cancer are advised not to take estrogen or progesterone.

Signs and symptoms that suggest a mass indicate breast cancer until proved otherwise: fixation of breast mass to the chest wall or overlying skin, satellite nodules or ulcers on the skin, lymphedema or peau d'orange, matted or fixed axillary lymph nodes, inflammatory skin changes (red, hot skin with enlargement of the breast caused by inflammatory cancer), prolonged unilateral scaling erosion of the nipple with or without discharge (may be Paget disease of the nipple, shown in Fig. 21-5), and *any new breast mass in a postmenopausal woman.*

The **conservative approach** is to biopsy every palpable breast mass in a woman older than 35 years when in doubt, especially if she has any risk factors. If the board question does not want you to biopsy the mass, it will give you clues that it is not cancer (e.g., bilateral, lumpy breasts that become symptomatic with every menses and have no dominant mass; age younger than 30 years).

Microcalcifications, spiculations, and irregular borders are suspicious findings on mammography. Coarse calcifications and smooth borders are benign findings. You are unlikely to be asked to read a mammogram on the USMLE, but you should be able to recognize these descriptions and handle them accordingly. You should also understand the Breast Imaging-Reporting and Data System (BI-RADS) system for mammography:

BI-RADS 0: Incomplete. Follow-up imaging is necessary.
BI-RADS 1: Completely negative. Regular follow-up.
BI-RADS 2: Definitely benign findings. Regular follow-up.
BI-RADS 3: Probably benign findings. Close follow-up at 6 month intervals for 1 year and then annual diagnostic mammogram and ultrasonography.
BI-RADS 4: Suspicious abnormality: Should be biopsied.
BI-RADS 5: Highly suggestive of malignancy. Must be biopsied.
BI-RADS 6: Biopsy proven malignancy.

Data From American College of Radiology (ACR) Breast Imaging Reporting and Data System Atlas (BI-RADS® Atlas). Reston, Va: © American College of Radiology; 2003. All rights reserved.

1. In women younger than 30 years, breast cancer is rare. With a discrete breast mass in this age group, think of fibroadenoma and observe the patient over a few menstrual cycles before considering biopsy. Fibroadenomas are usually roundish, rubbery feeling, and freely movable.
2. The most common histologic type of breast cancer is invasive ductal carcinoma.
3. In patients with a palpable breast mass, the decision to do a biopsy is a clinical one. A mammogram that looks benign (unless it is definitive) should not deter you from doing a biopsy if a lesion is clinically suspicious. On the other hand, a lesion that is detected on mammography and looks suspicious should be biopsied even if it is not palpable (needle localization biopsy).
4. Mammograms in women younger than age 30 years are rarely helpful (breast tissue is too dense to see cancer). Ultrasonography is often a more important way to image the breast in younger women. MRI is increasingly being used to screen high-risk women and evaluate masses found on mammography or ultrasonography.
5. Aromatase inhibitors (e.g., anastrozole, exemestane, and letrozole) are used for the treatment of hormone-sensitive breast cancer in postmenopausal women. Aromatase inhibitors generally are not used in premenopausal women. These medications have important side effects, including increased bone turnover and osteoporosis.
6. Tamoxifen (often with endocrine therapy) improves outcomes in premenopausal women with estrogen receptor–positive breast cancer. Tamoxifen has also been shown to decrease the risk of breast cancer in women at high risk of developing the disease. It is associated with vascular incidents and endometrial carcinoma.
7. Raloxifene has also been shown to be as effective as tamoxifen in reducing breast cancer risk in postmenopausal women at increased risk of the disease. However, raloxifene did not reduce the risk of noninvasive breast cancers, such as ductal carcinoma in situ (DCIS) and lobular carcinoma in situ (LCIS).
8. Trastuzumab is used after surgery and chemotherapy for HER-2/neu breast cancer and targets with HER-2 protein.
9. Total mastectomy and breast-conserving surgery plus radiation are considered equal in efficacy. In either case, do an axillary sentinel node biopsy or full dissection to determine spread to the nodes. If nodes are positive, chemotherapy (hormone therapy, traditional chemotherapy, or both) is given.

PROSTATE CANCER

Risk factors:
○ **Age** (rare in men younger than 40 years; the incidence increases with age; 60% of men older than 80 years have prostate cancer)
○ **Race:** Black > white > Asian

Patients often present late (in the absence of screening) because early prostate cancer is asymptomatic. Look for symptoms suggestive of benign prostatic hyperplasia (hesitancy, dysuria, frequency) with hematuria or elevated prostate-specific antigen (PSA), a test used for screening and monitoring of disease. Look for prostate irregularities (e.g., nodules) on rectal examination. Patients might present with back pain from vertebral metastases (osteoblastic).

Local prostate cancer is treated with surgery (prostatectomy) or radiation. Patients with metastases have several options for hormonal therapy, including orchiectomy, gonadotropin-releasing hormone agonist (leuprolide), androgen-receptor antagonist (flutamide), estrogen (diethylstilbestrol), and others (e.g., cyproterone). Chemotherapy does not work, and radiation therapy is used for local disease or pain from bony metastases.

COLORECTAL CANCER

Risk factors:
- **Age:** Incidence begins to increase after age 40 years; peak incidence is between 60 and 75 years
- **Family history:** Especially with familial polyposis or Gardner, Turcot, Peutz-Jegher, or Lynch syndrome
- **Inflammatory bowel disease:** Risk from ulcerative colitis is greater than risk from Crohn disease, but both increase risk
- **Low-fiber, high-fat diet** (weak evidence)

IMPORTANT POINTS

1. Patients might present with asymptomatic blood in the stool (visible streaks of blood in the stool or guaiac-positive stool), anemia with right-sided colon cancer, or a change in stool caliber (pencil stool) or frequency (alternating constipation and frequency) with left-sided colon cancer. As with any cancer, look for weight loss.
2. Occult blood in the stool of a patient older than 40 years should be considered colon cancer until proved otherwise. To rule out colon cancer, either do flexible sigmoidoscopy and a barium enema or do a total colonoscopy. If you see any lesions with a flexible sigmoidoscope or barium enema (Fig. 21-6), you need to do a total colonoscopy with removal and histologic examination of all polyps and lesions. For this reason, most physicians now start with colonoscopy.
3. Carcinoembryonic antigen (CEA) is often elevated with colon cancer, and a preoperative level is usually measured. After surgery to remove the tumor, CEA should return to normal levels. Periodic monitoring of CEA postoperatively helps to detect recurrence before it is clinically apparent. CEA is not used as a screening tool for colon cancer because it is neither sensitive nor specific; it is used only to follow known cancer.
4. Treatment is primarily surgical, with resection of involved bowel. Adjuvant chemotherapy is sometimes given (e.g., 5-fluorouracil with leucovorin, irinotecan, oxiliplatin, cetuximab and panitumumab, or bevacizumab) for lymph node involvement.
5. Colon cancer often metastasizes to the liver; if the metastasis is solitary, surgical resection may be attempted. With metastases elsewhere, chemotherapy is the only option, and prognosis is poor.
6. Colon cancer is a common cause of a large bowel obstruction in an adult.

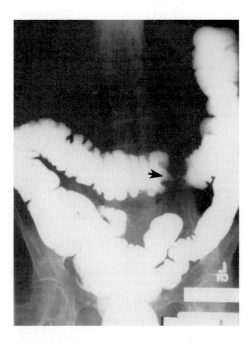

FIGURE 21-6 An apple-core lesion on barium enema (*arrow*).

PANCREATIC CANCER

The classic presentation for adenocarcinoma (most common type and reflects 85%–90% of cases; cell of origin is ductal epithelium) is a smoker between the ages of 40 and 80 years who has lost weight and is jaundiced. Other signs and symptoms include epigastric pain; migratory thrombophlebitis (**Trousseau syndrome,** which can also be seen with other visceral cancer); or a palpable, nontender gallbladder (**Courvoisier sign**). Pancreatic cancer is more common in men than in women, in diabetics than in nondiabetics, and in blacks than in whites. Surgery is rarely curative (Whipple procedure), and the prognosis is dismal (5% 5-year survival). Islet cell tumors (only 5%–10% of pancreatic cancer cases but classic on boards; often have a good prognosis):

○ **Insulinoma (beta cell tumor):** Most common islet cell tumor. Look for two-thirds of the Whipple triad: hypoglycemia (glucose <50 mg/dL) and central nervous system symptoms caused by hypoglycemia (confusion, stupor, loss of consciousness). As the good doctor, you will provide the third part of the Whipple triad: give glucose to relieve symptoms. Ninety percent of insulinomas are benign and can be cured with resection. In your workup, take a history and check the C-peptide level first to make sure that the patient is not a diabetic who accidentally took too much insulin or a patient with factitious disorder. C-peptide is high with insulinoma and low with other conditions.

○ **Gastrinoma:** Zollinger-Ellison syndrome is gastrinoma plus acid hypersecretion and peptic ulcer disease (gastrin causes acid secretion). Peptic ulcers are often multiple and resistant to therapy; they may be in an unusual location (distal duodenum or jejunum). More than half are malignant. Diagnosis is made with an elevated fasting serum gastrin level or a secretin stimulation test.

○ **Glucagonoma (alpha cell tumor):** Hyperglycemia with high glucagon level and migratory necrotizing skin erythema

○ **VIPoma:** Tumor that secretes vasoactive intestinal peptide (VIP), causing watery diarrhea, hypokalemia, and achlorhydria

On the USMLE Step 2, a patient with an islet cell tumor should prompt you to think of multiple endocrine neoplasia. See the Chapter 9 for more information on multiple endocrine neoplasia.

OVARIAN CANCER

Ovarian cancer usually manifests late, with weight loss, pelvic mass, ascites (Meigs syndrome), or bowel obstruction in a postmenopausal woman. Any ovarian enlargement in a postmenopausal woman is cancer until proved otherwise. In women of reproductive age, most ovarian enlargements are benign. Ultrasonography is a good first test to evaluate an ovarian lesion. Treatment includes debulking surgery and chemotherapy; prognosis is usually poor. Most ovarian cancer arises from ovarian epithelium. Serous cystadenocarcinoma, the most common ovarian cancer, often has psammoma bodies on histopathology.

 Oral contraceptives have been shown to reduce the incidence of ovarian cancer by 50% (also reduce endometrial cancer risk).

Germ cell tumors provide fodder for Step 2 questions:

○ **Teratoma or dermoid cyst:** Look for a description of the tumor to include skin, hair, or teeth or bone; it can show up as pelvic calcifications on radiographs

○ **Sertoli-Leydig cell tumor:** Causes virilization (hirsutism, receding hairline, deepening voice, clitoromegaly)

○ **Granulosa-theca cell tumor:** Causes feminization and precocious puberty.
Terms worth knowing:

○ **Meigs syndrome:** Ovarian fibroma, ascites, and right hydrothorax or pleural effusion

○ **Krukenberg tumor:** Stomach (or other gastrointestinal) cancer with metastases to the ovaries

CERVICAL CANCER

Papanicolaou (Pap) smears decrease the incidence and mortality of cervical cancer. Give female patients a Pap smear if they are due even if they present with an unrelated complaint. Screening should start at 21 years of age. The frequency of screening depends on whether human papillomavirus (HPV) testing is also being used as well as the patient's age and results of previous Pap smears.

The follow-up of an abnormal Pap smear depends on the age of the patient, pregnancy status, and cervical cytologic results. Lower grade lesions may be evaluated with repeat cytology, HPV testing, and colposcopy or endocervical curettage if needed. Higher grade lesions require colposcopy with biopsy or loop electrosurgical excision (LEEP). Invasive cancer requires surgery (at least a hysterectomy) and may include radiation with cisplatin-based chemotherapy.

Risk factors for cervical cancer:

○ Younger than 20 years old at first coitus, pregnancy, or marriage
○ Multiple sexual partners (role of HPV and possibly herpes) or coitus with a promiscuous person
○ Smoking
○ Low socioeconomic status
○ High parity (which protects against endometrial cancer)

IMPORTANT POINTS

1. Invasive cervical cancer begins in the transformation zone and usually manifests with vaginal bleeding or discharge (may be postcoital, intermenstrual spotting, or abnormal menstrual bleeding).
2. Maternal exposure to diethylstilbestrol increases the daughter's risk of developing clear cell cancer of the cervix or vagina.

UTERINE CANCER

Postmenopausal bleeding is cancer until proved otherwise; endometrial cancer is the most common cancer to manifest in this fashion (fourth most common cancer in women). Get an endometrial biopsy (generally preferred) for any patient with postmenopausal bleeding. Any woman with unexplained gynecologic bleeding that persists needs a Pap smear, endocervical curettage, and endometrial biopsy. Risk factors for endometrial cancer:

○ Chronic, unopposed estrogen stimulation, as in polycystic ovary syndrome, estrogen-secreting neoplasm (granulosa-theca cell tumor), and estrogen replacement (increases risk of cancer only if taken without progesterone)
○ Diabetes mellitus
○ Gallbladder disease
○ Hypertension
○ Late menopause
○ Nulliparity
○ Obesity

IMPORTANT POINTS

1. Oral contraceptives have been shown to reduce the incidence of endometrial as well as ovarian cancer.
2. Most uterine cancer is adenocarcinoma and spreads by direct extension.
3. Treat with surgery, radiation, or both.

MISCELLANEOUS NEOPLASMS

Adrenal Tumors

Adrenal tumors may be functional and cause primary hyperaldosteronism (Conn syndrome) or hyperadrenalism (Cushing disease). Patients also might have a pheochromocytoma; look for intermittent, severe hypertension with mental status changes, headaches, and diaphoresis. Check plasma metanephrines or 24-hour urine catecholamines (vanillylmandelic acid, homovanillic acid, or metanephrines). Most adrenal tumors are benign nonfunctional adenomas and can be diagnosed by CT or MRI. Percutaneous needle biopsy can be used in uncertain cases. Never use only a β-blocker to control blood pressure in a patient with suspected pheochromocytoma because this may cause a paradoxical increase in blood pressure because of unopposed α activity.

Bladder Cancer

Look for persistent, painless hematuria, especially in patients older than 40 years of age. Patients often are smokers or work in the rubber or dye industry (aniline dye exposure). Do CT scan with contrast first, but this is better for renal cancer than bladder cancer (both cause hematuria). Cystoscopy is usually done first to evaluate a potential bladder cancer. Local destructive therapy is done for noninvasive tumors, and cystectomy with adjuvant chemoradiotherapy is done for invasive disease.

Brain Tumors

In adults, two-thirds of primary tumors (metastases are more common than primary tumors) are supratentorial (i.e., cerebral hemispheres). In children two-thirds are infratentorial (posterior fossa, i.e., cerebellum and brainstem). In either group, look for new-onset seizures, neurologic deficits, and signs of intracranial hypertension (headache, blurred vision, papilledema, nausea and projectile vomiting). In children, also look for hydrocephalus (inappropriately increasing head circumference), ataxia, new clumsiness, loss of developmental milestones, or a change in school performance or personality.

The most common types of brain tumors in adults are gliomas (most are intraparenchymal astrocytomas with little or no calcification) and meningiomas (usually calcified, external to the brain substance). In children, the most common types are cerebellar astrocytoma and medulloblastoma followed by ependymoma.

Treatment is surgical removal, which may be followed by radiation and chemotherapy, depending on the tumor.

IMPORTANT POINTS

1. A young, obese woman who has headaches, papilledema, and vomiting with a negative CT or MRI result has pseudotumor cerebri, not a malignancy.
2. The most common primary posterior fossa tumors in children are astrocytoma and medulloblastoma; in adults, they are acoustic neuroma (watch for neurofibromatosis) and hemangioblastoma (watch for von Hippel-Lindau syndrome). Metastases are much more likely than primary tumors in adults.
3. Metastases (Fig. 21-7) are much more likely than primary brain tumors in adults. Lung cancer, breast cancer, and melanoma are the most common, together accounting for 75% of brain metastases.
4. Children can develop craniopharyngiomas (remnant of Rathke pouch), a classically calcified tumor in or around the sella turcica.

Carcinoid Tumors

The most common location is the small bowel, but carcinoid is the most common appendiceal tumor (other locations are uncommon). The liver breaks down serotonin and other vasoactive secreted substances to make the tumor initially asymptomatic, but when carcinoid metastasizes to the liver and vasoactive products reach the systemic circulation, symptoms begin (carcinoid syndrome); these include

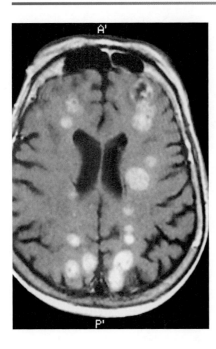

FIGURE 21-7 Axial T1-weighted magnetic resonance image of metastases from breast carcinoma are seen after administration of contrast (gadolinium). Multiple nodular enhancing masses of varying sizes are seen. Some have low signal intensity centers signifying necrosis.

episodic cutaneous flushing, abdominal cramps, diarrhea, and right-sided heart valve damage. Urinary 5-hydroxyindoleacetic acid (5-HIAA) is increased (a product of serotonin breakdown). Lung carcinoids also occur, but the tumor is rarely endocrinologically active.

Esophageal Cancer

Signs and symptoms of esophageal cancer include weight loss, possibly anemia, and complaints that "my food is sticking," which progresses to dysphagia for liquid. Patients present late because early cancer is often asymptomatic. The most common type in the United States is now adenocarcinoma, seen in obese whites and blacks with a long-term history of reflux or heartburn. Barrett esophagus (columnar metaplasia of esophageal squamous epithelium caused by chronic acid reflux) is a precursor to adenocarcinoma and, after it is found, routine endoscopic surveillance for cancer is indicated. Look for chronic smokers and drinkers (blacks more than whites) when the subtype is squamous cell carcinoma.

Histiocytosis

CD1-positive cells and electron microscopy showing Birbeck granules (cytoplasmic inclusion bodies that look like tennis rackets) within histiocytes are the two major cytologic clues for histiocytosis.

Kaposi Sarcoma

Kaposi sarcoma is mostly seen in HIV-positive patients. It is a vascular skin tumor that starts as a purple papule or plaque, commonly on the upper body or in the oral cavity. The classic description is a rash that does not respond to multiple treatments. Kaposi sarcoma is highly associated with human herpesvirus 8 (HHV8) infection.

Liver Tumors

Risk factors for hepatocellular carcinoma include alcohol abuse, chronic hepatitis (B or C), and anything else that causes cirrhosis (hemochromatosis is especially known to cause liver cancer). Alpha fetoprotein is often elevated and can be measured postoperatively to detect recurrences. Patients have a history of alcoholism, chronic hepatitis, hemochromatosis, or other causes of cirrhosis and present with weight loss, right upper quadrant pain, and an enlarged liver. Surgery is the only hope for cure; the prognosis is poor. Treatment options include percutaneous ethanol injection, transcatheter arterial chemoembolization, radiofrequency ablation, and sorafenib (a receptor tyrosine kinase inhibitor). Liver metastases are shown in Figure 21-8. Other tumors of the liver:

○ **Angiosarcoma:** Look for industrial exposure to vinyl chloride. Malignant.
○ **Cholangiosarcoma:** 50% of patients have a history of inflammatory bowel disease, especially ulcerative colitis; liver flukes (*Clonorchis* spp.) might be the cause in immigrants. Malignant.

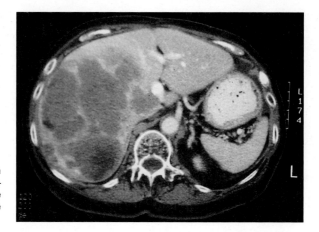

FIGURE 21-8 Large liver metastases from colon carcinoma. Contrast-enhanced computed tomography shows replacement of the right hepatic lobe and a portion of the left hepatic lobe by hypodense lesions.

○ **Hemangioma:** The most common primary tumor of the liver is benign and generally left alone. Definitive diagnosis is usually possible with CT, MRI, or nuclear medicine ("hemangioma scan"). Surgery is done only in the rare case of symptoms (e.g., pain, bleeding) because of the large size. Percutaneous needle biopsy can be done in uncertain cases.

○ **Hepatic adenoma:** A benign tumor in women of reproductive age taking oral contraceptives. Stop the pills! The tumor may then regress; if not, surgical removal is generally advocated (to prevent hemorrhage and rare malignant transformation) after establishing the diagnosis with percutaneous needle biopsy.

○ **Hepatoblastoma:** The main primary liver tumor in children. Malignant.

Nasopharyngeal Cancer
Nasopharyngeal cancer is typically seen in Asians; remember the association with Epstein-Barr virus.

Oral Cancer
Similar to other head and neck malignancies, oral cancer is usually the squamous cell type and is caused by smoking, chewing tobacco, or drinking alcohol; also look for poor oral hygiene. Oral cancer often starts as leukoplakia (know the appearance), which must be differentiated from oral hairy leukoplakia, a condition associated with Epstein-Barr virus that affects HIV-positive patients.

Osteosarcoma
Osteosarcoma most commonly is seen around the knee in 10- to 30-year-old individuals. The classic radiographic finding is a "sunburst" or Codman triangle appearance of periosteal reaction (Fig. 21-9) in the distal femur or proximal tibia associated with a mass.

Pituitary Tumors
The classic physical finding is bitemporal hemianopsia. Order an MRI of the brain in any patient with this finding. Patients also may have signs and symptoms of increased intracranial pressure. The most common type is a prolactinoma, which is associated with high prolactin levels, galactorrhea, and menstrual or sexual dysfunction. Other types of pituitary tumors may cause hyperthyroidism, Cushing disease, or acromegaly, or they may be nonfunctional (i.e., they do not secrete hormones).

Retinoblastoma
See Pediatrics chapter (Chapter 24).

Sarcoma Botryoides
See Pediatrics chapter (Chapter 24).

Skin Cancer
Ultraviolet light increases the risk of basal, squamous, and melanoma (Fig. 21-10) skin cancer. The **ABCDs** of melanoma should make you suspicious of malignancy. Biopsy any lesion with any of these characteristics: **a**symmetry, **b**orders (irregular), **c**olor (change in color or multiple colors), or **d**iameter. The bigger the lesion (especially a diameter >6 mm), the more likely that it is malignant. Melanoma commonly metastasizes.

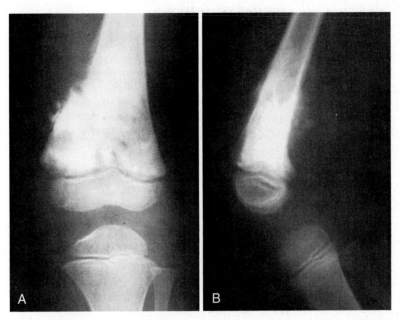

FIGURE 21-9 An aggressive osteosarcoma in the distal metaphysis of the femur. **A,** Anteroposterior radiograph showing bone destruction and extension into the adjacent soft tissues. **B,** Lateral radiograph showing the classic Codman triangle–type periosteal reaction proximal to the lesion. *(From Burke DL, Collins AJ: Musculoskeletal imaging. In Provenzale JM, Nelson RC (eds):* Duke Radiology Case Review. *Philadelphia, Lippincott, 1998, pp. 229–287; with permission.)*

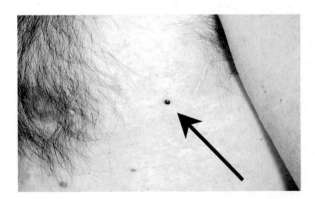

FIGURE 21-10 Skin melanoma *(arrow)* of the trunk.

Basal cell cancer is classically described as a pearly, umbilicated nodule with telangiectasias. Basal cell cancer is extremely common and almost never metastasizes.

Squamous cell cancer sometimes metastasizes and often has a red, scaly, inflamed appearance or presents as an area of skin ulceration. Biopsy is appropriate for all suspicious lesions.

Stomach Cancer

Risk factors for stomach cancer are Japanese race, increasing age, smoking, and consumption of smoked meat. *Helicobacter pylori* infection also is implicated. Symptoms and signs include anemia, weight loss, early satiety, abdominal pain, and a nonhealing gastric ulcer. All gastric ulcers must be biopsied to exclude malignancy. Consider follow-up endoscopy to document resolution of an ulcer. Krukenberg tumor is stomach cancer with bilateral ovarian metastases. Virchow node is left supraclavicular node enlargement caused by visceral cancer spread (classically stomach cancer).

Testicular Cancer

The most common solid malignancy in men younger than 30 years. The main risk factor is cryptorchidism. Transillumination and ultrasonography help to distinguish hydrocele (fluid-filled, transilluminates) from cancer (solid). Use ultrasonography to make the diagnosis. The most common type is seminoma, which is radiosensitive. Lymphatic drainage follows testicular veins to the retroperitoneal lymph nodes in the region of the abdominal aorta and inferior vena cava at the level of the renal veins.

Thyroid Cancer

In thyroid cancer, the patient presents with a nodule in the thyroid gland. Be suspicious of cancer in any of the following scenarios: cold nodule on nuclear scan, male patient, history of childhood irradiation, nodule described as "stony hard," recent or rapid enlargement, and increased calcitonin level (medullary thyroid cancer, usually in patients with multiple endocrine neoplasia type II). Hoarseness indicates recurrent laryngeal nerve involvement. To evaluate a nodule in the thyroid, get thyroid function tests and an ultrasound scan. Thyroid-stimulating hormone is the best screening test; "toxic" or functional nodules are unlikely to be cancer. On a nuclear scan, a cold nodule or area of decreased uptake is more suspicious than normal or increased uptake. Perform fine-needle aspiration for diagnosis.

Unicameral Bone Cyst

See Pediatrics chapter (Chapter 24).

Wilms Tumor and Neuroblastoma

See Pediatrics chapter (Chapter 24).

Note   *Patients with cancer, like all others, have the right to refuse treatment. However, watch for and treat depression, especially in terminal patients, before accepting a patient's refusal of treatment.*

QR CODE

The QR code includes three USMLE-style questions and answers. For more questions, redeem the PIN code on the inside cover for the Crush Step 2 question bank powered by USMLE Consult.

Please see the Introduction for instructions on how to access content using the QR codes.

Question

Which of the following tumors is matched properly with its most commonly used tumor marker?
(A) Liver cancer—CA 19-9
(B) Ovarian cancer—carcinoembryonic antigen (CEA)
(C) Choriocarcinoma—human chorionic gonadotropin (hCG)
(D) Pancreatic cancer—acid phosphatase
(E) Breast cancer—S-100

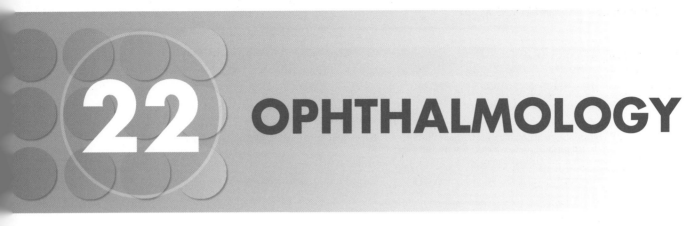

22 OPHTHALMOLOGY

CONJUNCTIVITIS

Conjunctivitis causes conjunctival vessel hyperemia. The three main causes are allergic (common), viral (common), and bacterial (rare) (Table 22-1). Conjunctivitis involves no loss of vision (other than transient blurriness caused by tear film debris that resolves with blinking). If loss of vision is present, think of other, more serious conditions. Neonatal conjunctivitis is usually attributable to one of three causes:

○ **Chemical:** Silver nitrate (or erythromycin) drops are given prophylactically to all newborns to prevent gonorrheal conjunctivitis. The drops can cause a chemical conjunctivitis (with no purulent discharge) that develops within 12 hours of instilling the drops and resolves within 48 hours (pick this answer if conjunctivitis occurs in the first 24 hours of life).

○ **Gonorrheal:** Look for symptoms of gonorrhea in the mother. The infant has an extremely purulent discharge at 2 to 5 days of age. Treatment is topical (e.g., erythromycin ointment) plus intravenous (IV) or intramuscular third-generation cephalosporin (e.g., ceftriaxone). Infants who are given prophylactic drops should not get gonorrheal conjunctivitis.

○ **Chlamydial** (inclusion conjunctivitis): The mother often reports no symptoms. The infant has mild to severe conjunctivitis beginning at 5 to 14 days of age. Patients must be treated with systemic antibiotics (oral erythromycin usually is used) to prevent chlamydial pneumonia (a common complication). Prophylactic eye drops do not effectively prevent chlamydial conjunctivitis.

For bacterial conjunctivitis in adults, treatment is with topical antibiotics (given as drops). Options include polymyxin B/trimethoprim or fluoroquinolones.

IMPORTANT POINT

○ If you forget everything else about neonatal conjunctivitis, remember the days after birth when the three causes occur.

GLAUCOMA

Glaucoma is best thought of as ocular hypertension with its resultant effects. The main risk factors are age older than 40 years, black race, and family history. Glaucoma is the number one cause of blindness in blacks of any age and the number three overall cause of blindness in the United States. There are two types: open-angle glaucoma and closed-angle glaucoma.

○ **Open-angle glaucoma:** Although it is traditional to talk about painful attacks, they are rare. Open-angle glaucoma causes 90% of cases of glaucoma, is painless, and does not involve acute attacks. The only signs are elevated intraocular pressure (IOP; usually 20–30 mm Hg) and optic nerve changes (increased cup-to-disc ratio on funduscopic examination). Symptoms may include a loss of peripheral vision, decreased night vision, or reduced clarity of colors. Treat with several different types of medications (β-blockers, prostaglandin α-adrenergic agonists [latanoprost] carbonic anhydrase inhibitors, cholinergic agonists) or laser therapy or surgery if medications fail.

TABLE 22-1 Conjunctivitis

ETIOLOGY	UNIQUE SIGNS AND SYMPTOMS	TREATMENT
Allergic	Itching, bilateral, seasonal, long duration	Vasoconstrictors or topical antihistamines or mast cell stabilizers
Viral*	Preauricular adenopathy, highly contagious (history of infected personal contacts); clear, watery discharge; often with recent URI symptoms	Supportive, hand washing (prevents spread)
Bacterial	Acute onset, purulent discharge; more common in neonates	Topical antibiotics ± systemic antibiotics

URI, upper respiratory infection.
*Number one cause is adenovirus (diarrhea may be present).

○ **Closed-angle glaucoma:** Closed-angle glaucoma manifests with sudden ocular pain; seeing haloes around lights; red eye; high IOP (>30 mm Hg); nausea and vomiting; sudden decreased vision; a hazy-appearing cornea; and a fixed, mid-dilated pupil. The globe may also feel firm to palpation. This is a medical emergency. Treat immediately with pilocarpine drops, topical β-blockers, mannitol, and acetazolamide to break the attack. Then obtain an emergency ophthalmologic consultation because ophthalmologists can use surgery to prevent further attacks (peripheral iridectomy).

In rare cases, anticholinergic medications or sympathomimetic medication (medications that can dilate the pupil) can cause an attack of closed-angle glaucoma in a susceptible, previously untreated patient. Medications do not cause glaucoma attacks in open-angle glaucoma or patients previously treated surgically for closed-angle glaucoma.

Corticosteroids, whether applied directly to the eye (i.e., topical) or systemic, can cause glaucoma and cataracts. Topical steroids can worsen ocular herpes and fungal infections. For board purposes, do not give topical ocular steroids, especially if the patient has a dendritic corneal ulcer stained green by fluorescein. Such an ulcer represents herpes.

 *The retinal and fundus changes seen in **diabetes** (dot-blot hemorrhages, microaneurysms, neovascularization; Fig. 22-1) and **hypertension** (arteriolar narrowing, copper or silver wiring, cotton wool spots, papilledema with severe hypertension) are fair game on Step 2. Make the diagnosis from the appearance of the fundus.*

LOSS OF VISION

Sudden Unilateral, Painless Vision Loss
A fairly short differential:
○ **Central retinal artery occlusion:** Presents with sudden (within a few minutes), painless, unilateral loss of vision. Funduscopic appearance is classic (a pale fundus with a cherry red spot in the center of the macula). The most common cause is emboli from carotid plaque or the

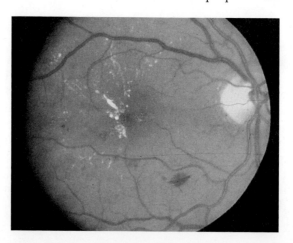

FIGURE 22-1 Background diabetic retinopathy with exudate, hemorrhages, and edema (dot and blot). (From Vander JF, Gault JA: Ophthalmology Secrets. Philadelphia, Hanley & Belfus, 1998.)

heart. Treatment consists of lowering the IOP (see acute closed-angle glaucoma above), digital massage of the globe in an attempt to dislodge the obstruction, and an emergency ophthalmologic consultation. High-dose steroids are used if the occlusion is suspected to be from temporal arteritis (discussed later).

○ **Central retinal vein occlusion:** Presents with sudden (within a few hours), painless, unilateral loss of vision. Funduscopic appearance is also classic (distended, tortuous retinal veins; retinal hemorrhages; and a congested, edematous fundus). No satisfactory treatment is available, although there occasionally may be spontaneous resolution. When seeing a patient like this, get an ophthalmology consultation. The most common causes are hypertension, diabetes, glaucoma, and increased blood viscosity (e.g., leukemia). Complications are related to neovascularization, which leads to vision loss and glaucoma.

○ **Retinal detachment:** The history usually includes a sudden (instant), painless, unilateral loss of vision with floaters and seeing flashes of light. Often described as a "curtain [or veil] coming down in front of my eye". This history should prompt immediate referral to an ophthalmologist because surgery to reattach the retina can save the patient's sight.

○ **Stroke or transient ischemic attack** (amaurosis fugax): See the discussion of visual pathways.

○ **Vitreous hemorrhage:** Patients complain of seeing dark spots ("floaters") and blurred vision. There may also be a loss of the red reflex, and it becomes very difficult to see the fundus. Usually caused by bleeding from areas of neovascularization, classically in patients with diabetes. Patients should be instructed to avoid exertion and should be on bedrest with the head of the bed elevated to prevent further hemorrhage. It sometimes resolves or can improve after surgical vitrectomy.

Sudden, Unilateral, Painful Vision Loss

Causes include:

○ **Closed-angle glaucoma:** See the discussion earlier for presenting signs and symptoms and treatment.

○ **Migraine headache:** Rare but can occur. Look for nausea and vomiting and aura.

○ **Optic neuritis or papillitis:** Usually takes at least a few hours (and more commonly a few days) to develop and is classically described as being painful, but it can occur quickly and be painless. Usually unilateral but is sometimes bilateral. If present in a 20- to 40-year-old woman, think multiple sclerosis. Worry about tumor if the patient is male, has signs of intracranial hypertension, or has other neurologic deficits. Lyme disease and syphilis are rare causes. Patients may complain of decreased perception of light and color, decreased depth perception, and painful eye movement. Disc margins might appear blurred on funduscopic exam, just as in papilledema (although intracranial pressure [ICP] is generally normal with papillitis). Treatment is IV steroids.

○ **Trauma:** History gives it away, and in almost all cases, an emergency ophthalmologic consultation is needed. Encourage use of goggles or safety glasses during athletics and work. With chemical burns to the eye (acid or alkali), the key to management is copious irrigation with closest source of water (tap water is fine). The longer you wait, the worse the prognosis (don't get additional history in this instance). Alkali burns have a worse prognosis because they tend to penetrate deeper into the eye. Patients also can suffer a ruptured globe from either blunt or penetrating trauma to the eye. If you find that the patient has ruptured the globe, defer the examination until the time of surgery because your examination may make things worse. While awaiting surgery, cover the eye with a shield.

Sudden Bilateral Vision Loss

This is rare. Consider:

○ **Conversion reaction or hysteria**

○ **Exposure to ultraviolet light:** Can cause keratitis (corneal inflammation) with resultant pain, foreign body sensation, red eyes, tearing, and decreased vision (usually some vision remains). The patient has a history of welding, using a tanning bed or sunlamp, or snow skiing (snow blindness). Treat with an eye patch (24 hours) and topical antibiotic, possibly also with an anticholinergic (cycloplegic agent, reduces pain).

○ **Toxins:** Classic is methanol poisoning, usually seen in people with alcoholism

Gradual-Onset Vision Loss, Unilateral or Bilateral

Longer differential but more common than sudden-onset vision loss:

○ **Cataracts:** The most common cause of a painless, slowly progressive loss of vision. Often bilateral, but one side may be worse than the other. Look for absent red reflex. Patient complains of "looking through a dirty windshield." Treatment is surgical. Surgery can be delayed until the patient's daily activities are affected. Cataracts in a neonate should make you think of TORCH infections (toxoplasmosis, other agents, rubella, cytomegalovirus, herpes simplex virus) or an inherited metabolic disorder (e.g., galactosemia).

○ **Diabetes:** Most common cause of blindness in adults younger than 50 years. Retinal and fundal changes in diabetes include dot-blot hemorrhages, microaneurysms, and neovascularization. The treatment for proliferative diabetic retinopathy (neovascularization present) is laser applied to the periphery of the whole retina (panretinal photocoagulation). Surgical or medical vitrectomy is used in some cases. Medical therapy for proliferative diabetic retinopathy is investigational but is used in some circumstances. The most promising are the vascular endothelial growth factor (VEGF) inhibitors (bevacizumab, ranibizumab, pegaptanib). Focal laser treatment is common for nonproliferative (background) retinopathy when macular edema is present; the laser is applied only to the affected area. In severe cases, panretinal photocoagulation may be used. Otherwise, nonproliferative retinopathy is treated supportively, primarily with tight control of blood glucose and follow-up eye examinations to watch for development of macular edema or neovascularization.

○ **Direct insult to the brain:** Tumor, trauma, or meningitis. See later section for visual pathway information.

○ **Eye infection:** Cornea (herpes keratitis, corneal ulcer [Fig. 22-2]), retina (cytomegalovirus retinitis in AIDS), orbital cellulitis (see later)

○ **Open angle glaucoma:** See earlier for specifics. Screen patients older than 40 years, especially if they are black or have diabetes or a positive family history. This is the most common cause of blindness in blacks.

○ **Macular degeneration:** Most common cause of blindness in adults older than 55 years. Often bilateral, but one side may be worse than the other. Patients experience progressive loss of central vision. The appearance of the fundus (macular drusen; Fig. 22-3) makes the diagnosis. There is no good treatment for the most common (90% of cases) dry type (high doses of vitamins A, C, and E and mineral zinc can slow progression). The wet type can be treated with VEGF inhibitors (e.g., pegaptanib) and laser therapy with or without verteporfin (a photosensitizing dye).

○ **Optic neuritis:** Classically from autoimmune-type conditions, infections (Lyme disease), or drugs (ethambutol)

○ **Papilledema:** Classically from hypertension or other cause of increased ICP (brain tumor, pseudotumor cerebri) (Fig. 22-4).

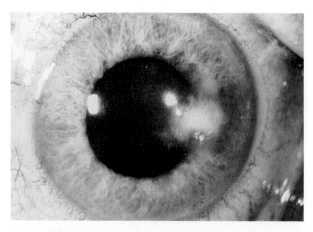

FIGURE 22-2 Infectious corneal ulcer caused by a filamentous fungus. Note the indistinct, feathery borders.

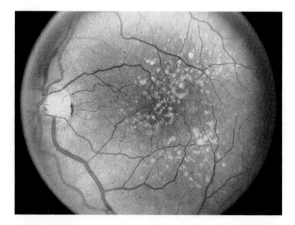

FIGURE 22-3 Drusen are the by-products of retinal metabolism and manifest as focal yellow-white deposits deep to the retinal pigment epithelium. They serve as a marker of non-exudative age-related macular degeneration. *(From Vander JF, Gault JA: Ophthalmology Secrets. Philadelphia, Hanley & Belfus, 1998.)*

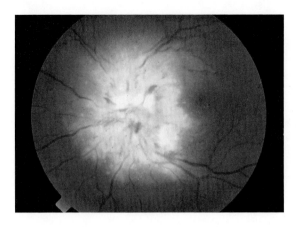

FIGURE 22-4 Papilledema, caused by cryptococcal meningitis in this case, is characterized by optic disc swelling and blurring of the disc margins.

○ **Presbyopia:** Between ages 40 and 50 years, the lens loses its ability to accommodate, and people need bifocals or reading glasses for near vision. This is a normal part of aging and not a disease.

○ **Uveitis:** Look for association with autoimmune-type diseases. Screen children with juvenile rheumatoid arthritis regularly to detect uveitis (a classic rheumatoid arthritis presentation in kids is uveitis with or without joint symptoms). Usually treated with corticosteroids (by an ophthalmologist).

*Be able to differentiate **orbital cellulitis** from **preorbital cellulitis** (preseptal cellulitis). Both can involve swollen eyelids; fever; chemosis; and a history of facial laceration, trauma, insect bite, or sinusitis. Ophthalmoplegia, proptosis, severe eye pain, or decreased visual acuity indicates orbital cellulitis (a **medical emergency**). The most common bugs in both are Streptococcus pneumoniae, Haemophilus influenzae type b, and staphylococci or streptococci with a history of trauma. Orbital cellulitis can extend into the skull with resulting meningitis, vein thromboses, and blindness. Treat either condition with blood cultures and administration of broad-spectrum antibiotics to cover the likely bugs until culture results are known. Computed tomography (CT) scan can help determine the extent of the infection (i.e., preorbital vs. orbital) and exclude complications such as an abscess. Inpatient IV antibiotics are needed for orbital cellulitis.*

OTHER OPHTHALMOLOGIC CONDITIONS AND COMPLICATIONS

Hordeolum (stye) is a painful red lump along the eyelid margin that is the result of acute glandular obstruction resulting in inflammation. These can become secondarily infected, most commonly with *Staphylococcus aureus*. Treat with warm compresses, and in severe cases, incision and drainage. You also can use topical antibiotic ointment to prevent secondary infection. Chalazion is a painless lump along the eyelid margin that is from chronic granulomatous inflammation. Treat with warm compresses. Refractory cases can be managed with intralesional steroid injection or incision and drainage.

Herpes simplex keratitis (Fig. 22-5) usually starts with conjunctivitis and a vesicular eyelid eruption and then progresses to the classic dendritic keratitis (seen with fluorescein). Treat with topical antivirals (e.g., idoxuridine, trifluridine). Corticosteroids are contraindicated with dendritic keratitis because they can make the condition worse.

Ophthalmic herpes zoster should be suspected with involvement of the tip of the nose or medial eyelid in a typical zoster dermatomal pattern (Fig. 22-6). Treat with oral famciclovir, valacyclovir, or acyclovir. Complications include uveitis, keratitis, and glaucoma.

When you have a patient with central retinal artery occlusion, look for coexisting symptoms of temporal arteritis, including an elderly patient with jaw claudication, tortuous temporal artery (as seen or palpated on examination), markedly elevated erythrocyte sedimentation rate, and coexisting polymyalgia rheumatica (in 50%; causes proximal muscle pain and stiffness). If temporal arteritis is

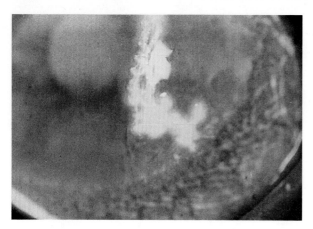

FIGURE 22-5 Classic herpes simplex dendrite staining brightly with fluorescein.

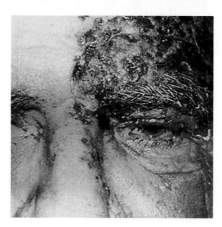

FIGURE 22-6 Characteristic appearance and location of herpes zoster skin lesions with involvement of the V1 distribution of the trigeminal nerve.

suspected in the setting of vision complaints, administer corticosteroids immediately before confirming the diagnosis with a temporal artery biopsy. Withholding treatment until a formal diagnosis can be made may cause the patient to lose vision in the other eye.

Children with a lazy eye or strabismus (deviation of the eye, usually inward) that persists beyond 3 months need ophthalmologic referral. The condition generally does not resolve on its own at this point and can cause blindness (amblyopia) in the affected eye. For this reason, visual screening must be done in pediatric patients; the visual system is still developing after birth until the age of 7 or 8 years. If one eye does not see well or is turned outward, the brain cannot fuse the two different images that it sees and suppresses the bad eye, which will not develop the proper neural connections. Thus, the eye will never see well, and vision cannot be corrected with glasses (it is a neural rather than a refractive problem).

OPHTHALMOLOGIC CRANIAL NERVE PALSIES

Ophthalmologic cranial nerve (CN) palsies are most commonly caused by vascular complications of diabetes and hypertension. Most cases resolve on their own within 2 months. CN palsies can also be the result of increased ICP from trauma or a mass, so in patients younger than 40 years, patients who have sustained head trauma, patients with other neurologic deficits or severe pain, and any patient who does not improve within 8 weeks, you will need to get imaging studies of the brain (magnetic resonance imaging [MRI] with contrast) to rule out serious intracranial pathology.

○ **Oculomotor (CN III):** The eye is down and out and can move only laterally. In cases caused by hypertension or diabetes mellitus, the pupil is normal. Close observation is all that is needed; the condition resolves on its own in several weeks. A pupil that is "blown" (dilated, nonreactive) is a medical emergency resulting from increased ICP from masses, aneurysms, or bleeding. Get imaging immediately (noncontrast CT in the case of trauma or if you suspect bleeding; otherwise, MRI).

○ **Trochlear (CN IV):** When the gaze is medial, the patient cannot look down, leading to vertical diplopia. Patients may tilt the head forward to compensate for this.

○ **Abducens (CN VI):** The patient cannot look laterally with the affected eye, leading to horizontal diplopia. This is the most common isolated nerve palsy.

○ **CN V and VII:** These also affect the eye because of corneal drying (loss of corneal blink reflex).

VISUAL PATHWAYS

The visual pathways (Fig. 22-7) make for classic board questions, just as on Step 1. The most commonly tested example is bitemporal hemianopsia, which usually is caused by a pituitary tumor. The visual field defects are listed in Table 22-2.

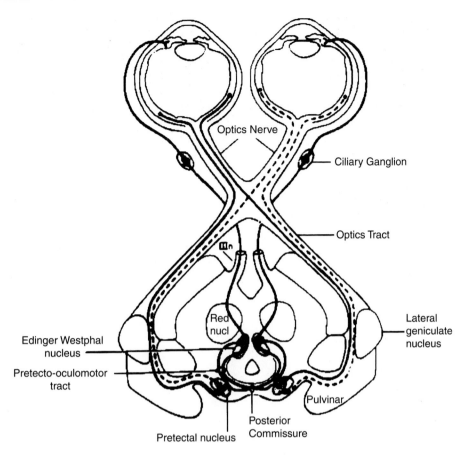

FIGURE 22-7 Light reflex pathway.

TABLE 22-2 Localization of Visual Field Defects

VISUAL FIELD DEFECT	LOCATION OF LESION
Right anopsia (monocular blindness)	Right optic nerve
Bitemporal hemianopsia	Optic chiasm (classically caused by a pituitary tumor)
Left homonymous hemianopsia	Right optic tract
Left upper quadrant anopsia	Right optic radiations in the right temporal lobe
Left lower quadrant anopsia	Right optic radiations in the right parietal lobe
Left homonymous hemianopsia with macular sparing	Right occipital lobe (from posterior cerebral artery occlusion)

QR CODE

The QR code includes three USMLE-style questions and answers. For more questions, redeem the PIN code on the inside cover for the Crush Step 2 question bank powered by USMLE Consult.

Please see the Introduction for instructions on how to access content using the QR codes.

Question

A 72-year-old woman complains of loss of vision in the right eye that happened suddenly this morning while she was eating breakfast. The woman relates a history of pain and stiffness in her shoulders as well as jaw muscle pain and fatigue after chewing for the past 2 weeks. Vital signs are remarkable only for a temperature of 100.9°F. There are no skin rashes. The right pupil does not respond well to light, although there is an intact consensual response in the right pupil. Funduscopic examination reveals a pale fundus and optic disk on the right with a small red spot in the area of the fovea. The patient has scalp tenderness to palpation, more on the right than the left side. Musculoskeletal examination shows intact strength but some tenderness in the shoulder muscles with movement against resistance. Laboratory tests reveal the following:

White blood cell count	4500/μL
Sedimentation rate	100 mm/h (reference range, 1–20)
AST	15 U/L
Creatinine	0.8 mg/dL
Potassium	4.2 mEq/L

What is the best thing to do next?
(A) Administer corticosteroids.
(B) Check an antinuclear antibody (ANA) titer.
(C) Refer the patient for a temporal artery biopsy.
(D) Refer the patient for a muscle biopsy.
(E) Order blood and urine cultures.

23 ORTHOPEDIC SURGERY

FRACTURE AND DISLOCATION

Fractures

Pelvic fracture is the fracture with the highest mortality rate. Patients can bleed to death. If the patient is unstable, consider heroic measures such as military antishock trousers and an external fixator.

For any fracture, always do a neurologic and vascular examination (Table 23-1) distal to the fracture site to see if there is neurologic or vascular compromise. Either may be an emergency. Also, get two radiographic views (usually anteroposterior and lateral) of the site and consider radiographs of the joint above and below the fracture site.

In an open fracture (compound fracture), the skin is broken (lacerated) over the fracture site. Give antibiotics with coverage for gram-positive and gram-negative organisms (cefuroxime is appropriate; fluoroquinolones are an alternative). If the patient is at risk for methicillin-resistant Staphylococcus aureus (MRSA) infection, add vancomycin. Debride surgically, give tetanus vaccine, lavage fresh wounds (<8 hours old), and do an open reduction and internal fixation. The main complication in open fractures is infection.

In a closed fracture, the skin is intact over the fracture site. Reasons to do open reduction include:
○ Intraarticular fractures or articular surface malalignment
○ Open (compound) fractures
○ Nonunion or failed closed reduction
○ Compromise of blood supply
○ Multiple trauma (to allow mobilization at earliest possible point)
○ Extremity function requiring perfect reduction (e.g., professional athlete)
○ Closed reduction can be done for most other fractures.

Anterior shoulder dislocations are more common than posterior dislocations and usually result from trauma. Patients present with the shoulder held high in slight abduction and external rotation. This type of dislocation is associated with axillary nerve damage. Posterior dislocations are much less common, but the classic history is a patient who has had a seizure and presents with the shoulder held in slight adduction and internal rotation. Posterior dislocations usually are not associated with neurologic deficits.

Compartment syndrome

Compartment syndrome usually occurs after a fracture, crush injury, burn, or other trauma, or it can occur as a reperfusion injury (e.g., after revascularization procedure). The most common site is the anterior distal lower extremity. Symptoms and signs include pain on passive movement (out of proportion to the injury), paresthesias, cyanosis or pallor, a firm-feeling muscle compartment, hypesthesia or numbness (decreased sensation and two-point discrimination), paralysis (late, ominous sign), and elevated compartment pressure (>30–40 mm Hg). The diagnosis usually is made clinically without a need to measure pressure. Compartment syndrome is an emergency, and quick action can save an otherwise doomed limb. Pulses are usually palpable or detectable with Doppler ultrasonography. Lack of pulses is an ominous, late sign.

Treatment is an immediate fasciotomy; incising the fascial compartment relieves the pressure. Untreated, the condition progresses to permanent nerve damage and muscle necrosis.

TABLE 23-1 Peripheral Nerve Examination

NERVE	MOTOR	SENSORY	WHEN CLINICALLY DAMAGED
Radial	Wrist extension	Back of forearm, back of hand (first three fingers)	Humeral fracture (wrist drop)
Ulnar	Finger abduction	Front and back of last two fingers	Elbow dislocation (claw hand)
Median	Pronation, thumb opposition	Palmar surface (first three digits)	Carpal tunnel syndrome, humeral fracture
Axillary	Abduction, lateral rotation	Lateral shoulder	Upper humeral dislocation or fracture
Peroneal	Dorsiflexion/eversion	Dorsal foot and lateral leg	Knee dislocation (foot drop)

The classic clinical scenarios associated with compartment syndrome are supracondylar elbow fractures in children, proximal or midshaft tibial fractures, electrical burns, arterial or venous disruption, and revascularization procedures.

KNEE LIGAMENT INJURIES

Ligament injuries in the knee commonly cause pain, joint effusions, instability of the joint, and patient history of the joint "popping," "buckling," or "locking up."

- **Anterior cruciate ligament (ACL):** Most common. Perform the anterior drawer test. Place the knee in 90 degrees of flexion and pull it forward (like opening a drawer). If the tibia pulls forward more than normal, the test result is positive, and the patient has an ACL tear.
- **Posterior cruciate ligament (PCL):** Perform the posterior drawer test. Push the tibia back with the knee in 90 degrees of flexion. If the tibia pushes back more than normal, the test result is positive, and the PCL is torn.
- **Medial collateral ligament (MCL):** Perform an abduction or valgus stress test. With the knee in 30 degrees of flexion, abduct the ankle while holding the knee. If the knee joint abducts to an abnormal degree, the test result is positive, and the MCL is injured.
- **Lateral collateral ligament (LCL):** Perform an adduction or varus stress test. Adduct the ankle while holding the knee. If the knee joint adducts to an abnormal degree, the test result is positive, and LCL injury is present.

Magnetic resonance imaging (MRI) is routinely performed to evaluate and confirm suspected clinical injuries. Arthroscopy is used for injury repair or when MRI results are clinically suspected to be falsely negative.

Treatment for all ligament injuries can be nonsurgical (older patient, nonathlete, minor injury) or surgical (young patient, athlete, severe injury).

DEGENERATIVE DISC DISEASE

Lumbar disc disease and herniation is a common correctable cause of low back pain. However, also consider other possibilities such as muscle strain or spasm, vertebral compression fracture secondary to osteoporosis, degenerative arthritis with or without spinal stenosis and the "red flag" associations with low back pain such as malignancy (e.g., metastatic prostate cancer), cauda equine syndrome, and osteomyelitis.

Keep these associations in mind when evaluation low back pain:

- **Disc herniation** with nerve root impingement results in sciatica as well as motor or sensory deficits of the affected lower extremity. Lumbar disc herniation may cause low back pain without nerve root impingement, so the absence of sciatica and motor or sensory deficits does not rule out disc herniation.
- **Muscle strain or muscle spasm** typically is associated with tenderness to palpation of the affected paraspinal muscles.

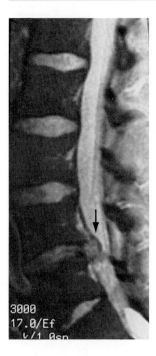

FIGURE 23-1 Large herniated disk at L4–L5. The gelatinous material from the nucleus pulposus becomes extruded from the disk, resulting in root compression and spinal stenosis (*arrow*).

○ **Osteoporotic compression fractures** occur most commonly in postmenopausal women and are associated with kyphosis and loss of height.

○ **Spinal stenosis** causes pain with walking and may present with symptoms similar to claudication, although peripheral arterial pulses will be intact. Spinal stenosis may result from osteoarthritis or malignancy and may require surgical decompression.

○ **Cauda equine syndrome** results in bowel or bladder dysfunction. If caused by malignancy, treatment options may include resection and radiation therapy.

○ **Osteomyelitis or discitis** usually results in fever and an insidious onset of back pain. Examination reveals tenderness to spinal percussion.

Points to remember about disc herniation:

○ The most common site of disc herniation is the L5–S1 disc. Herniation affects the S1 nerve root. Look for decreased ankle jerk, weakness of plantar flexors in the foot, pain from the midgluteal area to the posterior calf, and sciatica with the straight-leg raise test.

○ The second most common site is L4–L5 (Fig. 23-1). Herniation affects the L5 nerve root. Look for decreased biceps femoris reflex, weakness of foot extensors, and pain in the hip or groin.

The diagnosis is made by MRI (preferred), computed tomography (CT), or myelography. Plain radiographs can show disc space narrowing, which is nonspecific, and cannot visualize the disc itself, so they are rarely helpful. Conservative treatment, including bedrest and analgesics, usually is tried first, because roughly 90% of cases resolve with conservative management. Epidural steroid injection may help. Surgery (discectomy) may be required if conservative treatment fails or significant neurologic deficit is present (to prevent permanent nerve damage).

Cervical disc disease (classic symptom = neck pain) is less common than lumbar disease. The C6–C7 disc is the most common site (C5–C6 is the second most common cervical disc). Herniation at the C6–C7 level affects the C7 nerve root. Look for decreased reflex and strength of the triceps and weakness of forearm extension.

OTHER ORTHOPEDIC PROBLEMS

Avascular necrosis describes local intravascular coagulation with subsequent bone ischemia and necrosis of cancellous bone and marrow. Patients present with pain in the affected area. There are many potential causes and associations, including trauma (usually in the setting of fracture), corticosteroid excess (endogenous or iatrogenic), sickle cell disease or other hemoglobinopathy, alcohol abuse, lupus and other connective tissue disorders, Caisson disease (i.e., decompression sickness), slipped capital femoral epiphysis, and pancreatitis. The best test to make the diagnosis is MRI because results become positive before regular radiographs.

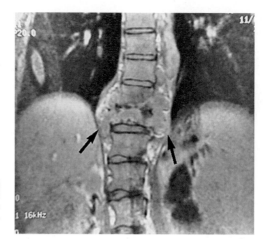

Figure 23-2 Septic spondylitis of the lumbar spine. The pyogenic infection in this case results in narrowing and destruction of the involved disk space and osteomyelitis of the adjacent vertebral bodies. *Arrows* indicate the mass-like paraspinal extension of infectious spondylodiskitis.

Charcot joints and neuropathic joints are seen most commonly in patients with diabetes mellitus and other conditions causing peripheral neuropathy (e.g., vitamin B12 deficiency, tertiary syphilis). Lack of proprioception causes gradual arthritis and arthropathy and joint deformity. Do radiography for any (even minor) trauma in neuropathic patients, who might not feel even a severe fracture. Treatment includes protective padded shoes to help prevent the development of pressure ulcers and infection. If nonoperative treatment fails, then surgical debridement, resection of bony prominences, or both may be necessary.

The most common cause of osteomyelitis is *S. aureus*, but think of gram-negative organisms in immunocompromised patients and IV drug abusers, and think of *Salmonella spp.* in sickle cell disease. Think *Pseudomonas aeruginosa* if there is a puncture wound through a tennis shoe. Aspirate or biopsy the affected bone and do Gram stain, cultures and sensitivities, blood cultures, and complete blood cell count with differential if you are suspicious. Also check a serum erythrocyte sedimentation rate or C-reactive protein. MRI or bone scan can also help confirm the diagnosis (Fig. 23-2).

Septic arthritis also is most commonly caused by infection with *S. aureus*, but in a sexually active adult (especially a promiscuous one), suspect *Neisseria gonorrheae*. Aspirate the joint and do Gram stain, culture and sensitivities, cell counts, and blood cultures if you are suspicious.

IMPORTANT POINTS

1. With a true posterior knee dislocation, check pulses and perform CT angiography (or MR or conventional angiography) if pulses are asymmetric or decreased (vascular injury commonly associated).

2. The most common type of bone tumor is metastatic (remember the cancers that commonly metastasize to bone with the mnemonic "BLT with a kosher pickle": **b**reast, **l**ung, **t**hyroid, **k**idney, and **p**rostate).

3. The most common primary bone tumor is multiple myeloma followed by osteosarcoma.

4. The most common cause of a pathologic fracture is osteoporosis (Fig. 23-3), especially in elderly, thin women. Osteoporosis typically leads to hip or spine (compression) fractures, which are diagnosed with plain radiographs. Use CT or MRI if the diagnosis or age of the fracture is in doubt or if a nonosteoporotic pathologic cause of bone weakening is suspected.

5. A hip dislocation, fracture, or inflammation can cause referred pain to the knee (classic in children).

6. Pain in the anatomic snuff box after trauma (fall on an outstretched hand, especially in young adults) usually is caused by a scaphoid bone fracture.

7. After a fall on an outstretched hand, the most likely fracture in older adults is a Colles fracture (distal end of radius; Fig. 23-4).

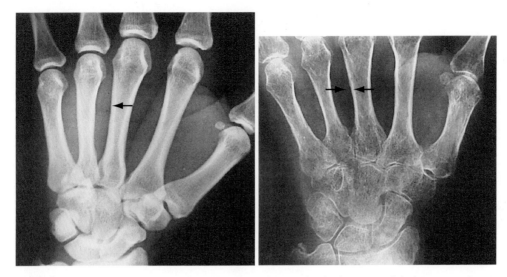

FIGURE 23-3 Osteoporosis. **A,** Note the normal cortical thickness at the third metacarpal shaft (*arrow*) in this 30-year-old patient. **B,** The cortices of this elderly woman with osteoporosis are markedly thinned (*arrows*).

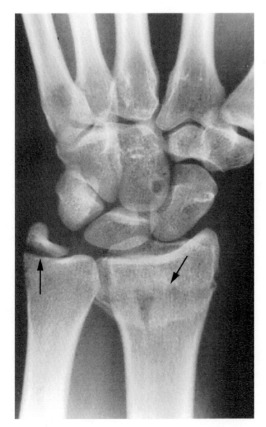

FIGURE 23-4 Colles fracture (*arrow* on *right side of figure*) with associated ulnar styloid fracture (*arrow* on *left side of figure*).

PEDIATRIC ORTHOPEDICS

See Pediatrics chapter (Chapter 24).

QR CODE

The QR code includes three USMLE-style questions and answers. For more questions, redeem the PIN code on the inside cover for the Crush Step 2 question bank powered by USMLE Consult.

Please see the Introduction for instructions on how to access content using the QR codes.

Question

Which of the following is true concerning slipped capital femoral epiphysis?
(A) Treatment generally involves surgical pinning.
(B) It rarely affects obese children for unknown reasons.
(C) It usually occurs in children between the ages of 4 and 7 years.
(D) Patients usually complain of contralateral knee pain.
(E) Plain radiographs are not helpful in making the diagnosis.

24 PEDIATRICS

MILESTONES

There are a million milestones during an infant's development, but concentrate on the common ones listed in Table 24-1. Rough average ages are given; the exact age is not as important as the overall pattern when you are looking for dysfunctional development. When in doubt, use a formal developmental test.

SCREENING AND PREVENTIVE CARE

Screening and preventive care are important parts of well-baby exams that also can help answer parents' questions. For example, a mother complains that her 4-year-old child sleeps 11 hours every night (this is normal). The answer to the question, "What should you do next?" may be to get an objective hearing exam, which is a routine screening procedure in a 4-year-old child. Height, weight, blood pressure, developmental and behavioral assessment, history and physical exam, and anticipatory guidance (counseling and discussion about age-appropriate concerns) should be done at every visit.

Anemia
Recommendations for routine screening for anemia (with a complete blood count [CBC] or hemoglobin or hematocrit) vary and are changing. Hemoglobin or hematocrit measurement is recommended at 12 months of age but may be required at other times as dictated by history and risk assessment. Recommendations for screening during adolescence vary, but adolescents should be screened at least once. If any risk factors for iron deficiency are present during infancy (prematurity, low birth weight, ingestion of cow's milk before 1 year of age, low dietary intake, low socioeconomic status), screen with a CBC or hemoglobin and hematocrit if given the option. Exclusively breastfed infants do not require supplementation. All other children should receive supplementation. Start iron supplements in full-term infants at 4 to 6 months of age and in preterm infants at 2 months of age. Most infant formulas and cereals contain iron, so separate supplements are usually not required.

Anticipatory Guidance
Tell parents to:
○ Keep the water heater set below 110°F to 120°F.
○ Use car restraints.
○ Put baby to sleep on the side or back to help prevent sudden infant death syndrome (most common cause of death in children ages 1–12 months).
○ Do not use infant walkers (which cause injuries).
○ Watch out for small objects (risk of aspiration).
○ Do not give cow's milk before 1 year of age.
○ Introduce solid foods gradually, starting at 6 months.
○ Supervise children in bathtubs and swimming pools.

Apgar Score
The Apgar score is a general measure of well-being in newborns and is commonly assessed at 1 and 5 minutes after birth. *Do not* wait until the 1-minute mark to evaluate the newborn; you may have to suction or intubate the infant 3 seconds after delivery. The Apgar score includes five categories with a

TABLE 24-1 Developmental Milestones	
MILESTONE	**AGE***
Social smile	1–2 mo
Cooing	2–4 mo
While prone, lifts head up 90 degrees	3–4 mo
Rolls front to back	4–5 mo
Voluntary grasp (no release)	5 mo
Stranger anxiety	6–9 mo
Sits with no support	7 mo
Pulls to stand	9 mo
Plays pat-a-cake	9–10 mo
First words	9–12 mo
Imitates others' sounds	9–12 mo
Voluntary grasp with voluntary release	10 mo
Waves "bye-bye"	10 mo
Separation anxiety	12–15 mo
Walks without help	13 mo
Can build tower of two cubes	13–15 mo
Good use of cup and spoon	15–18 mo
Understands one-step commands (no gesture)	15 mo
Can build tower of six cubes	2 y
Runs well	2 y
Rides a tricycle	3 y
Skips	4 y
Ties shoelaces	5 y

*When the development of a premature infant is assessed, the infant's age is reduced in the first 2 years. For example, subtract 3 months from the chronologic age of an infant born prematurely after 6 months' gestation; therefore, the infant is expected to perform at the 6-month-old interval at the age of 9 months.

maximum score of 2 points per category and a total maximum of 10 points. Remember the APGAR pneumonic: appearance (skin color), pulse (heart rate), grimace (reflex irritability), activity (muscle tone), and respiration (breathing).

○ Appearance (skin color): 0 = pale, blue; 1 = body pink and extremities blue; 2 = completely pink
○ Pulse (heart rate): 0 = absent; 1 = rate <100 beats/min; 2 = rate >100 beats/min
○ Grimace (reflex irritability: response to stimulation of sole of foot or catheter put in nose): 0 = none; 1 = grimace; 2 = grimace and strong cry, cough, or sneeze
○ Activity (muscle tone): 0 = limp; 1 = some flexion of extremities; 2 = active motion
○ Respiration (breathing): 0 = none; 1 = slow, weak cry; 2 = good, strong cry
   Continue to score every 5 minutes until the infant reaches a score of 7 or more (while resuscitating).

Fluoride

Start supplementation in the first few years of life if water is inadequately fluoridated (rare) or if the patient is fed exclusively from a premixed, ready-to-eat formula (nonfluoridated water is used in such products). Most children need no supplementation.

Hearing and Vision

Hearing and vision should be measured objectively at least once by 4 years of age. Measure every few years until adulthood, more often if history dictates.

   After a bout of meningitis, all children should be screened objectively for hearing loss (the most common neurologic complication of meningitis). Hearing screening is also important after congenital TORCH (toxoplasmosis, other agents, rubella, cytomegalovirus, herpes simplex virus) infections, measles and mumps, and chronic middle ear effusions, otitis media, and if the child is meeting all developmental milestones except verbal abilities.

Check the red reflex at birth and routinely thereafter to detect congenital cataracts (usually caused by congenital rubella, other TORCH infections, or galactosemia) or retinoblastoma (look for leukocoria). When a penlight is shined at the pupil, you usually see red because of the underlying fundus. If a cataract (or tumor) is present in the eye, the red reflex disappears, and you see black (with a cataract) or white (known as leukocoria and classically caused by retinoblastoma).

It is normal for children to have occasional ocular misalignment (strabismus) until 3 months of age; after that, strabismus should be evaluated further by an ophthalmologist to prevent possible blindness in the affected eye.

Height, Weight, and Head Circumference

Head circumference should be measured routinely in the first 2 years; height and weight should be measured routinely until adulthood. All are markers of general well-being. The pattern of growth along plotted growth curves (which you need to know how to read) tells you more than any raw number. If a patient's measurements have always been low or high compared with peers, this pattern is generally benign. Parents commonly bring in a child with delayed physical growth or delayed puberty, and you must know when to reassure and follow up and when to do further testing and questioning. If a patient goes from a normal curve to an abnormal curve, this is a much more worrisome pattern.

○ **Failure to thrive:** There is no consensus definition for failure to thrive, but commonly used definitions include a head circumference, height, or weight less than the fifth percentile for age; a weight less than 80% of ideal weight for age; or a weight gain that causes a decrease in two or more major percentage lines on the growth curve. Failure to thrive is most commonly caused by psychosocial or functional problems. Watch for signs of neglect and child abuse. Organic causes usually have specific clues to trigger your suspicion.

○ **Obesity** is usually caused by overeating and too little activity; fewer than 5% of cases are attributable to organic causes (Cushing or Prader-Willi syndrome).

○ **Increased head circumference** can mean hydrocephalus or tumor, and decreased head circumference can mean microcephaly (e.g., from congenital TORCH infection).

Immunizations

When to give normal immunizations (Table 24-2) is constantly being updated, so the administration schedule for common vaccines is often given, but of course, this material is still fair game on Step 2. High yield: special patient populations (pneumococcal vaccine for patients with sickle cell disease or splenectomy) and vaccine contraindications (no measles, mumps, and rubella or influenza vaccine for egg-allergic patients; no live vaccines to pregnant women or immunocompromised patients) (Table 24-3).

TABLE 24-2 Pediatric Vaccine Recommendations

VACCINE	WHEN TO GIVE IN ROUTINE CASES
Hepatitis B	Birth, 2 mo, and 6 mo (three doses)
Diphtheria, tetanus, pertussis (DTP)	2, 4, 6, 15–18 mo, and 4–6 y (five doses) plus tetanus, diphtheria, and pertussis (Tdap) booster at 11–12 y
Haemophilus influenzae type b	2, 4, 6, 12–15 mo (four doses)
Pneumococcus spp. (heptavalent)	2, 4, 6, 12–15 mo (four doses)
Polio, inactivated (IPV)	2, 4, 6–18 mo and 4–6 y (four doses)
Measles, mumps, rubella (MMR)	12–15 mo and 4–6 y (two doses)
Hepatitis A	12–18 mo; second dose 6 mo after first (two doses)
Varicella	12–18 mo and 4–6 y (two doses)
Meningococcal	11–12 y (or at high school entry)
Rotavirus	2, 4, and 6 mo (three doses)
Influenza	Every fall
Human papillomavirus	Three doses beginning around age 11 y and up to age 26 y in girls and women HPV4 may be given in a three-dose series to boys and men ages 9–26 y to reduce the likelihood of acquiring genital warts

Table 24-3 Who Should Receive Pediatric Vaccinations

VACCINE	INDICATIONS AND CONTRAINDICATIONS
Hepatitis B	Give first dose at birth with hepatitis B immune globulin if mother has active hepatitis B
Influenza	Give to children >6 mo with immunodeficiency, heart or lung disease (including asthma), or on chronic aspirin therapy (to prevent Reye syndrome)
Measles, mumps, rubella (MMR)	Avoid in children with anaphylactic reaction to eggs or neomycin; avoid in those with immunodeficiency other than HIV/AIDS
Meningococcal	Give to children >2 y with terminal complement deficiencies or functional or anatomic asplenia
Pneumococcus spp.	Give to children >2 y who have not been vaccinated if they have immunodeficiency of any kind, are asplenic, or lack splenic function (sickle cell disease)
Polio, inactivated (IPV)	Avoid in children with anaphylaxis to neomycin or streptomycin
Varicella	Avoid in children with immunodeficiency or anaphylaxis to neomycin

Lead

Screening for lead toxicity is controversial. Routine screening is no longer recommended. However, all Medicaid-eligible children must be screened. In children with risk factors, screening is very important because chronic low-level exposure may lead to permanent neurologic sequelae. Screening should start at age 6 months in children with risk factors, such as a sibling or playmate with lead toxicity, pica (especially paint chips and dust in old buildings that may have lead paint), residence in an old or neglected building, or residence near or family members who work at a lead-smelting or battery-recycling plant. Screen and measure symptomatic exposure with serum lead levels (normal value, <10 μg/dL). If the initial lead level is abnormally high, closer follow-up and intervention are needed. The best first step is to repeat the lead level and stop the exposure, if known. Mildly elevated lead levels can be repeated in 1 to 3 months, but lead levels greater than 45 μg/dL should be repeated in 1 to 2 days. Lead chelation therapy should be initiated for lead levels greater than 45 μg/dL and hospitalization with intravenous (IV) chelation therapy for lead levels >70 μg/dL (succimer is preferred in children; dimercaprol is used in more severe cases).

Metabolic and Congenital Disorders

States vary widely in their policies regarding newborn screening. All states mandate screening for hypothyroidism and phenylketonuria at birth (within the first month). Most mandate screening for galactosemia and sickle cell disease. If any of the screen results are positive, the first step is a confirmatory test to make sure that the screen gave you a true positive.

Tuberculosis

Universal screening for tuberculosis recommended. However, you should screen for tuberculosis immediately if it is suggested by history; screen annually at any age if risk factors are present (HIV, incarceration). Risk assessment should occur regularly until 2 years of age and then annually. Test those at high risk (family member with tuberculosis, family member with a positive tuberculosis test result, a child born in a high-risk country, a child who has traveled to a high-risk country, or a child who has consumed unpasteurized milk or cheese). If the only risk factor is living in a high-risk area or immigrant parents, screen once at 4 to 6 years old and once at 11 to 16 years old. If no risk factors are present, do not screen.

Urinalysis

Universal screening is not recommended. However, you should screen for congenital and anatomic abnormalities (e.g., vesicoureteral reflux) after a urinary tract infection in children 2 months to 2 years of age by getting an ultrasound scan and voiding cystourethrogram (VCUG). Screening after the age of 2 years is more controversial and likely won't be asked on the USMLE.

Vitamin D

The American Academy of Pediatrics recommends that exclusively and partially breastfed infants receive vitamin D supplements shortly after birth and continue until they are weaned and consume formula or whole milk. Formula-fed infants do not require supplements in the United States because all formulas contain vitamin D supplements.

Other

The first dental referral should be made around 2 to 3 years old.

 Children have different normal laboratory and physiology values (normal values usually are given): lower blood pressure, higher heart and respiratory rates, and different hemoglobin and hematocrit values (higher at birth; lower throughout childhood). The renal, pulmonary, hepatic, and central nervous systems (CNS) are still not fully mature and functional at birth.

CHILD ABUSE

Watch for failure to thrive; multiple fractures, bruises, or injuries in different stages of healing; shaken baby syndrome (subdural hematomas and retinal hemorrhages with no external trauma signs); behavioral, emotional, and interaction problems; sexually transmitted diseases (STDs); and multiple personality disorder (classically caused by sexual abuse). Metaphyseal "bucket handle" and metaphyseal "corner" fractures on radiographs (Fig. 24-1) are essentially pathognomonic of child abuse. Consider abuse whenever the injury does not fit the story.

 Reporting all child abuse suspicion is mandatory. You do not need proof and cannot be sued for reporting your suspicion.

CYSTIC FIBROSIS

Cystic fibrosis (CF) occurs via autosomal recessive inheritance. It is the most common lethal genetic disease in white children. Always suspect it in children when the mother says the child tastes salty or with recurrent pulmonary infections, rectal prolapse, meconium ileus, esophageal varices, or failure to thrive. Some states perform routine neonatal screening. The **diagnosis** can be made by an abnormal increase in sweat electrolytes (sodium and chloride), immunoreactive trypsinogen assay, and the confirmatory DNA probe test.

Treatment includes chest physiotherapy (to loosen viscous mucus); immunizations, including influenza and pneumococcus; treatment for pancreatic insufficiency (give pancreatic enzyme replacements and fat-soluble vitamin supplements); dornase alfa to reduce sputum viscosity; and as-needed antibiotics and bronchodilators. In addition, 98% of male and many female patients are infertile; those who aren't need genetic counseling. Many eventually develop cor pulmonale (right heart failure). Look for *Staphylococcus aureus* and *Pseudomonas* spp. to cause respiratory infections and treat these infections aggressively.

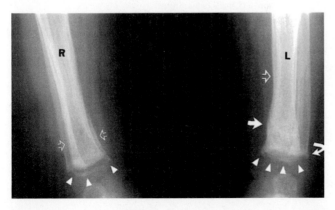

FIGURE 24-1 Metaphyseal bucket handle fractures of the distal tibias (*arrowheads*). Note the periosteal reaction extending proximally along both tibial shafts (*open arrows*). In addition, there is a corner fracture of the left distal fibula (*curved arrow*) and a healing transverse fracture of the left distal tibia (*heavy arrow*).

CARDIOLOGY

Table 24-4 lists congenital heart defects.

IMPORTANT POINTS

1. A heart rate greater than 100 beats/min may be normal in young children.
2. In the presence of a ventricular septal defect, think about the possibility of fetal alcohol syndrome, TORCH syndrome, or Down syndrome.
3. Hypertrophic obstructive cardiomyopathy classically appears in a boy who passes out on exertion (watch for collapse or sudden death in an athlete) and often is associated with a family history of sudden death. This condition causes an asymmetric ventricular hypertrophy that reduces cardiac output (diastolic dysfunction). Treat with β-blockers to give the heart more time to fill. Calcium channel blockers can be used if β-blockers are not tolerated. Positive inotropic agents (e.g., digoxin), diuretics, and vasodilators are *contraindicated* because they make the condition worse.
4. Oxygen content in the fetal circulation is highest in the umbilical vein (the blood coming from the mother) and lowest in the umbilical arteries. Oxygen content is higher in blood going to upper extremities than in blood going to lower extremities.
5. Understand the changes in the circulation from intra- to extrauterine life. The first breaths inflate the lungs and cause decreased pulmonary vascular resistance, which increases blood flow to the pulmonary arteries. This and the clamping of the cord increase left-sided heart pressures, which functionally close the foramen ovale. Increased oxygen concentration shuts off prostaglandin production in the ductus arteriosus, causing gradual closure.

TABLE 24-4 Congenital Heart Defects*

DEFECT	SYMPTOMS	TREATMENT	OTHER INFORMATION
Patent ductus arteriosus	Constant, machine-like murmur in the upper left sternal border; dyspnea and possible CHF	Close with indomethacin (or surgery if indomethacin fails); keep open with prostaglandin E1	Associated with congenital rubella and high altitudes
Ventricular septal defect	Holosystolic murmur next to sternum	Most cases resolve on their own	Most common congenital heart defect
Atrial septal defect	Often asymptomatic until adulthood; fixed, split S2 and palpitations	Most defects do not need correction (unless very large)	Secundum type is most common (80%)
Tetralogy of Fallot	Ventricular septal defect, right ventricular hypertrophy, pulmonary stenosis, and overriding aorta	Surgery	Most common cyanotic congenital heart defect; look for "tet" spells (squatting after exertion; associated with Down syndrome; can present a few years after birth
Coarctation of aorta	Upper extremity hypertension only; radiofemoral delay; systolic murmur heard over mid upper back; rib notching on radiographs	Surgery	Associated with Turner syndrome
Transposition of the great vessels	Cyanotic newborn	Surgery	Associated with diabetic mothers; most common cause of cyanotic heart disease on the first day of life

*Endocarditis prophylaxis is required for all of these cardiac defects except asymptomatic secundum-type atrial septal defect.
CHF, congestive heart failure.

GASTROENTEROLOGY

Pediatric gastrointestinal (GI) malformations are listed in Table 24-5. Esophageal atresia is shown in Figure 24-2. Other pediatric GI conditions are shown in Table 24-6.

Omphalocele versus gastroschisis:

○ **Omphalocele** is in the midline. The sac contains multiple abdominal organs; the umbilical ring is absent; and other anomalies are common.

○ **Gastroschisis** is to the right of the midline. Only small bowel is exposed (no true hernia sac), the umbilical ring is present, and other anomalies are rare.

Henoch-Schönlein purpura: A vasculitis that may present with GI bleeding and abdominal pain. Look for history of upper respiratory infection, a characteristic rash on the lower extremities and buttocks, swelling in hands and feet, arthritis, and hematuria or proteinuria. Treat supportively.

Children (more than adults) can develop nausea and vomiting or diarrhea with any systemic illness. They also can develop inflammatory bowel disease or irritable bowel syndrome. Diarrhea, fever, bloody stools, anemia, joint pains, and poor growth are more concerning for inflammatory bowel disease.

Children often have GI complaints with anxiety (e.g., separation anxiety, reluctance to go to school), psychiatric problems (e.g., depression), or child abuse.

Diaphragmatic hernia is more common in boys. Ninety percent are on the left side. The main point to know is that bowel herniates into the thorax through the diaphragmatic defect, compressing the lung and impeding lung development (pulmonary hypoplasia develops). Patients present with respiratory distress and have bowel sounds in the chest and bowel loops in the thorax on chest radiographs. Treat with surgical correction of the diaphragm.

TABLE 24-5 Gastrointestinal Malformations Seen in Children

NAME	PRESENTING AGE	DESCRIPTION OF VOMITING	FINDINGS AND KEY WORDS
Pyloric stenosis	0–3 mo	Nonbilious, projectile	M >> F; palpable olive-shaped mass in epigastrium, low potassium, metabolic alkalosis
Intestinal atresia	0–1 wk	Bilious	Double-bubble sign, Down syndrome
Tracheoesophageal fistula	0–2 wk	Food regurgitation	Respiratory compromise with feeding, aspiration pneumonia, inability to pass nasogastric tube, gastric distension (air)
Hirschsprung disease	0–1 y	Feculent	Abdominal distension, obstipation, no ganglia seen on rectal biopsy, M >> F
Anal atresia	0–1 wk	Late, feculent	Detected on initial exam in nursery, M > F
Choanal atresia	0–1 wk	—	Cyanosis with feeding that is relieved by crying; inability to pass nasogastric tube through the nose
Diaphragmatic hernia	Prenatal or at birth	—	Difficulty breathing, tachycardia, cyanotic; initial management is orogastric tube to decompress the intestines; *do not* bag-mask ventilate or intestinal distension may occur

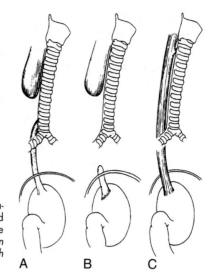

FIGURE 24-2 Esophageal atresia. **A,** The most common form of esophageal atresia (85%) consists of a dilated proximal esophageal pouch and a connection of the distal esophagus to the carina of the trachea. **B,** Pure esophageal atresia. **C,** Fistula of the H-type without atresia. *(From Coran AG (ed): Surgery of the Neonate. Boston, Little, Brown, 1978, p. 46, with permission.)*

TABLE 24-6 Other Gastrointestinal Conditions Seen in Children

NAME	PRESENTING AGE	DESCRIPTION OF VOMITING	FINDINGS AND KEY WORDS
Intussusception	3 mo–2 y	Bilious	Currant-jelly stools (blood and mucus), palpable sausage-shaped mass; diagnose and treat with air-contrast radiographic enema; most common at the ileocolic junction
Necrotizing enterocolitis	0–2 mo	Bilious	Premature babies, fever, rectal bleeding, air in bowel wall; treat with NPO, orogastric tube, IV fluids, antibiotics
Meconium ileus	0–1 wk	Feculent, late	CF manifestation (as is rectal prolapse); a meconium plug has a similar presentation (also consider CF)
Midgut volvulus	0–2 y	Bilious	Caused by malrotation; sudden onset of pain, vomiting, rectal bleeding; diagnose with upper GI series (look for the classic "bird's beak"); treat with immediate surgery
Meckel's diverticulum	0–2 y	Varies	Rule of twos*; GI ulceration or bleeding; use Meckel scan to detect; treat with surgery; caused by incomplete obliteration of the omphalomesenteric duct
Strangulated hernia	Any age	Bilious	Physical exam detects bowel loops in inguinal canal

*Rule of twos for Meckel's diverticulum: 2% of population affected (most common gastrointestinal [GI] tract abnormality—remnant of the omphalomesenteric duct), roughly 2 inches long, within 2 feet of ileocolic junction, and manifests in first 2 years of life. Meckel's diverticulum can cause intussusception, obstruction, or volvulus.
CF, cystic fibrosis; IV, intravenous; NPO, nothing by mouth.

Neonatal Jaundice

○ **Neonatal jaundice:** May be physiologic or pathologic. The first step is to measure total, direct, and indirect bilirubin. The main concern is kernicterus, which is attributable to high levels of unconjugated bilirubin and subsequent deposit into the basal ganglia. Look for poor feeding, seizures, flaccidity, opisthotonos, or apnea in the setting of severe jaundice. Severe hyperbilirubinemia is suggested by jaundice in the first 24 to 36 hours, bilirubin rising faster than 5 mg/dL in 24 hours (0.2 mg/dL/h), total serum bilirubin greater than the age-in-hours specific 95th percentile, conjugated bilirubin greater than 1 mg/dL if the total bilirubin is less than 5 mg/dL or conjugated bilirubin greater than 20% of the total bilirubin if the total is greater than 5 mg/dL, or jaundice after 2 weeks of age in a term newborn.
○ **Physiologic jaundice:** Present in 50% of normal infants; even more common in premature infants. Bilirubin is mostly unconjugated because of incomplete maturation of liver function. In preterm infants, bilirubin is less than 15 mg/dL, peaks at 3 to 5 days, and may be elevated for up to 3 weeks. In full-term infants, bilirubin is less than 12 mg/dL, peaks at 2 to 4 days, and returns to normal by 2 weeks.

○ **Pathologic jaundice:** Bilirubin levels rise higher than normal and continue to rise or fail to decrease appropriately. Any jaundice present at birth is pathologic.

○ **Breast milk jaundice:** Breastfed infants with peak bilirubin of 10 to 20 mg/dL occurring at 2 to 3 weeks of age. Treat with temporary cessation of breastfeeding (switch to bottle) until jaundice resolves.

○ **Illness:** Infection or sepsis, hypothyroidism, liver insult, CF, and other illnesses can prolong neonatal jaundice and lower the threshold for kernicterus. The youngest, sickest infants are at greatest risk for hyperbilirubinemia and kernicterus.

○ **Hemolysis:** From Rh incompatibility or congenital red cell diseases that cause hemolysis in the neonatal period. Look for anemia, peripheral smear abnormalities, family history, and higher level of unconjugated bilirubin.

○ **Metabolic:** Crigler-Najjar syndrome, an autosomal recessive illness, causes severe unconjugated hyperbilirubinemia. Type 1 is manifested by a pure unconjugated hyperbilirubinemia and is associated with kernicterus and death if liver transplant is not performed. Type 2 is associated with lower serum bilirubin concentrations, so kernicterus does not occur. Type 2 can be treated with phenobarbital. Gilbert disease causes mild unconjugated hyperbilirubinemia caused by decreased glucuronidation enzyme. Rotor and Dubin-Johnson syndromes cause conjugated hyperbilirubinemia. Both are benign conditions.

○ **Biliary atresia:** Usually term infants with clay- or gray-colored stools and high levels of conjugated bilirubin. Treat with surgery.

○ **Medications:** Avoid sulfa drugs in neonates (displaces bilirubin from albumin and can precipitate kernicterus).

Treatment for unconjugated hyperbilirubinemia that persists, rises higher than 15 mg/dL, or rises rapidly is phototherapy to convert the unconjugated bilirubin to a water-soluble form that can be excreted. The last resort is exchange transfusion (but don't even *think* about it unless the level of unconjugated bilirubin is >20 mg/dL).

 Any infant born to a mother with active hepatitis B should get the first immunization shot and hepatitis B immunoglobulin at birth.

GENETICS

See the Genetics chapter (Chapter 9) for a thorough discussion of this topic.

GYNECOLOGY

In a child with **ambiguous genitalia,** look for congenital adrenal hyperplasia (also called adrenogenital syndrome), which usually is caused by 21-hydroxylase deficiency (90% of cases). Patients are female; boys with this disease show precocious sexual development. Patients with 21-hydroxylase deficiency have salt wasting (low sodium levels), hyperkalemia, hypotension, and elevated 17-hydroxyprogesterone. Treat with corticosteroids and IV fluids immediately to prevent death. No patient with ambiguous genitalia should be assigned a gender until the workup is complete. A karyotype must be done.

IMPORTANT POINTS

1. Any child with a "bunch of grapes" protruding from her vagina probably has sarcoma botryoides, a malignant tumor (rhabdomyosarcoma subtype).

2. Premature or precocious puberty is usually idiopathic but may be caused by a hormone-secreting tumor or CNS disorder, which must be ruled out. By definition, the patient must be younger than 8 years (9 years for boys). Treat the underlying cause or, if idiopathic, treat with gonadotropin-releasing hormone analogue (e.g., leuprolide) to prevent premature epiphyseal closure and to arrest or reverse puberty until the appropriate age.

(Continued)

IMPORTANT POINTS—Cont'd

3. Most cases of pediatric vaginitis or vaginal discharge are nonspecific or physiologic. But look for foreign body, sexual abuse (especially with STD), or candidal infection (as a presentation of diabetes; measure serum glucose or check for glycosuria).
4. Imperforate hymen is seen in a patient of menarche age with hematocolpos (blood in the vagina) that cannot escape (the hymen bulges outward). Treatment is surgical opening of the hymen.
5. Vaginal bleeding in neonates is usually physiologic as a result of maternal estrogen withdrawal and resolves by itself.
6. Pap smears should be performed beginning at age 21 years. Sexually active teenage girls need screening for chlamydial infection and gonorrhea.

INFECTIOUS RASHES

Infectious rashes occur most often in children. Treatment is supportive only unless otherwise specified.

Chickenpox (Varicella)

The description and progression of the rash itself should lead to the diagnosis: Discrete macules (usually on the trunk) turn into papules, which turn into vesicles that rupture and crust over. These changes occur within 1 day. The lesions appear in successive crops; therefore, the rash is in different stages of progression in different areas. The patient is infectious until the last lesion crusts over. A Tzanck smear of tissue from the base of a vesicle shows multinucleated giant cells (Fig. 24-3).

A complication is infection of the lesions (streptococci, staphylococci [erysipelas], cellulitis, sepsis). The patient should be instructed to keep clean to avoid infection. Other complications include pneumonia (especially in very young children and immunocompromised adults), encephalitis, and Reye syndrome. *Do not* give aspirin to any child with a fever unless the diagnosis requires its use.

Varicella zoster immunoglobulin is available for prophylaxis in patients with debilitating illness (e.g., leukemia, AIDS) if you see them within 4 days of exposure or in newborns of mothers with chickenpox. Acyclovir may be used in severe cases. The varicella zoster virus can reactivate years later to cause shingles (zoster), which is characterized by a dermatomal distribution of rash. Pain and paresthesias often precede the rash.

Erythema Infectiosum (Fifth Disease)

Classic "slapped-cheek" rash (confluent erythema over the cheeks) appears around the same time as mild constitutional symptoms (low fever, malaise). One day later, a maculopapular rash appears on the arms, legs, and trunk. It is caused by parvovirus B19 (the same virus that causes aplastic crisis in sickle cell disease).

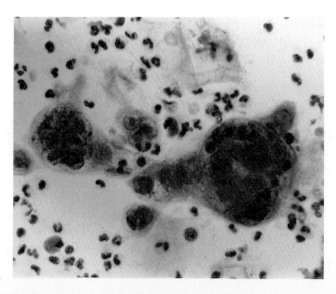

FIGURE 24-3 Positive Tzanck preparation.

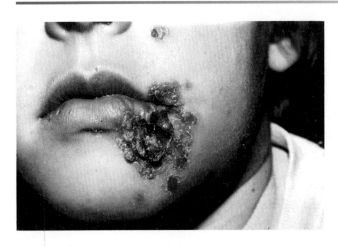

Figure 24-4 Impetigo.

Impetigo

Look for history of skin break (e.g., previous chickenpox, insect bite, scabies, cut). The rash starts as thin-walled vesicles that rupture and form yellowish crusts (Fig. 24-4). The skin often is described as "weeping." Classically, lesions are on the face and tend to be localized. Impetigo is infectious; look for sick contacts. Treat with oral antistaphylococcal penicillin (e.g., dicloxacillin), cephalexin, or clindamycin to cover streptococci and staphylococci, the most common causative bugs. Topical mupirocin also may be used.

Infectious Mononucleosis (Epstein-Barr Virus Infection)

Look for fatigue, fever, pharyngitis, and cervical lymphadenopathy (similar to streptococcal pharyngitis, but malaise tends to be more prolonged and pronounced). To differentiate from streptococcal disease, look for splenomegaly; hepatomegaly; atypical lymphocytes (bizarre forms that can resemble leukemia) with lymphocytosis, anemia, or thrombocytopenia; and positive serology (heterophile antibodies [e.g., Monospot test] or specific Epstein-Barr virus [EBV] antibodies, such as the viral capsid antigen). Patients can develop splenic rupture and should avoid contact sports and heavy lifting. Include HIV in the differential diagnosis. Remember the association of EBV with nasopharyngeal cancer and African Burkitt lymphoma.

Kawasaki Disease (Mucocutaneous Lymph Node Syndrome)

Kawasaki disease is rare and usually occurs in patients younger than 5 years. Diagnostic criteria include fever longer than 5 days (mandatory for diagnosis); bilateral conjunctival injection; changes in the lips, tongue, or oral mucosa (strawberry tongue, fissuring, injection); changes in the extremities (desquamation, edema, erythema); a polymorphous truncal rash (usually begins one day after the fever starts); and cervical lymphadenopathy. Also look for arthralgia and arthritis. The most feared complications involve the heart (coronary artery aneurysms, congestive heart failure, arrhythmias, myocarditis, myocardial infarction). Think of Kawasaki disease in the differential diagnosis of any child who has a myocardial infarction. If Kawasaki disease is suspected, give aspirin and IV immunoglobulin, both of which reduce the risk of developing cardiac lesions. Follow up with echocardiography to detect heart involvement.

Measles (Rubeola)

Look for a reason for the patient not to be immunized. Koplik spots (tiny white spots on buccal mucosa) are seen 3 days after high fever. Other symptoms include a cough, runny nose, and conjunctivitis and photophobia. On the next day, the rash (maculopapular) begins on the head and neck and spreads downward to cover the trunk (cephalocaudal progression). Complications include pneumonia (giant cell pneumonia, especially in very young and immunocompromised patients), otitis media, and encephalitis (which may be acute or cause subacute sclerosing panencephalitis, which usually occurs years later). Vitamin A can help reduce morbidity and mortality, particularly in areas where vitamin A deficiency is prevalent.

Rocky Mountain Spotted Fever (*Rickettsia Rickettsii* Infection)

Look for history of a tick bite (especially on the East Coast) 1 week before the development of high fever or chills, severe headache, and prostration or severe malaise. Roughly 4 days after these symptoms, the rash appears on the palms and wrists and the soles and ankles, rapidly spreading to the trunk and face (unique pattern of spread). Patients often look very sick (disseminated intravascular coagulation, delirium). Treat with doxycycline; chloramphenicol is a second choice.

Roseola Infantum (Exanthem Subitum)

Roseola infantum is easy to recognize because of its progression: high fever (may be >40°C) with no apparent cause for 4 days (patient may get febrile seizures) and then an abrupt return to normal temperature as a diffuse macular and maculopapular rash appears on the chest and abdomen. It is rare in children older than 3 years, it is caused by human herpesvirus type 6 (a DNA virus).

Rubella (German Measles)

Rubella is important mainly because infection in pregnant women can cause severe birth defects in fetuses. Screen and immunize any woman of reproductive age *before* she becomes pregnant; the vaccine is contraindicated in pregnant women. Rubella is milder than measles, with low-grade fever, malaise, tender swelling of the suboccipital and postauricular nodes, and arthralgias. After a 2- to 3-day prodrome, the rash (maculopapular, faint) starts on the face and neck and spreads to the trunk (cephalocaudal progression). Complications include encephalitis and otitis media.

Scarlet Fever

Look for a history of untreated streptococcal pharyngitis (caused only by *Streptococcus* spp. that produce erythrogenic toxin) followed by a sandpaper-like rash on the abdomen and trunk with classic circumoral pallor and strawberry tongue. The rash tends to desquamate after the fever subsides. Treat with penicillin to prevent rheumatic fever.

KIDNEY AND HEMATOLOGIC DISORDERS IN CHILDREN

Table 24-7 shows the differential diagnosis of pediatric kidney and hematologic disorders.

TABLE 24-7 Kidney and Hematologic Disorders in Children				
CHARACTERISTIC	**HUS**	**HSP**	**TTP**	**ITP**
Most common age	Children	Children	Young adults	Children or adults
Previous infection	Diarrhea (*Escherichia coli*)	URI	None	Viral (especially in children)
RBC count	Low	Normal	Low	Normal
Platelet count	Low	Normal	Low	Low
Peripheral smear	Hemolysis	Normal	Hemolysis	Normal
Treatment	Supportive*	Supportive*	Plasmapheresis, NSAIDs; no platelets†	Steroids; splenectomy if medications fail‡
Kidney manifestations	ARF, hematuria	Hematuria	ARF, proteinuria	None
Key differential points	Age, diarrhea	Rash, abdominal pain, arthritis, melena	CNS changes, age	Antiplatelet antibodies

*In HUS and HSP, patients might need dialysis and transfusions.
†Do not give platelet transfusions to patients with TTP (can form clots).
‡Give steroids only if the patient is symptomatic (bleeding) or platelets are less than 20,000/mm³.
ARF, acute renal failure; CNS, central nervous system; HSP, Henoch-Schönlein purpura; HUS, hemolytic uremic syndrome; ITP, idiopathic thrombocytopenic purpura; NSAID, nonsteroidal antiinflammatory drug; RBC, red blood cell; TTP, thrombotic thrombocytopenic purpura; URI, upper respiratory infection.

Potter Syndrome

Bilateral renal agenesis causes oligohydramnios in utero (the fetus swallows fluid but cannot excrete it). It is also associated with limb deformities, abnormal facies, and hypoplasia of the lungs. It is generally incompatible with life.

NEUROLOGY

Floppy Baby Syndrome

Infants have hypotonia or flaccidity. It can be caused by two disorders:

○ **Werdnig-Hoffmann disease:** Autosomal recessive degeneration of anterior horn cells in the spinal cord and brainstem (lower motor neurons). Most infants are hypotonic at birth, and all are affected by age 6 months. Look for a positive family history and a long and slowly progressive course of disease. Treatment is supportive.

○ **Infant botulism:** Look for a sudden onset and a history of honey ingestion (or other home-canned foods). Diagnosis is made by finding *Clostridium botulinum* toxin or organisms in the feces. Treat on an inpatient basis with close monitoring of respiratory status. Patients might need intubation for respiratory muscle paralysis. Spontaneous recovery usually occurs within 1 week.

Muscular Dystrophy

Muscular dystrophy is most commonly caused by **Duchenne muscular dystrophy**, an X-linked recessive disorder of dystrophin that usually manifests in boys ages 3 to 7 years. Look for muscle weakness, markedly elevated creatine kinase, and pseudohypertrophy of the calves (caused by fatty and fibrous infiltration of the degenerating muscle). IQ often is less than normal. The Gowers sign is classic (in trying to rise from a prone position, the patient walks the hands and feet toward each other). Muscle biopsy establishes the diagnosis. Treatment is supportive. Most patients die by age 20 years.

Seizures

Seizures (including febrile seizures) are discussed in detail in the Neurology chapter (Chapter 18).

ONCOLOGY

Brain Tumors

In children, two-thirds of brain tumors are infratentorial (posterior fossa; i.e., cerebellum and brainstem). Look for new-onset seizures, neurologic deficits, or signs of intracranial hypertension (headache, blurred vision, papilledema, nausea, and projectile vomiting). In children particularly, look for hydrocephalus (inappropriately increasing head circumference), ataxia, new clumsiness, loss of developmental milestones, or a change in school performance or personality. In children, the most common types of brain tumor are cerebellar astrocytoma and medulloblastoma followed by ependymoma. Children can develop craniopharyngiomas (remnant of Rathke pouch), a classically calcified tumor in or around the sella turcica.

Osteosarcoma

See the Oncology chapter (Chapter 21).

Retinoblastoma

Retinoblastoma manifests as leukocoria (the papillary red reflex is white; Fig. 24-5) or unilateral exophthalmos in a young child (typically younger than 3 years of age); the inherited form may be bilateral.

Sarcoma Botryoides

Sarcoma botryoides is a rhabdomyosarcoma subtype that manifests in a girl with a "bunch of grapes" coming out of the vagina.

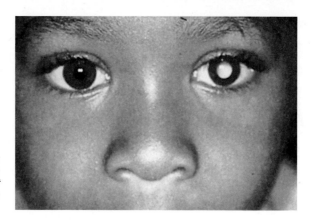

FIGURE 24-5 Leukocoria in the left eye caused by retinoblastoma. *(From Rubin R, Strayer DS, Rubin E (eds): Pathology, 6th ed. Philadelphia, Lippincott Williams & Wilkins, 2012, Figure 29-22A, with permission.)*

Unicameral Bone Cyst

A unicameral bone cyst is an expansile, lytic, well-demarcated lesion in the proximal portion of the humerus in children and adolescents. It is benign but can weaken bone enough to cause a pathologic fracture.

Wilms Tumor and Neuroblastoma

Both Wilms tumor and neuroblastoma manifest as flank masses in children at a peak age of around 2 years old. Whereas neuroblastomas occur at a slightly younger age, usually arise from the adrenal gland, and classically contain calcifications, Wilms tumor arises from the kidney and rarely calcifies; thus, imaging tests (e.g., computed tomography [CT] scan or magnetic resonance imaging [MRI]) can usually tell the two apart. Rarely, neuroblastomas regress spontaneously (for unknown reasons).

PEDIATRIC ORTHOPEDICS

Pediatric hip problems (Table 24-8) give referred pain to the knee, but the patient has no knee swelling or pain with palpation of the knee.

Congenital hip dysplasia, Legg-Calvé-Perthes disease (idiopathic avascular necrosis of the femoral head), and slipped capital femoral epiphysis all may manifest in an adult as arthritis of the hip. Given the correct history (especially age of onset of symptoms!), you should be able to tell which disorder the patient had. Radiographs may be taken, but history gives it away.

Osgood-Schlatter disease is osteochondritis of the tibial tubercle. It is often bilateral and usually manifests in boys 10 to 15 years old with pain, swelling, and tenderness in the knee. Treat with rest, activity restriction, and nonsteroidal antiinflammatory drugs (NSAIDs). The disease usually resolves on its own.

TABLE 24-8 Pediatric Hip Problems				
NAME	**AGE**	**EPIDEMIOLOGY**	**SYMPTOMS AND SIGNS**	**TREATMENT**
CHD	At birth	First-born girl with breech delivery	Barlow and Ortolani signs	Observation, abduction splint, or open or closed reduction
LCP disease	4–10y	Short boy with delayed bone age	Knee, thigh, and groin pain, limp	Orthoses
SCFE	9–13y	Overweight male adolescent	Knee, thigh, and groin pain, limp	Surgical pinning

CHD, congenital hip dysplasia; LCP, Legg-Calvé-Perthes disease; SCFE, slipped capital femoral epiphysis.

Scoliosis usually affects prepubertal girls and most commonly is idiopathic. Ask the patient to touch her toes and look at the spine. With scoliosis, a lateral curvature is seen. Radiographs are confirmatory and can be used to follow the progression. Treat with a brace unless the curvature is minor (<15 degrees). Consider surgery if the deformity is severe (with rapid progression or respiratory compromise).

PREADOLESCENCE AND PUBERTY

Tanner Stages
The Tanner stages measure the stages of puberty. Stage 1 is preadolescent, and stage 5 is adult. Increasing stages are assigned for testicular and penile growth in boys and breast growth in girls; pubic hair development is used for both sexes. Puberty = changes from stage 1 status.
○ **Boys:** The average age of puberty is 11.5 years. The first event usually is testicular enlargement.
○ **Girls:** The average age of puberty is 10.5 years. The first event usually is breast development.

Delayed Puberty
Delayed puberty is defined as no testicular enlargement in boys by age 14 years or no breast development or pubic hair in girls by age 13 years. The usual cause is *constitutional delay*. Parents often have a similar history of being "late bloomers." In this normal variant, the growth curve lags behind others of the same age but is parallel to the normal growth curve. Delayed puberty is rarely caused by primary testicular failure (Klinefelter syndrome, cryptorchidism, history of chemotherapy, gonadal dysgenesis) or ovarian failure (Turner syndrome, gonadal dysgenesis). Other rare causes include hypothalamic and pituitary defects, such as Kallmann syndrome, and tumors.

Precocious Puberty
True precocious puberty is defined as activation of the hypothalamic–pituitary axis with sexual maturation before the age of 8 years in girls and before the age of 9 years in boys. In pseudoprecocious puberty, secondary sex characteristics develop prematurely because of high circulating levels of androgen or estrogen.

True precocious puberty is usually idiopathic but can be caused by CNS lesions. A general rule of thumb is that true precocious puberty causes testicular or ovarian enlargement, which does not occur with pseudoprecocious puberty (ovarian cysts are not considered true ovarian enlargement). All patients with suspected precocious puberty should have a gonadotropin-releasing hormone (GnRH) stimulation test. If a dose of GnRH produces the typical pubertal response of increased follicle-stimulating hormone (FSH) and luteinizing hormone (LH), true precocious puberty is diagnosed. An MRI of the brain should be obtained to rule out CNS disease (e.g., hamartomas, tumors, cysts, trauma) as the cause.

Pseudoprecocious puberty may be caused by exogenous hormones, adrenal tumors, congenital adrenal hyperplasia (e.g., 21-hydroxylase deficiency), hormone-secreting tumors, or McCune-Albright syndrome in girls (ovarian cysts, pseudoprecocious puberty, polyostotic fibrous dysplasia of bone, and café-au-lait spots).

Because premature puberty causes premature fusion of growth plates in the bone and can cause serious social problems for affected children, treatment is indicated. Treatment of any underlying disorders is indicated for pseudoprecocious puberty. For true idiopathic precocious puberty, treatment with long-acting GnRH agonists is indicated to suppress the pituitary–hypothalamic axis and to delay the onset of puberty until an appropriate age.

PSYCHIATRY

Many psychiatric illnesses have overlap between the pediatric and adult populations. For a discussion of pediatric psychiatry topics such as attention-deficit/hyperactivity disorder, autism, conduct disorder, encopresis, enuresis, learning disorder, mental retardation, oppositional defiant disorder, separation anxiety disorder, and Tourette disorder, please see the Psychiatry chapter (Chapter 27).

PULMONOLOGY

Asthma

Look for wheezing in children. Treat with β_2-agonists in the emergency department. As-needed β_2-agonists (e.g., albuterol) are all that is needed for mild intermittent asthma. Inhaled glucocorticoids, leukotriene receptor antagonists (zafirlukast, zileuton), cromolyn, nedocromil, and long-acting β-agonists are used in asthma maintenance, not for acute attacks. Do not use a long-acting β-agonist without concomitant use of an inholed glucocorticoid because of the risk of death. Use oral steroids, magnesium, or both if asthma is severe or does not respond to β_2-agonists. Wheezing in children younger than age 2 years is often attributable to **respiratory syncytial virus (RSV),** especially in the winter. Look for coexisting fever.

Bronchiolitis

Look for a 0- to 18-month-old patient; bronchiolitis usually occurs in fall or winter. More than 75% of cases are caused by the RSV; other causes are parainfluenza and influenza. Patients start with symptoms of viral upper respiratory infection followed 1 to 2 days later by rapid respirations, intercostal retractions, and expiratory wheezing. The patient also might have crackles on auscultation of the chest. Diffuse hyperinflation of the lungs is classic on chest radiographs; look for flattened diaphragms. Treat supportively (oxygen, mist tent, bronchodilators, IV fluids). Use ribavirin in patients with severe symptoms or increased risk (cyanosis, other health problems).

Croup or Acute Laryngotracheitis

Look for the patient to be 1 to 2 years old; croup usually occurs in fall or winter. About 50% to 75% of cases are caused by parainfluenza virus; the other causative agent is influenza virus. Patients start with symptoms of a viral upper respiratory infection (rhinorrhea, cough, and fever) and roughly 1 or 2 days later develop a barking cough, hoarseness, and inspiratory stridor. The "steeple sign" (subglottic tracheal narrowing) is classic on frontal radiography of the neck. Treat supportively with a mist tent, humidified oxygen, and racemic epinephrine.

Diaphragmatic Hernia

Diaphragmatic hernia commonly causes respiratory problems right after birth because bowel herniates into the chest in utero, pushing on the developing lung and causing lung hypoplasia on the affected side. Look for a scaphoid abdomen and bowel sounds in the chest. Herniated bowel also may be seen in the chest on radiography. Ninety percent of hernias are *left sided,* and they are more common in boys.

Diphtheria and Pertussis

Diphtheria (infection with *Corynebacterium diphtheriae*) and pertussis (infection with *Bordetella pertussis*) should be considered if the patient is not immunized. Diphtheria is associated with grayish pseudomembranes (necrotic epithelium and inflammatory exudate) on the pharynx, tonsils, or uvula, and myocarditis. Treat with antitoxin and penicillin G or erythromycin. Pertussis is associated with severe paroxysmal coughing and a high-pitched whooping inspiratory noise (classically called "whooping cough"). Treat with a macrolide antibiotic; close contacts should also be given prophylactic treatment with a macrolide.

Epiglottitis

The patient usually is 2 to 5 years old. The main cause by far used to be *Haemophilus influenzae* type b, but with widespread vaccination, *H. influenzae* and *S. aureus* are equally frequent. Pick *H. influenzae* if you have to choose. Look for little or no prodrome with rapid progression to high fever, toxic appearance, drooling, and respiratory distress with no coughing. The "thumb sign" (enlarged, swollen epiglottis) is classic on lateral neck radiographs (Fig. 24-6). *Do not* examine the throat or irritate the patient in any way—you might precipitate airway obstruction. When a case of epiglottitis is presented, the first step is to be prepared to establish an airway. Treat with a combination of (1) oxacillin or cefazolin or clindamycin or vancomycin plus (2) cefotaxime or ceftriaxone.

Meconium Aspiration

Look for meconium aspiration if the infant is covered with meconium when delivered. Suction secretions first from the mouth (oropharynx) and then from the nose with a bulb syringe or catheter immediately after the head is delivered. Intubate if necessary.

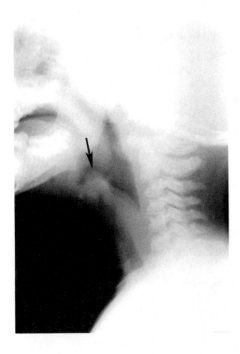

FIGURE 24-6 Classic thumb sign of an enlarged, swollen epiglottis.

Peritonsillar Abscess

Peritonsillar abscess typically presents in patients older than the age of 10 years with a "hot potato" voice, drooling, and trismus. Exam reveals a very swollen and fluctuant tonsil with deviation of the uvula to the opposite side. Group A streptococcus is the most common pathogen, though *S. aureus*, *Streptococcus pneumoniae*, and anaerobes are possible. Surgical intervention (needle aspiration, incision and drainage, or tonsillectomy) and broad-spectrum antibiotic therapy (typically ampicillin-sulbactam or clindamycin) are the cornerstones of treatment.

Pneumonia

Symptoms such as fever, cough, tachypnea, and respiratory distress are suggestive of pneumonia. However, neonates and young infants may have subtle symptoms such as difficulty feeding or restlessness. Examination may reveal tachypnea or respiratory distress, and lung auscultation may reveal crackles, decreased breath sounds, or wheezing. Look for infiltrate(s) on chest radiographs. Elevated white blood cell count and elevated C-reactive protein are also suggestive of pneumonia (particularly bacterial) in the setting of pulmonary symptoms.

S. pneumoniae is the most common cause of pneumonia in children. Give the vaccine to all children. *H. influenzae* is now uncommon in children because of vaccination. In children younger than 1 year, also think of RSV. In children 2 to 5 years of age, also think of parainfluenza (croup) or epiglottitis. Don't forget to think about *B. pertussis* infection, especially in acutely ill infants, because rates of this infection are rapidly increasing.

Mycoplasma spp. infection is most common in adolescents and young adults (the classic case is a college student who lives in a dorm and has sick contacts). This is called "atypical" pneumonia because the clinical course is different from that of *S. pneumoniae* infection with a long prodrome and gradual worsening of malaise, headaches, dry nonproductive cough, and sore throat. Chest radiographs show a patchy, diffuse bronchopneumonia (the radiograph classically looks terrible, although the patient does not feel that bad). Look for positive cold-agglutinin antibody titers (can cause hemolysis and anemia). *Chlamydia pneumonia* is second only to *Mycoplasma* spp. as the cause of pneumonia in adolescents and young adults. It manifests similarly but has negative cold-agglutinin antibody titers.

Children with pneumonia may need to be hospitalized, particularly if they are young or the symptoms are significant. The empiric treatment of pediatric pneumonia is as follows:

○ **Neonates (early onset):** ampicillin and gentamicin to cover maternal genital organisms
○ **Neonates (after 3–5 days of life in a term infant):** vancomycin and gentamicin to add coverage for staphylococcus, particularly methicillin-resistant *S. aureus* (MRSA)

○ **Infants 1 to 4 months:** macrolide
○ **Children 4 months to 4 years:** amoxicillin if bacterial infection is suspected, though viral etiologies predominate in this age group
○ **Children older than 5 years:** macrolide

Recurrent pediatric pneumonia in the same lung segment is classically attributable to **foreign body aspiration,** especially when in the right middle or lower lobe (a foreign body is more likely to go down the right mainstem bronchus). Other possibilities include reflux with aspiration, congenital lung malformation, and immunodeficiency. Patients with immunodeficiency have other signs (e.g., other types of infections, CF symptoms; should not always be the same lung segment involved).

Respiratory Distress Syndrome

Respiratory distress syndrome (RDS), which is caused by atelectasis from deficiency of surfactant, almost always occurs in premature infants and infants of diabetic mothers. Look for rapid, labored respirations; substernal retractions; cyanosis; grunting; or nasal flaring. Arterial blood gases show hypoxemia and hypercarbia. Radiographs show a diffuse granular pattern in the lungs (Fig. 24-7). Treat with O_2, give surfactant, and intubate if needed (often). Complications include pneumothorax or **bronchopulmonary dysplasia** (acute or chronic mechanical ventilation complications) and intraventricular hemorrhage.

Measurement of amniotic fluid in the pregnant mother can determine whether the fetus is producing adequate surfactant. A lecithin-to-sphingomyelin ratio greater than 2:1 or the presence of phosphatidylglycerol in the amniotic fluid indicates fetal lung maturity and a low likelihood of infant RDS. The fluorescence polarization test reflects the ratio of surfactant to albumin in amniotic fluid and is a direct measurement of surfactant concentration. An elevated ratio indicates fetal lung maturity.

Retropharyngeal Abscess

Retropharyngeal abscess typically presents in patients 6 months to 6 years of age who have a fever, odynophagia, a "hot potato" voice, and drooling. Examination typically reveals an ill-appearing child with cervical lymphadenopathy (usually unilateral) and may reveal a mass in the posterior pharyngeal wall (although examination in the operating room may be necessary to permit controlled placement of an airway if needed). Patients with retropharyngeal abscess demonstrate an unwillingness to move the neck because of pain and particularly avoid extension of the neck. Group A streptococcus is the most common pathogen, although *S. aureus* and *Bacteroides* spp. also may cause retropharyngeal abscess. Lateral neck radiographs or contrast-enhanced CT of the neck can be used to help make the diagnosis. Lateral neck radiographs demonstrate a prevertebral space that is increased in depth compared with the

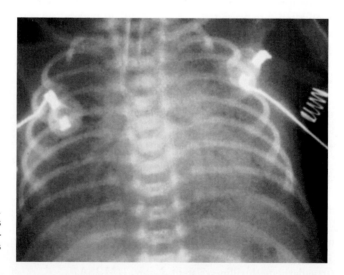

FIGURE 24-7 Respiratory distress syndrome. Chest radiograph in a premature infant shows fine, uniform granularity distributed symmetrically throughout both lung fields. The baby is intubated.

anteroposterior measurement of the adjacent vertebral body. Treatment is surgical drainage and broad-spectrum antibiotics.

Tracheoesophageal Fistula

The most common type (85%) of tracheoesophageal fistula is an esophagus with a blind pouch proximally (i.e., esophageal atresia) and a fistula between a bronchus or the carina and the distal esophagus. Look for a neonate with excessive oral secretions, coughing and cyanosis with attempted feedings, abdominal distension (because breaths transmit air to the GI tract), and aspiration pneumonia. Diagnosis is made by inability to pass a nasogastric tube; air-contrast radiography shows the proximal esophagus only. Treatment is early surgical correction.

VIRILIZATION IN CHILDREN

In female neonates, congenital adrenal hyperplasia is a likely cause of virilization. The classic example is a female infant born with ambiguous genitalia. However, the patient also may be a male child with precocious puberty. At least 90% of cases are attributable to 21-hydroxylase deficiency. Because 21-hydroxylase is involved in the production of both aldosterone and cortisol, children develop signs of hypoadrenalism with salt wasting, hypotension, hyperkalemia, hyponatremia, hypoglycemia, acidosis, and nausea and vomiting. Abnormally high levels of serum 17-hydroxyprogesterone or urinary 17-ketosteroids (dehydroepiandrosterone [DHEA], DHEA sulfate, and androsterone) along with decreased free cortisol in the serum clinch the diagnosis. Give corticosteroids to prevent death. In older children, worry about a testosterone-secreting gonadal neoplasm.

OTHER PEDIATRIC DISORDERS

Cavernous hemangioma is a benign vascular tumor that is first noticed a few days after birth. Lesions increase in size after birth and gradually resolve within the first 2 to 5 years of life in at least 50% of patients. The best treatment in most cases is to do nothing but observe and follow up.

Caput succedaneum is diffuse swelling or edema of the scalp that crosses the midline and is benign. **Cephalohematomas** are subperiosteal hemorrhages that are sharply limited by sutures and do not cross the midline. Cephalohematomas are usually benign and self-resolving, but rarely, they indicate an underlying skull fracture; get a CT scan to rule it out.

A **large anterior fontanelle** can indicate hypothyroidism, hydrocephalus, rickets, or intrauterine growth retardation. The anterior fontanel usually is closed by 18 months; delayed closure may be attributable to the same factors.

IMPORTANT POINTS

1. Reye syndrome can cause encephalopathy, liver failure, or both in children taking aspirin. The syndrome usually develops after influenza or varicella infection. Avoid aspirin in children; use acetaminophen instead.
2. The Moro and palmar grasp reflex should disappear by 6 months.
3. Check the umbilical cord at birth for two arteries, one vein, and the absence of the urachus. If there is only one artery, consider the possibility of congenital renal malformations (get a renal ultrasonography to check).
4. Female infants might have a milky white (and possibly blood-tinged) vaginal discharge in the first week of life. This discharge is physiologic and caused by maternal hormone withdrawal.

QR CODE

The QR code includes three USMLE-style questions and answers. For more questions, redeem the PIN code on the inside cover for the Crush Step 2 question bank powered by USMLE Consult.

Please see the Introduction for instructions on how to access content using the QR codes.

Question

A woman brings in her 3-month-old daughter because she noticed the child does not seem to be gaining much weight. The woman also notices a salty taste when she kisses her infant and read in a magazine that this could mean the infant has cystic fibrosis (CF). She vehemently denies any family history of CF in her or her husband's family. She wants to know whether or not the infant has CF and the likelihood she has "defective DNA" because this is her first child. Which of the following is true regarding CF?

(A) It is an autosomal dominant disease; either the woman's or her husband's DNA could be "at fault."

(B) It is an X-linked recessive disease; the woman and her husband must have genetic mutations for the child to get the disease.

(C) If the child has CF, there is a 50% chance that the next child the woman has will develop CF.

(D) The diagnosis can be made presumptively if the potassium concentration in sweat is elevated markedly.

(E) If the child has CF, she still may be able to give her mother normal, healthy grandchildren if she survives to adulthood.

25 PHARMACOLOGY

GENERAL PHARMACOLOGY

Side Effects

Bizarre, unique, and fatal side effects are tested as well as common side effects of common drugs (Table 25-1). These questions are very common, so knowing side effects is key!

The side effects of diuretics are high yield:

○ Thiazides cause hyperglycemia, hyperlipidemia, hyperuricemia, and hypercalcemia (which you can remember as hyperGLUC). They also cause hyponatremia, hypokalemic metabolic alkalosis, and hypovolemia. Because they are sulfa drugs, thiazides should be avoided in patients with sulfa allergy.

○ Loop diuretics cause hypokalemic metabolic alkalosis, hypovolemia, ototoxicity, and calcium excretion. All loop diuretics except ethacrynic acid are also sulfa drugs.

○ Carbonic anhydrase inhibitors cause metabolic acidosis. This side effect can be used as prophylaxis for altitude sickness.

Antihypertensives are notorious for causing sedation, depression (the worst is methyldopa), and sexual dysfunction. β-Blockers also cause bradycardia and heart block and can acutely worsen an exacerbation of congestive heart failure. Calcium channel blockers also should be avoided in some cardiac patients for the same reasons. Because β-blockers can precipitate asthmatic attacks and mask the symptoms of hypoglycemia, they should be avoided in people with asthma and used with caution in people with diabetes (the benefits often outweigh risks, such as with a prior myocardial infarction). $\alpha 1$-Antagonists are notorious for severe first-dose orthostatic hypotension. Rebound hypertension is commonly seen after discontinuation of methyldopa.

The side effects of psychiatric medications are also high yield. See the chapter on Psychiatry (Chapter 27).

Antidotes

Antidotes to drug poisoning or overdose are listed in Table 25-2.

Drug Interactions

A few drug–drug interactions are high yield. Do not give the following drugs together:

○ Monoamine oxidase inhibitors and selective serotonin reuptake inhibitors or meperidine (can cause the serotonin syndrome: hyperthermia, rigidity, myoclonus, autonomic instability)

○ Aminoglycosides and loop diuretics (enhanced ototoxicity)

○ Thiazides and lithium (lithium toxicity)

IMPORTANT POINTS

1. Barbiturates, antiepileptics, isoniazid, alcohol, and rifampin induce the P450 hepatic enzyme system; cimetidine, amiodarone, macrolide antibiotics (e.g., erythromycin), metronidazole, cyclosporine, and ketoconazole and other azole antifungals inhibit these hepatic enzymes (important for drug–drug interactions).

2. If a patient responds to placebo, it does not mean that the disease is psychosomatic; it means simply that the patient responded to placebo! Normal people with real diseases often have an improvement in symptoms with placebo. Never give placebo to patients as an experiment.

TABLE 25-1 Drug Side Effects

DRUG	SIDE EFFECT(S)
Anesthesia and Pain Management	
Acetaminophen	Liver toxicity (in high doses)
Aspirin	GI bleeding, hypersensitivity
Halogen anesthetics	Malignant hyperthermia
Halothane	Liver necrosis
Local anesthetics	Seizures, arrhythmias
Methoxyflurane	Diabetes insipidus
Morphine	Sphincter of Oddi spasm
Opiates	SIADH, respiratory depression, pinpoint pupils, decreased GI motility, nausea, itching
Succinylcholine	Malignant hyperthermia, increased intracranial pressure, hyperkalemia
Infectious Diseases	
Aminoglycosides	Hearing loss, renal toxicity
Chloramphenicol	Aplastic anemia, gray baby syndrome
Clindamycin	Pseudomembranous colitis (may be caused by any broad-spectrum antibiotic)
Ethambutol	Optic neuritis
Isoniazid	Vitamin B_6 deficiency, lupus-like syndrome, liver toxicity
Metronidazole	Disulfiram-like reaction with alcohol
Penicillins	Anaphylaxis, rash with Epstein–Barr virus (particularly amoxicillin or ampicillin)
Quinolones	Teratogens (cartilage damage), Achilles tendon rupture in adults
Rifampin	Hepatotoxicity
Tetracyclines	Photosensitivity, teeth staining in children
Vancomycin	Red man syndrome (with rapid infusion)
Zidovudine (AZT)	Bone marrow suppression (always produces macrocytic anemia)
Internal Medicine	
Acetazolamide	Metabolic acidosis
Amiodarone	Thyroid dysfunction, pulmonary fibrosis, skin discoloration
Angiotensin-converting enzyme inhibitors	Cough, angioedema, hyperkalemia, teratogenic to fetal kidneys
Chlorpropamide	SIADH
Clofibrate	Increased GI neoplasms
Demeclocycline	Diabetes insipidus
Digitalis	GI disorders, vision changes (yellow vision), arrhythmias
Heparin	Thrombocytopenia, thrombosis
HMG CoA reductase inhibitors	Liver and muscle toxicity
Hydralazine	Lupus-like syndrome
Methyldopa	Hemolytic anemia (Coombs positive)
Niacin	Skin flushing, pruritus
Phenytoin	Folate deficiency, teratogen, hirsutism, gingival hyperplasia
Procainamide	Lupus-like syndrome
Quinine	Cinchonism (e.g., tinnitus, vertigo)
Trimethadione	Terrible teratogen
Valproic acid	Neural tube defects in offspring
Warfarin	Skin necrosis, teratogen, bleeding

TABLE 25-1 Drug Side Effects—Cont'd

Oncology

Bleomycin	Pulmonary fibrosis
Busulfan	Pulmonary fibrosis, adrenal failure
Cisplatin	Nephrotoxicity
Cyclophosphamide	Hemorrhagic cystitis
Doxorubicin	Cardiomyopathy
Vincristine	Peripheral neuropathy

Psychiatry

Bupropion	Seizures (particularly in bulimic patients)
Clozapine	Agranulocytosis
Lithium	Diabetes insipidus, thyroid dysfunction
Monoamine oxidase inhibitors	Tyramine crisis (cheese, wine)
Selective serotonin reuptake inhibitors	Anxiety, agitation, insomnia, suicidality, sexual dysfunction
Thioridazine	Retinal deposits, cardiac toxicity
Trazodone	Priapism

Miscellaneous

Cyclosporine	Renal toxicity
Isotretinoin	Terrible teratogen
Minoxidil	Hirsutism
Oxytocin	SIADH
Sulfa drugs	Allergies, kernicterus in neonates

GI, gastrointestinal; HMG CoA, 3-hydroxy-3-methylglutaryl-coenzyme A; SIADH, syndrome of inappropriate secretion of antidiuretic hormone.

TABLE 25-2 Antidotes

POISONING OR OVERDOSE	ANTIDOTE
Acetaminophen	Acetylcysteine
Benzodiazepines	Flumazenil
β-Blockers	Glucagon
Carbon monoxide	Oxygen (hyperbaric if severe)
Cholinesterase inhibitors	Atropine, pralidoxime
Copper or gold	Penicillamine
Digoxin	Normalize potassium and other electrolytes, digoxin antibodies
Iron	Deferoxamine
Lead	Edetate
Methanol or ethylene glycol	Fomepizole, ethanol
Muscarinic receptor blockers	Physostigmine
Opioids	Naloxone
Quinidine or tricyclic antidepressants	Sodium bicarbonate (cardioprotective)

HORMONE REPLACEMENT THERAPY AND ORAL CONTRACEPTIVES

Hormone Replacement Therapy and Oral Contraceptives

See Chapter 11 for a complete discussion of these topics.

ANALGESICS AND ANTIINFLAMMATORIES

Effects

Aspirin and nonsteroidal antiinflammatory drugs (NSAIDs) inhibit cyclooxygenase (COX) centrally and peripherally, giving them antiinflammatory, antipyretic, analgesic, and antiplatelet properties. Whereas aspirin inhibits COX irreversibly and thus for the life of the platelet, other NSAIDs inhibit COX reversibly. COX-2 inhibitors only inhibit the COX-2 isozyme and thus have no antiplatelet effects. Acetaminophen is mostly central acting; thus, it is only an analgesic and antipyretic with no platelet or antiinflammatory effects. Toxicity and side effect issues:

○ Aspirin and other NSAIDs can cause gastrointestinal (GI) upset, GI bleeding, and gastric ulcers; aspirin can aggravate gout. Always consider GI bleeding and ulcer in any patient taking aspirin or NSAIDs. COX-2 inhibitors (e.g., celecoxib) or an NSAID–prostaglandin E1 combination can help prevent GI damage, although the COX-2 inhibitors may not be as protective against GI bleeding as initially thought.

○ NSAIDs also can cause renal damage (interstitial nephritis and papillary necrosis), especially in patients who are dehydrated, who take them chronically, and who have preexisting renal disease. Renal insufficiency can be seen with long-term use of NSAIDs and can occur acutely in patients with significant renal artery stenosis.

○ Higher aspirin doses cause tinnitus, vertigo, respiratory alkalosis and metabolic acidosis, hyperthermia, coma, and death.

○ Aspirin can be removed by dialysis in severe overdose.

○ Do not give aspirin to people with asthma and nasal polyps. Hypersensitivity reactions are extremely common in this group; look for nasal polyps in anyone with an asthmatic-type reaction to aspirin (people with asthma can have an asthma attack after taking aspirin—even those without nasal polyps).

○ Do not give aspirin to children younger than 19 years who have fever or viral infection; it can cause Reye syndrome (look for encephalopathy and liver dysfunction).

○ Acetaminophen causes liver toxicity in high doses because of depletion of glutathione. Treat with acetylcysteine.

Low-dose aspirin has been proved to be of benefit in reducing the risk of myocardial infarction in patients who have had a previous myocardial infarction and patients with stable or unstable angina who have not had an infarction. The 2008 American College of Chest Physicians clinical practice guidelines on antithrombotic and thrombolytic therapy recommends that all patients with chronic stable angina or other clinical or laboratory evidence of coronary artery disease receive aspirin indefinitely.

The data on the use of aspirin for primary prevention of myocardial infarction are inconclusive. However, aspirin is recommended in all people with diabetes who have cardiovascular disease and for primary prevention in people with diabetes with one or more risk factors (e.g., age older than 40 years, cigarette smoking, hypertension, hyperlipidemia, obesity, albuminuria, or family history of cardiovascular disease). The risks of aspirin prophylaxis may outweigh the benefits in patients with a history of liver disease, kidney disease, peptic ulcer disease or GI bleeding, poorly controlled hypertension, or a bleeding disorder.

Low-dose aspirin is of proven benefit in reducing strokes in patients with transient ischemic attacks (TIAs), previous stroke, or known carotid artery stenosis. However, the risks may outweigh the benefits, as mentioned in the paragraph above, especially in patients with uncontrolled hypertension, which, coupled with aspirin, can increase the risk of a hemorrhagic stroke.

IMPORTANT POINTS

1. Give aspirin to any patient in the emergency department who has unstable angina, myocardial infarction, or transient ischemic attack (if computed tomography of the brain shows no hemorrhage).

2. Stop aspirin 1 week before surgery; stop other NSAIDs on the day before surgery.

QR CODE

The QR code includes three USMLE-style questions and answers. For more questions, redeem the PIN code on the inside cover for the Crush Step 2 question bank powered by USMLE Consult.

Please see the Introduction for instructions on how to access content using the QR codes.

Question

Which of the following medications is most likely to cause a clinically significant induction of liver enzymes, potentially resulting in increased metabolism of other drugs?

(A) Cimetidine

(B) Penicillin

(C) Phenobarbital

(D) Lansoprazole

(E) Fluoxetine

26 PREVENTIVE MEDICINE, EPIDEMIOLOGY, AND BIOSTATISTICS

PREVENTIVE MEDICINE

Guidelines for cancer screening are given in Table 26-1. Table 26-2 gives vaccination guidelines for adults. For guidelines regarding general health screening in adults, please see the Internal Medicine chapter (Chapter 15). For guidelines regarding general health screening in children, please see the Pediatrics chapter (Chapter 24).

In general, urinalysis (screening for urinary tract cancer that results in hematuria), alpha fetoprotein (liver and testicular cancer), and other serum markers are not appropriate for screening asymptomatic patients with no physical findings, but look for these abnormal lab values to show up in Step 2 questions as a clue to diagnosis. Prostate-specific antigen (PSA) is somewhat controversial as a prostate cancer screening test, and it does not replace a rectal exam.

EPIDEMIOLOGY

○ **Incidence:** The number of new cases of disease in a unit of time (generally 1 year, but any time frame can be used). Incidence rate also equals the absolute risk (to be differentiated from relative or attributable risk).
○ **Prevalence:** The total number of cases of disease that exist (new or old)

IMPORTANT POINTS

1. The classic question about incidence and prevalence: When a disease can be treated and people can be kept alive longer but the disease cannot be cured, what happens to the incidence and prevalence? Answer: Nothing happens to incidence, but prevalence will increase as people live longer. In short-term diseases, such as the flu, incidence may be higher than prevalence, but in chronic diseases, such as diabetes mellitus, prevalence is greater than incidence.
2. An epidemic occurs when the observed incidence greatly exceeds the expected incidence.

Per-year rates commonly used to compare groups:
○ **Birth rate:** Live births per 1000 population
○ **Fertility rate:** Live births per 1000 population of women ages 15 to 45 years
○ **Death rate:** Deaths per 1000 population
○ **Neonatal mortality rate:** Neonatal deaths (in the first 28 days) per 1000 live births; the rate in the United States is roughly six in 1000 (higher in blacks)

TABLE 26-1 American Cancer Society Guidelines for Cancer Screening in Asymptomatic Patients*

CANCER	PROCEDURE	AGE (Y)	FREQUENCY
Colorectal	Colonoscopy or Flexible sigmoidoscopy or Double contrast barium enema or CT colonography or Fecal occult blood test or Fecal immunochemical test or Stool DNA test	>50 for all studies†	Every 10 years Every 5 years Every 5 years Every 5 years Annually Annually Interval uncertain
Colon, prostate	Digital rectal exam	>40	Annually
Prostate	Prostate specific antigen test	>50‡ Do not screen if life expectancy is <10 years	Offer to patients annually (still controversial)
Cervical	Pap smear	Beginning at age 21 years regardless of sexual activity	If conventional Pap test is used, test annually, then every 2–3 y for women ≥30 years old who have had three negative cytology tests results. If Pap and HPV testing are used, test every 3 years if both HPV and cytology results are negative.
Gynecologic	Pelvic examination	21–64	Annually; every 2–3 y after three normal exams
		≥65	Annually; when to stop is not clearly established
Endometrial	Endometrial biopsy		No recommendation for routine screening in the absence of symptoms
Breast	Breast self-examination	>20	Benefits and limitations should be discussed, but breast self-examination is no longer recommended by the American Cancer Society
Breast	Physician exam	20–40	Every 3 y
		>40	Annually
Breast	Mammography	>40	Annually
Lung	Sputum, chest radiography, CT scan		Testing is not recommended for asymptomatic individuals even if they are at high risk

*This table is for screening of asymptomatic, healthy patients. Other guidelines exist, but you'll be fine if you follow this table for boards (controversial areas are not generally tested).
†Individuals with a family history of colon cancer, a personal history of inflammatory bowel disease, and certain inheritable syndromes such as familial adenomatous polyposis should be screened earlier.
‡Start at age 45 years in African Americans and at age 40 years for patients with a first-degree relative diagnosed with prostate cancer at an early age.
CT, computed tomography; HPV, human papillomavirus.

○ **Perinatal mortality rate:** Neonatal deaths plus stillbirths and deaths in the first 7 days of life per 1000 total births. A stillbirth (fetal death) is defined as a prenatal or natal death after 20 weeks' gestation. In the United States, the major cause is prematurity and the rate is higher in nonwhites.
○ **Infant mortality rate:** Deaths (from 0–1 year old) per 1000 live births. The top three causes in the United States, in descending order, are congenital abnormalities, low birth weight, and sudden infant death syndrome.
○ **Maternal mortality rate:** Maternal pregnancy-related deaths (deaths during pregnancy or in the first 42 days after delivery) per 100,000 live births. The top three causes in the United States are pulmonary embolism, pregnancy-induced hypertension, and hemorrhage. The risk increases with age and is higher in blacks.

Insurance and the government:
○ Medicare is health insurance run by the federal government for people who are eligible for Social Security (primarily people older than 65 years as well as the permanently and totally disabled and patients with end-stage renal disease).
○ Medicaid is state-run health insurance that covers indigent people who are deemed eligible by the individual states.

TABLE 26-2 Immunizations in Adults

VACCINE	WHICH ADULTS SHOULD RECEIVE THE VACCINATION
Hepatitis B	Adolescents through 18 years of age and adults at increased risk of hepatitis B virus infection (including health care workers).
Herpes zoster	Approved for adults ≥60 years of age to help reduce the risk of developing zoster (shingles).
Human papillomavirus	Quadrivalent human papillomavirus (HPV) recombinant vaccine is FDA approved in girls and women ages 9–26 years to prevent cervical cancer, vaginal and vulvar cancer, precancerous genital lesions, and genital warts. It is also approved for use in boys and men ages 9–26 years to prevent genital warts.
Influenza	Anyone who wants to reduce their chances of getting the flu can get vaccinated. It is recommended for people who are at high risk of having serious flu complications or people who live with or care for those at high risk for serious complications. People who should get vaccinated each year are children ages 6 months to 18 years, women who will be pregnant during the flu season, people who are immunosuppressed, adults ages ≥50 years, people with chronic medical conditions (pulmonary, cardiovascular, renal, hepatic, hematologic, or metabolic disorders [including diabetes]), people who live in nursing homes and other long-term care facilities, health care personnel, household contacts and caregivers of children ages <5 years and adults >50 years, and household contacts and caregivers for those at high risk of serious flu complications.
Pneumococcus	All adults ≥65 years of age; people ages 2–64 years with chronic cardiovascular disease, COPD, or diabetes mellitus; people ages 2–64 years with functional or anatomic asplenia; people ages 2–64 years with alcoholism, chronic liver disease, or CSF leak.
Rubella	All women of childbearing age who lack immunity or history of immunization. Do not give to pregnant women. Women should avoid pregnancy for 4 weeks after the vaccine. Also give to health care workers (to protect pregnant women's unborn children). Give to susceptible adolescents and adults without evidence of immunity. Do not give to immunocompromised patients (except HIV-positive patients).
Tetanus (Td and Tdap)	All people should be given a tetanus booster every 10 years. Give tetanus prophylaxis for any wound if vaccination history is unknown or patient has received less than three total doses. Give tetanus booster in people with full vaccination history if more than 5 years have passed since the last dose for all wounds other than clean, minor wounds (including burns). Give tetanus immunoglobulin with vaccine for patients with unknown/incomplete vaccination and nonclean or major wounds. Adults (ages 11–64) should receive a single dose of Tdap to replace a single dose of Td if they received their last dose of Td ≥10 years earlier. Adults who have or anticipate having close contact with an infant age <12 months should receive a single dose of Tdap. When possible, women should receive Tdap before conception. Pregnant women should receive Tdap in the immediate postpartum period. Health care workers should receive Tdap. Tdap is preferred to Td if prophylaxis is indicated for a wound. Adults ≥65 years of age should get Td (not Tdap) every 10 years.
Varicella	May be given to any person ≥12 months (including adults and adolescents) with no reliable history of previous vaccination or previous infection with the varicella virus. Contraindications include pregnancy, immunosuppressant therapy, leukemia, lymphoma, active untreated tuberculosis, and immunodeficiency states such as AIDS.

COPD, chronic pulmonary disease; CSF, cerebrospinal fluid; HPV, human papillomavirus; Td, diphtheria and tetanus; Tdap, diphtheria, pertussis, tetanus.

BIOSTATISTICS

The 2 × 2 table and its derivatives

Review this section of Step 1 material for some easy (hopefully) points.

When faced with these types of questions, get in the habit of drawing a 2 × 2 table to make calculations easier:

		DISEASE		TEST NAME	FORMULA
		(+)	(−)	Sensitivity	$A/(A + C)$
				Specificity	$D/(B + D)$
Test or	(+)	A	B	PPV	$A/(A + B)$
Exposure	(−)	C	D	NPV	$D/(C + D)$
				Odds ratio	$(A \times D)/(B \times C)$
				Relative risk	$[A/(A + B)]/[C/(C + D)]$
				Attributable risk	$[A/(A + B)]−[C/(C + D)]$

Sensitivity and Specificity

Sensitivity is the ability to detect disease. Mathematically, sensitivity is calculated by dividing the number of true positives by the number of people with the disease. Tests with high sensitivity are used for screening. They might have false positives but do not miss many people with the disease (low false-negative rate).

Specificity is the ability to detect health (or nondisease). Mathematically, specificity is calculated by dividing the number of true negatives by the number of people without the disease. Tests with high specificity are used for disease confirmation. They might have false negatives but do not call anyone sick who is actually healthy (low false-positive rate). The ideal confirmatory test must have high sensitivity and high specificity; otherwise, people with the disease may be called healthy.

The trade-off between sensitivity and specificity is a classic statistics question. Understand how changing the cut-off glucose value in screening for diabetes (or changing the value of any of several screening tests) will change the number of true and false negatives and true and false positives. For example, if the cut-off value of glucose is raised, fewer people will be called diabetic (more false negatives, fewer false positives), but if the cut-off value is lowered, more people will be called diabetic (fewer false negatives, more false positives).

 The sensitivity and specificity of a test is an innate characteristic of the test and cannot be altered by the composition of a certain population. In contrast, the positive predictive value and negative predictive value can change depending on the prevalence of a disease in a given population.

Predictive Values

When a test result comes back positive for disease, the positive predictive value (PPV) measures how likely it is that the patient has the disease (probability of having a condition, given a positive test). Mathematically, PPV is calculated by dividing the number of true positives by the number of people with a positive test result. PPV depends on the prevalence of a disease (the higher the prevalence, the greater the PPV) and the sensitivity and specificity of the test (e.g., an overly sensitive test that gives more false positives has a lower PPV).

When a test comes back negative for disease, the negative predictive value (NPV) measures how likely it is that the patient is healthy and does not have the disease (probability of not having a condition, given a negative test result). Mathematically, NPV is calculated by dividing the number of true negatives by the number of people with a negative test result. NPV depends on prevalence and the sensitivity and specificity, just like PPV. The higher the prevalence, the lower the NPV. In addition, an overly sensitive test with lots of false positives will make the NPV higher.

Risk

Odds ratio (OR) is used only for retrospective studies (e.g., case-control). OR compares disease in exposed and nondisease in unexposed populations with disease in unexposed and nondisease in exposed populations to determine whether there is a difference between the two. Of course, there should be more disease in exposed than unexposed populations and more nondisease in unexposed than exposed populations. OR is a less than perfect way to estimate relative risk.

Relative risk (RR) compares the disease risk in the exposed population with the disease risk in the unexposed population. RR can be calculated only after prospective or experimental studies; it cannot be calculated from retrospective data. RR greater than 1 is clinically significant.

Attributable risk is the number of cases attributable to one risk factor; in other words, it is the amount by which you can expect the incidence to decrease if a risk factor is removed. For example, if the incidence rate of lung cancer in the general population is 1 in 100 and in smokers it is 10 in 100, the attributable risk of smoking in causing lung cancer is nine in 100 (assuming a properly matched control).

Accuracy and Precision

Reliability of a test (synonymous with precision) measures the reproducibility and consistency of a test (e.g., the concept of interrater reliability: If two different people administer the same test, they will get the same score if the test is reliable). Random error reduces reliability and precision (e.g., limitation in significant figures).

Validity of a test (synonymous with accuracy) measures the trueness of measurement—whether the test measures what it claims to measure. For example, if you give a valid IQ test to a genius, the test should not indicate that he or she is retarded. Systematic error reduces validity and accuracy (e.g., miscalibrated equipment).

The Bell Curve and its Variations

Standard deviation (SD): With a normal or bell-shaped distribution, 1 SD holds 68% of values, 2 SD holds 95% of values, and 3 SD holds 99.7% of values centered around the mean. The classic question gives you the mean and SD and asks you what percentage of values will be above a given value. For example, if the mean score on a test is 80 and the SD is 5, 68% of the scores will be within 5 points of 80 (scores of 75–85), and 95% of the scores will be within 10 points of 80 (scores of 70–90). The question may ask what percentage of scores are over 90. The answer is 2.5% because 2.5% of the scores fall below 70, and 2.5% of the scores are over 90. Variations on this question are also common.

In a normal distribution, the mean = median = mode. The mean is the average value, the median is the middle value, and the mode is the most common value. Questions might give you several numbers and ask for their mean, median, and mode. For example, if the question gives you the numbers 2, 2, 4, and 8:

○ The **mean** is the average of the 4 numbers: 2 + 2 + 4 + 8/4 = 16/4 = 4.
○ The **median** is the middle value. Because there are four numbers, there is no true middle value. Therefore, take the average between the two middle numbers (2 and 4). The median = 3.
○ The **mode** is 2, because the number 2 appears twice (more times than any other value).

Skewed distribution: A positive skew is asymmetry with an excess of high values (tail on right, mean > median > mode); a negative skew is asymmetry with an excess of low values (tail on left, mean < median < mode). These are not normal distributions; thus, the SD and mean are less meaningful values.

HYPOTHESIS TESTING, DATA COMPARISONS, AND CONFIDENCE INTERVAL

Correlation Coefficient

The correlation coefficient measures the degree of relationship between two values. The range of the coefficient is −1 to +1. Zero equals no association whatsoever, +1 equals a perfect positive correlation (when one variable increases, so does the other), and −1 equals a perfect negative correlation (when one variable increases, the other decreases). Use the absolute value to give you the strength of the correlation (e.g., −0.3 is a stronger correlation than +0.2).

Comparison of Data

○ Chi-square test: Used to compare percentages or proportions (nonnumeric data, also called nominal data)
○ T-test: Used to compare two means
○ Analysis of variance (ANOVA): Used to compare three or more means

Confidence Interval

When you take a set of data and calculate a mean, you want to say that it is equivalent to the mean of the whole population, but usually they are not exactly equal. The confidence interval (CI; usually set at 95%) says that you are 95% confident that the population mean is within a certain range (usually within two SDs of the experimental or derived mean). For example, if you sample the heart rate of 100 people and calculate a mean of 80 beats/min and an SD of 2 beats/min, your CI (confidence limits) would be written as 76 < X < 84 = 0.95. This means that you are 95% certain that the mean heart rate of the whole population (X) is between 76 and 84 beats/min.

P Value

The board exam always contains one or more questions about the significance of the P value. If someone tells you P <.05 for a given set of data, there is less than a 5% chance (because 0.05 = 5%) that these data were obtained by random error or chance. If P <.01, the chance that the data were obtained by random error or chance is less than 1%. For example, if I tell you that the blood pressure in my controls is 180/100 mm Hg but decreases to 120/70 mm Hg after administration of drug X and that P <.10, there is less than a 10% chance that the difference in blood pressure was attributable to random error or chance. However, there is up to a 9.99% chance that the result is attributable to random error or chance. Somewhat arbitrarily chosen, P <.05 is commonly used as the cutoff number for statistical significance in medicine.

Three points to remember:

○ The study might still have serious flaws.
○ A low P value does not imply causation.
○ A study that has statistical significance does not necessarily have clinical significance.

For example, if I tell you that drug X can lower the blood pressure from 130/80 to 128/80, P <.00001, you still would not use drug X (because of cost and potential side effects relative to the minimal clinical benefit).

The P value also ties into the null hypothesis (the hypothesis of no difference). For example, in a drug study about hypertension, the null hypothesis is that the drug does not work; any difference in blood pressure is attributable to random error or chance. When the drug works beautifully and lowers the blood pressure by 60 points, we don't accept (i.e., we reject) the null hypothesis because clearly the drug works. If that lowering of blood pressure is accompanied by a calculated P value <.05, we can confidently reject the null hypothesis because the P value tells us that there is less than a 5% chance that the null hypothesis is correct. If the null hypothesis is incorrect, the difference in blood pressure is not attributable to chance and must be attributable to the new drug. In other words, the P value represents the chance of making a type I error (claiming an effect or difference when none exists, rejecting the null hypothesis when it is true). If P <.07, there is less than a 7% chance that you are making a type I error. A type II error is to accept the null hypothesis when it is false (e.g., the hypertension drug works, but you say that it does not).

Power

Power is the probability of rejecting the null hypothesis when it is false (a good thing). The best way to increase power (and thus reduce the risk of making a type II error) is to increase sample size.

Study Types and Errors

Different types of studies (listed in decreasing order of quality and desirability):

○ **Experimental:** The gold standard, which compares two equal groups in which one variable is manipulated and its effect is measured. Remember to use double blinding (or at least single blinding) and well-matched controls.
○ **Prospective** (aka longitudinal, cohort, incidence, or follow-up): Choose a sample and divide it into two groups based on presence or absence of a risk factor and follow the group over time to see what diseases they develop (e.g., follow people with and without asymptomatic hypercholesterolemia to see whether people with hypercholesterolemia have a higher incidence of myocardial infarction [MI] later in life). This approach is sometimes called an observational study because all you do is observe. Relative risk and incidence can be calculated. Whereas prospective studies are time consuming, expensive, and good for common diseases, retrospective studies are less expensive, less time consuming, and good for rare diseases.
○ **Retrospective or case control:** Samples are chosen after the fact based on presence (cases) or absence (controls) of disease. Information can then be collected about risk factors; for example, look at people with lung cancer versus people without lung cancer and see if the people with lung cancer smoke more. An OR can be calculated, but you cannot calculate a true relative risk or measure incidence from a retrospective study.
○ **Case series:** Good for extremely rare diseases (as are retrospective studies). Case series simply describe the clinical presentation of people with a certain disease and might suggest the need for a retrospective study.
○ **Prevalence survey or cross-sectional survey:** Looks at prevalence of a disease and the prevalence of risk factors. When comparing two different cultures, you might get an idea about the cause of a disease, which can be tested with a prospective study (e.g., more colon cancer and higher-fat diet in the United States vs. less colon cancer and low-fat diet in Japan).

Experimental Conclusions and Errors

The exam might give you data and the experimenter's conclusion and ask you to explain why the conclusion should not be drawn or to point out flaws in the experimental design.

○ **Confounding variables:** An unmeasured variable affects both the independent (manipulated, experimental variable) and dependent (outcome) variables. For example, an experimenter measures the number of ashtrays owned and the incidence of lung cancer and finds that people with lung cancer have more ashtrays. He or she concludes that ashtrays cause lung cancer. Smoking tobacco is the confounding variable because it causes the increase in both ashtrays and lung cancer.

○ **Nonrandom or nonstratified sampling:** City A and city B can be compared but might not be equivalent. For example, if city A is a retirement community and city B is a college town, of course city A will have higher rates of mortality and heart disease if the groups are not stratified into appropriate age-specific comparisons.

○ **Nonresponse bias:** People fail to return surveys or answer the phone for a phone survey. If nonresponse is a significant percentage of the results, the experiment will suffer. The first strategy is to visit or call the nonresponders repeatedly in an attempt to reach them and get their responses. If this strategy is unsuccessful, list the nonresponders as unknown in the data analysis and see if any results can be salvaged. Never make up or assume responses!

○ **Lead time bias:** Caused by time differentials. The classic example is a cancer screening test that claims to have prolonged survival compared with old survival data when in fact the measured difference in survival (i.e., elapsed time from diagnosis until death) is attributable only to earlier detection, not to improved treatment or prolonged survival.

○ **Admission rate bias:** In comparing hospital A with hospital B for mortality from MI, you find that hospital A has a higher mortality rate. But this finding may be because of tougher hospital admission criteria at hospital A, which admits only the sickest patients with MI and thus has higher mortality rates, although their care may be superior. The same bias can be found in a surgeon's mortality and morbidity rates if the surgeon takes only tough cases.

○ **Recall bias:** Risk for retrospective studies. When patients cannot remember, they might inadvertently over- or underestimate risk factors. For example, whereas John died of lung cancer, and his angry wife remembers him as smoking "like a chimney," Mike died of a non–smoking-related cause, and his loving wife denies that he smoked "much." In fact, both men smoked 1 pack per day.

○ **Interviewer bias:** Caused by a lack of blinding. A scientist gets big money to do a study and wants to find a difference between cases and controls. Thus, he or she inadvertently labels the same patient comment or outcome as "no significance" in controls and "serious difference" in treated cases.

○ **Unacceptability bias:** Patients in experiments want to be "acceptable" to the person conducting the study; thus, they might not admit to embarrassing behavior or might claim to take experimental medications when in fact they spit them out.

QR CODE

The QR code includes three USMLE-style questions and answers. For more questions, redeem the PIN code on the inside cover for the Crush Step 2 question bank powered by USMLE Consult.

Please see the Introduction for instructions on how to access content using the QR codes.

Question

An experimenter does a prospective study after placing 50,000 subjects who are equally matched for demographic and lifestyle variables into one of two groups based on the number of pills they take each day (<three pills, >three pills). He measures only the number of pills subjects take and their mortality data over a 5-year period. He notes that subjects who take more pills are more likely to die and concludes that medications cause an unacceptable number of deaths. Which of the following is the most likely reason for his conclusion to be invalid?
(A) Nonrandom bias
(B) Lead-time bias
(C) Confounding variables
(D) Type II error
(E) Interviewer bias

27 PSYCHIATRY

ANTIPSYCHOTIC MEDICATIONS

Features of antipsychotic medications are listed in Table 27-1. Extrapyramidal side effects:

○ **Acute dystonia:** First few hours or days of treatment. The patient has muscle spasms or stiffness (e.g., torticollis, trismus), tongue protrusions and twisting, opisthotonos, and oculogyric crisis (forced sustained deviation of the head and eyes). Most common in young men. Treat by giving anticholinergics (benztropine, trihexyphenidyl). Diphenhydramine acts as both an antihistamine and an anticholinergic, so it is frequently used as well.

○ **Akathisia:** First few days of treatment. The patient has a subjective feeling of restlessness. Look for constant pacing, alternate sitting and standing, and an inability to sit still. β-Blockers can be tried for treatment.

○ **Parkinsonism:** First few months of treatment. The patient has stiffness, cogwheel rigidity, shuffling gait, masklike facies, and drooling. Parkinsonism is most common in older women. Treat by giving antihistamines (diphenhydramine) or anticholinergics (benztropine, trihexyphenidyl).

○ **Tardive dyskinesia:** Occurs after years of treatment. Most commonly, the patient has perioral movements (darting, protruding movements of the tongue; chewing; grimacing; puckering). The patient also can have involuntary, choreoathetoid movements of the head, limbs, and trunk. There is no known treatment for tardive dyskinesia. If you have to make a choice when the patient develops tardive dyskinesia, discontinue the antipsychotic and consider switching to a newer antipsychotic (e.g., risperidone, clozapine). Drug holidays (periods of time when the patient is off medication) may be helpful, too.

○ **Neuroleptic malignant syndrome:** Life-threatening condition (≤20% mortality rate) that can develop **at any time** during treatment. The patient has rigidity, mutism, obtundation, agitation, **high fever** (up to 107°F), **high creatine phosphokinase** (often >5000 U/L), sweating, and myoglobinuria. Treatment: **First** discontinue the antipsychotic; then administer benzodiazepines and provide supportive care for fever. Watch for renal failure caused by myoglobinuria. Finally, consider giving **dantrolene** (as in malignant hyperthermia).

Other antipsychotic medication pearls:

○ **Dopamine blockade** causes increases in prolactin (dopamine is a prolactin-inhibiting factor in the tuberoinfundibular tract), which can cause galactorrhea, impotence, menstrual dysfunction, and decreased libido.

○ **Classic antipsychotic side effects:** Thioridazine causes retinal pigment deposits, clozapine causes agranulocytosis (white blood cells counts must be monitored), and chlorpromazine causes jaundice and photosensitivity.

○ **Side effects of the atypical antipsychotics:**
  ○ Olanzapine causes weight gain, sedation, hypotension, and dry mouth.
  ○ Quetiapine causes sedation, orthostatic hypotension, akathisia, weight gain, and dry mouth.
  ○ Ziprasidone causes nausea, weakness, and mild QT prolongation.
  ○ Aripiprazole causes headache, nausea, akathisia, tremor, and constipation.
  ○ Paliperidone causes parkinsonism, dystonia, dyskinesia, akathisia, and QT prolongation.
  ○ Clozapine causes orthostatic hypotension, weight gain, metabolic syndrome, sedation, and constipation (in addition to the agranulocytosis mentioned above).

TABLE 27-1 Features of Antipsychotic Medications

FEATURE	ANTIPSYCHOTIC MEDICATION		
	High Potency	**Low Potency**	**Atypical***
Example(s)	Haloperidol	Chlorpromazine	Risperidone, olanzapine, aripiprazole, paliperidone, quetiapine, ziprasidone
Extrapyramidal side effects	High incidence	Low incidence	Low incidence
Autonomic side effects†	Low incidence	High incidence	Medium incidence
Positive symptoms	Works well	Works well	Works well
Negative symptoms	Works poorly	Works poorly	Works somewhat well

*Atypical, newer agents are the drugs of choice for maintenance therapy because of reduced extrapyramidal side effects and potential effect on negative symptoms. Choose them over older agents.
†Autonomic side effects include anticholinergic (dry mouth, urinary retention, blurry vision, mydriasis), α_1-blockade (orthostatic hypotension), and antihistamine (sedation) effects.

SCHIZOPHRENIA

The five main diagnostic criteria (Box 27-1) provide clues: delusions, hallucinations, disorganized speech, grossly disorganized or catatonic behavior, and negative symptoms (flat affect, refusal to talk, avolition, apathy). Factors indicating prognosis are listed in Table 27-2.
- **Time period** is important: Less than 1 month = acute psychotic episode; 1 to 6 months = schizophreniform disorder; longer than 6 months = schizophrenia
- Typical **age of onset** is 15 to 25 years for men (look for someone going to college and deteriorating) and 25 to 35 years for women.
- **Suicide:** Up to 10% of schizophrenics eventually commit suicide (past attempt is the best predictor of eventual success).
  Subtypes: Schizophrenia can be divided into five subtypes:
- **Paranoid:** Patients have delusions and hallucinations but do not exhibit disorganized behavior or affective flattening.
- **Disorganized:** Patients have very disorganized thoughts and behaviors with poor functional status.
- **Catatonic:** Patients have little interaction with the environment and maintain odd postures (called waxy flexibility).
- **Residual:** Patients experience something like a partial remission with periods of decreased symptoms.
- **Undifferentiated:** This includes patients who don't fit into one of the first four groups.
  Antipsychotic medications are the mainstay of therapy, but psychosocial treatment has been shown to improve outcome. Medications are used first, but the best treatment (as in most of psychiatry) is medications plus therapy.

 Roughly 1% of people have schizophrenia (in all cultures).

 In the United States, most patients with schizophrenia are born in the winter (not known why).

 Psychiatric patients can be hospitalized against their will if they are a danger to themselves (suicidal or unable to take care of themselves) or others (homicidal).

Schizoaffective disorder is a combination of mood disorder (bipolar disorder, depression) and schizophrenia. To make the diagnosis, patients must have exhibited periods of psychosis without mood symptoms in addition to periods of mood symptoms while psychotic.

BOX 27-1 SYMPTOMS OF SCHIZOPHRENIA

Positive Symptoms	**Negative Symptoms**
Delusions	Flat affect
Hallucinations	Alogia (no speech)
Bizarre behavior	Avolition (apathy)
Thought disorder	Anhedonia
Poor attention	

TABLE 27-2 Prognosis for Schizophrenia

GOOD PROGNOSTIC FACTORS	POOR PROGNOSTIC FACTORS
Good premorbid functioning	Poor premorbid functioning
Late onset	Early onset
Obvious precipitating factors	No precipitating factors
Married	Single, divorced, widowed
Family history of mood disorders	Family history of schizophrenia
Positive symptoms	Negative symptoms
Good support system	Poor support system

BIPOLAR DISORDER

○ **Mania** is the only symptom required for a diagnosis of bipolar disorder, but a history of mania alternating with depression is classic.
○ **Mania symptoms:** Decreased need for sleep, pressured speech, sexual promiscuity, shopping sprees, and exaggerated self-importance or delusions of grandeur.
  ○ **Mnemonic: DIGFAST**—distractibility, indiscretion (i.e., promiscuity), grandiosity, flight of ideas, activity increase, sleep (decreased need), talkative
  ○ To make the diagnosis, the patient must meet three of these seven criteria if they have an elevated mood or four of these seven criteria if they are irritable.
○ Look for an initial onset between 16 and 30 years of age.
○ Lithium and valproic acid are first-line treatments. Typical antipsychotics (haloperidol), atypical antipsychotics (risperidone, quetiapine, clozapine, ziprasidone, aripiprazole), carbamazepine, and gabapentin are second-line agents. Lithium can cause renal dysfunction (e.g., diabetes insipidus), thyroid dysfunction, tremor, and central nervous system (CNS) effects at toxic levels. Valproic acid can cause liver dysfunction, and carbamazepine can cause bone marrow depression. Antipsychotics may be needed if the patient becomes psychotic; use at the same time as a mood stabilizer.
○ **Bipolar II disorder** is **hypomania** (mild mania without psychosis that does not cause occupational dysfunction) plus major depression. **Cyclothymia** is at least 2 years of **hypomania** alternating with dysthymia (see below). There is *no* full-blown mania or depression.

DEPRESSION

Patients might not directly say, "I'm depressed." You have to watch for clues, such as a change in sleep habits (classically insomnia), vague somatic complaints, anxiety, low energy or fatigue, a change in appetite (classically decreased appetite), poor concentration, psychomotor retardation, or anhedonia (loss of pleasure).

The most commonly used mnemonic for the symptoms of depression is SIGECAPS: sleep (poor), interest (poor), guilt, energy (little), concentration (poor), appetite (poor), psychomotor retardation, and suicidal thoughts. To make the diagnosis, patients must have five or more of these during the same 2-week period.

Patients might or might not have obvious precipitating factors in the history, such as loss of a loved one, divorce or separation, unemployment or retirement, or chronic or debilitating disease. Depression is more common in women.

Adjustment Disorder with Depressed Mood

When a bad situation occurs, the patient does not handle it well and feels "bummed out" for less than 6 months but does not meet criteria for full-blown depression. For example, the patient gets a divorce, seems to cry a lot for the next few weeks, and leaves work early on most days.

 Antidepressants can trigger mania or hypomania, especially in bipolar patients. Always ask about any history of manic or hypomanic episodes before prescribing an antidepressant.

Dysthymia

Depressed mood on most days for more than 2 years with no episodes of major depression, mania, hypomania, or psychosis. Usually difficult to treat.

Treatment

Treat with both antidepressants and psychotherapy (combination works better than medications alone). Selective serotonin reuptake inhibitors (SSRIs) usually are the preferred first-line agents. Other options include serotonin–norepinephrine reuptake inhibitors (SNRIs) and the tricyclic antidepressants. Bupropion and mirtazapine have unique modes of action.

Antidepressants:

○ The **SSRIs** (e.g., fluoxetine, paroxetine, citalopram) prevent reuptake of serotonin only and have less serious side effects (e.g., insomnia, anorexia, **sexual dysfunction**).

○ The **SNRIs** (e.g., venlafaxine, duloxetine, desvenlafaxine) are a newer group of antidepressants that prevent reuptake of serotonin and norepinephrine. The side effects of SNRIs are similar to those of SSRIs but also include noradrenergic symptoms such as sweating and dizziness. Watch for orthostatic hypotension, nausea, fatigue, and dry mouth.

○ The **tricyclic antidepressants** (TCAs; e.g., nortriptyline, amitriptyline) prevent reuptake of norepinephrine and serotonin. They also block α-adrenergic receptors (watch for orthostatic hypotension, dizziness, and falls) and muscarinic receptors (watch for anticholinergic effects such as dry mouth, blurred vision, constipation, and urinary retention), cause sedation, and lower the seizure threshold (especially bupropion, which technically is not a TCA). TCAs are dangerous in overdose primarily because of **cardiac arrhythmias** (look for a widened QRS interval and QT prolongation), which might respond to bicarbonate.

○ **Monoamine oxidase inhibitors** (MAOIs; e.g., phenelzine, tranylcypromine) are older medications and are rarely used. They may be good for atypical depression (look for hypersomnia and hyperphagia, the opposite of classic depression). When patients eat tyramine-containing foods (especially wine and cheese), they may get a hypertensive crisis. *Do not* give MAOIs at the same time as SSRIs or meperidine; severe reactions can occur, possibly including death (serotonin syndrome).

○ **Trazodone** is a notorious cause of priapism (persistent, painful erection without sexual arousal or desire). It is seldom used anymore for depression, but it is used as a sleep aid for insomnia.

○ Keep in mind that antidepressants can increase suicidality in patients. As patients respond to the medication, they get more energy before an improvement in mood, which makes them more likely to act on their feelings of sadness, guilt, and suicidality.

GRIEF

Normal versus pathologic grief, mourning, and bereavement:

○ **Initial grief after a loss** (e.g., death of a loved one) can include a state of shock, a feeling of numbness or bewilderment, distress, crying, sleep disturbances, decreased appetite, difficulty with concentrating, weight loss, and guilt (survivor guilt) **for up to 1 year**—in other words, the same symptoms as depression.

○ It is **normal** to have an illusion or hallucination about the deceased person, but a normal grieving person *knows* that it is an illusion or hallucination, but a depressed person believes that the illusion or hallucination is real.

○ **Intense yearning** (even years after the death) and even searching for the deceased are normal.
○ Feelings of worthlessness, psychomotor retardation, and suicidal ideation *are not* normal expressions of grief; they are signs of depression.

PERSONALITY DISORDERS

Personality disorders are lifelong disorders with no real treatment, although psychotherapy may be tried. They can be divided into 3 clusters: A, B, and C. A good way to remember which cluster is which is the following: A (weird), B (wild), C (worried). It is important to note that personality disorders represent an enduring pattern of behavior that deviates markedly from societal expectations.

Cluster A:
○ **Paranoid:** Patients think that everyone is out to get them (friends, too) and often start lawsuits. Characterized by an inherent and excessive mistrust for the rest of the world. Don't confuse this with paranoid schizophrenia, in which patients have delusions that make them paranoid (e.g., there is a chip in my head that the government placed there to watch me).
○ **Schizoid:** The classic loner; no friends and **no interest** in having friends. Don't confuse this with avoidant personality disorder in which patients want friends but are too afraid to seek them out.
○ **Schizotypal:** Bizarre beliefs (extrasensory perception, cults, superstition, illusions) and manner of speaking but no psychosis. When you are given a sample patient who comes into the office wearing a cape, makes references to tarot cards, and mentions that he or she chose you as a doctor because the letters of your name have a favorable energy, think schizotypal. Don't confuse this with schizophrenia in which patients are frankly delusional.

Cluster B:
○ **Antisocial:** Most frequently tested personality disorder. Patients have a long criminal record (con artists) and torture animals or set fires as children (a history of conduct disorder is required for this diagnosis). They are aggressive, do not pay bills or support children, often lie, and have no remorse or conscience. Strong association with alcoholism and drug abuse as well as somatization disorder. Most patients are male.
○ **Borderline:** Unstable mood, behavior, relationships (many bisexual), and self-image. Look for splitting (people are all good or all bad and may frequently change categories), suicide attempts, micropsychotic episodes (2 minutes of psychosis), impulsiveness, and constant crisis (see Glenn Close in the movie *Fatal Attraction*).
○ **Histrionic:** Overly dramatic, attention seeking, and inappropriately seductive; the patient must be the center of attention. More commonly occurs in women.
○ **Narcissistic:** Egocentric and lacking empathy; patients use others for their own gain or have a sense of entitlement.

Cluster C:
○ **Avoidant:** Patients have no friends but want them; they are afraid of criticism or rejection and avoid others (inferiority complex). Don't confuse with schizoid personality disorder in which patients have no desire to have friends.
○ **Dependent:** Patients cannot be (or do anything) alone; highly dependent on others (e.g., a wife who stays with a severely abusive husband).
○ **Obsessive-compulsive:** Patients are obsessed with rules, perfection, and organization, but they lack true obsessions or compulsions. They may seem anal retentive and stubborn. Rules are more important than objectives. Affect is restricted. Money is a frequent concern and is often hoarded. Patients with this personality disorder are not aware that their habits are excessive. More common in medical students (seriously!). Don't confuse with obsessive-compulsive disorder in which patients do know that their habits are excessive.

SUICIDE

The major risk factors are age older than 45 years; alcohol or substance abuse; history of rage or violence; prior suicide attempts; male sex (men successfully commit suicide three times more often than women, but women attempt it four times more often than men); prior psychiatric history; depression; recent loss or separation; loss of health; unemployment or retirement; and single, widowed, or divorced status.

Always ask patients about suicide (it does not make them more likely to commit the act). For patients who appear to be on the verge of committing suicide or have just unsuccessfully attempted suicide, acutely hospitalize these patients against their will. For patients who are more chronically suicidal, you can get the patient to agree to a "contract for safety" in which you and your patient come to an agreement that the patient will seek help before attempting suicide.

When patients come out of a deep depression, they are at increased risk for suicide. The antidepressant begins to work, and the patient gets more energy—just enough to carry out suicide plans.

If you have to choose on Step 2, the best predictor of future suicide is a past attempt.

Suicide rates are rising the fastest in 15- to 24-year-old individuals, but the greatest risk is in people older than 65 years.

OTHER PSYCHIATRIC DISORDERS

○ **Adjustment disorder:** Normal life experience (e.g., relationship breakup, failing grade, loss of job) is not handled well. Patients often are depressed (adjustment disorder with depressed mood) but *do not* meet the criteria for full-blown depression. For example, a high school girl who breaks up with her boyfriend may mope around the house, crying and not wanting to attend school or go out with her friends for a few weeks.

○ **Anorexia:** See child psychiatry section but note that anorexia can be present in adults as well.

○ **Dissociative fugue (also called psychogenic fugue or fugue state):** A reversible amnesia for personal identity including the memories, personality, and other identifying characteristics of individuality. It usually involves unplanned travel or wandering. There is complete amnesia for the fugue episode. The classic patient develops amnesia, travels, and assumes a new identity but does remember the event upon returning.

○ **Dissociative identity disorder** (old name: **multiple personality disorder**): This is the disorder most likely to be associated with childhood sexual abuse.

○ **Generalized anxiety disorder:** Patients worry about everything (e.g., career, family, future, relationships, money) at the same time. Symptoms are not as dramatic as in panic disorder; patients are just severe worriers. Treat with cognitive behavioral therapy and buspirone or SSRIs (both nonaddictive and nonsedating). Second-line treatment is benzodiazepines (addictive, sedating).

○ **Narcolepsy:** Daytime sleepiness; decreased rapid eye movement (REM) latency (patients go into REM as soon as they fall asleep); cataplexy (loss of muscle tone, falls); hypnopompic (as patient wakes up) and hypnagogic (as patient falls asleep) hallucinations. Treat with modafinil (a nonamphetamine stimulant), methylphenidate, or amphetamines.

○ **Obsessive-compulsive disorder:** Patients have recurrent thoughts or impulses (obsessions) or recurrent behavior or acts (compulsions) that cause marked dysfunction in their occupational or interpersonal lives. Look for **washing rituals** (e.g., wash hands 30 times a day) and **checking rituals** (check to see if door is locked 30 times a day). Onset usually is in adolescence or early adulthood. Treat with SSRIs (especially fluvoxamine) or clomipramine. Behavioral therapy also may be effective (e.g., flooding).

○ **Panic disorder:** Characterized by recurrent severe panic attacks. Attacks are usually short lived (1–5 minutes) and may include symptoms of rapid heart rate, perspiration, dizziness, and trembling. Look for 20- to 40-year-old patient who thinks that he or she is dying or having a heart attack (chest pain and dyspnea are very common symptoms) but is healthy and has a negative workup for organic disease. Patients often hyperventilate and are extremely anxious. A common association is agoraphobia (fear of leaving the house). Treat with SSRIs (e.g., fluoxetine) over benzodiazepines (which are addicting and sedating). Remember, do not assume a patient is having a panic attack unless the medical workup is complete.

○ **Posttraumatic stress disorder:** Look for someone who has been through a life-threatening event (Vietnam or Iraq war veteran, victim of severe accident or rape) who recurrently experiences the event in nightmares or flashbacks, tries to avoid thinking about it, and has depression or poor concentration as a result. Treat with group therapy, SSRIs, or both.

○ **Simple phobias:** Examples include fear of needles, blood products, animals, or heights. Treat with behavioral therapy such as flooding, systematic desensitization, biofeedback, and mental imagery if the patient desires treatment.

  ○ **Flooding:** The patient is placed in a room with the feared stimulus, and the psychiatrist or psychologist works with the patient to relax and control emotion.

  ○ **Systematic desensitization:** Gradual and progressive exposure of the patient to the feared stimulus.

  ○ **Biofeedback:** Monitoring the patient's vital signs and activity in response to the feared stimulus to learn to control responses to the feared stimulus.

  ○ **Mental imagery:** The patient thinks about him- or herself being exposed to the feared stimulus.

○ **Social anxiety disorder** (social phobia): A specific simple phobia that is best treated with behavioral therapy. β-Blockers may be used to reduce symptoms before a public appearance that cannot be avoided. SSRIs are increasingly being used as primary treatment, although SNRIs and benzodiazepines also may be used.

○ **Somatoform disorders:** A patient with somatoform disorder experiences psychiatric stress and expresses it through physical symptoms. Patients do not do so on purpose. Treat with frequent return clinic visits, psychotherapy, or both.

  ○ **Somatization disorder:** Multiple *different* complaints in multiple *different* organ systems (at least three systems, commonly neurologic, gynecologic, musculoskeletal, or gastrointestinal) over many years with extensive workups in the past.

  ○ **Conversion disorder:** Obvious precipitating factor (fight with boyfriend) followed by unexplainable neurologic symptoms (blindness, stocking-and-glove numbness). Classically, patients are not concerned by their symptoms ("la belle indifference").

  ○ **Hypochondriasis:** Patients keep believing that they have the *same* specific disease despite an extensive negative workup.

  ○ **Body dysmorphic disorder:** Preoccupation with an imagined physical defect (e.g., a teenager who thinks that his or her nose is too big when it is of normal size)

Somatoform disorders versus factitious disorder versus malingering:

  ○ **Somatoform disorders:** Patients *do not* intentionally create symptoms.

  ○ **Factitious disorders:** Patients *intentionally* create their illnesses or symptoms (e.g., inject themselves with insulin to provoke hypoglycemia) and subject themselves to procedures to assume the role of a patient (no financial or other secondary gain).

  ○ **Malingering:** Patients intentionally create their illnesses for *secondary gain* (e.g., money, to get out of work or jail).

  ○ **Substance abuse:** See later discussion in this chapter.

PSYCHOLOGICAL TESTS

Many different psychological tests are available to aid in a difficult diagnosis; they are not used for a straightforward case. There are two types of tests: objective (multiple choice, scored by a computer) and subjective (no right answers, scored by the test giver).

○ **Beck Depression Inventory:** Objective test to screen for depression

○ **Halstead-Reitan Battery:** Used to determine the location and effects of specific brain lesions

○ **Luria-Nebraska Neuropsychological Battery:** Objective test that assesses a wide range of cognitive functions and tells you the patient's cerebral dominance (left or right)

○ **Minnesota Multiphasic Personality Inventory:** Objective test designed to measure personality type

○ **Rorschach test:** Subjective test in which patients describe what they see in an inkblot

○ **Stanford-Binet:** Objective IQ test for adults

○ **Thematic Apperception Test:** Subjective test in which the patient describes what is going on in a cartoon drawing of people

○ **Wechsler Intelligence Scale for Children:** Objective IQ test for children (4–17 years old)

CHILD PSYCHIATRY

Anorexia

Look for a female adolescent who is a good athlete or student with a perfectionistic personality. Patients have body weight at least 15% below normal, intense fear of gaining weight (or "feel fat" even though they are emaciated), and amenorrhea (all three are required for diagnosis). Death occurs in roughly 10% to 15% of patients as a result of complications of starvation and/or bulimia (electrolyte imbalances, cardiac arrhythmias, infections). Some patients are hospitalized against their will for intravenous (IV) nutrition. Roughly half of people with anorexia also have bulimia. Use caution when refeeding patients who have been severely malnourished. There is a "refeeding syndrome" that can result in death, most commonly from hypophosphatemia.

Attention-Deficit/Hyperactivity Disorder

In attention-deficit/hyperactivity disorder (ADHD), as the name implies, affected children are hyperactive and have short attention spans. Three subtypes exist: predominantly hyperactive-impulsive, predominantly inattentive, and combined hyperactive-impulsive/inattentive. Boys are affected more often than girls. Boys are more likely to be hyperactive, but girls more commonly have attention problems. Look for a fidgety child who is impulsive and cannot pay attention but is not cruel. To make the diagnosis, behavioral disturbances must be present in two or more settings (i.e., school and home). Treat with stimulants (paradoxical calming effect) such as modafinil, methylphenidate (Ritalin), or dextroamphetamine, all of which can cause insomnia, abdominal pain, anorexia, and weight loss or growth suppression. This is a hot topic because of concerns about overdiagnosis and treatment. Use drug holidays (temporarily stop the drug) to combat side effects.

Autism Spectrum

Autistic symptoms can begin as early as 6 months, becoming well established by age 2 or 3 years. Look for impaired social interaction (isolative, unaware of surroundings), impaired verbal and non-verbal communication (strange words, babbling, repetition), and restricted activities and interests (head banging, strange movements, focus on small details). Autism can be thought of as a spectrum of disorders in which patients may range from very highly functioning (e.g., Asperger syndrome) to severely mentally retarded. Most individuals with autism manifest some degree of mental retardation, which typically is moderate in severity. No single cause has been identified for the development of autism. Genetic origins are suspected by twin studies and an increased incidence among siblings. Possible contributing factors include fetal alcohol exposure, infections (congenital rubella infection), other perinatal factors, or immunologic causes. If you get a patient with normal language development who has impaired social interactions and restricted activities, think Asperger syndrome.

Bulimia

Look for a female adolescent who is of normal weight or overweight (unless anorexia coexists). Patients have binge-eating episodes during which they feel a lack of control and then engage in purging behavior (vomiting, laxatives, exercise, fasting). Patients might require hospitalization for electrolyte disturbances. In the classic patient, the tooth enamel has been eroded because of frequent vomiting; the skin over the knuckles may also be eroded from putting the fingers into the throat. Look for swollen parotid glands ("chipmunk cheeks").

Conduct Disorder

Conduct disorder is the pediatric form of antisocial disorder. Look for fire setting, cruelty to animals, lying, stealing, or fighting. As adults, patients often have antisocial disorder. Note: Conduct disorder in childhood is required to make a diagnosis of antisocial personality disorder in an adult.

Encopresis and Enuresis

Encopresis and enuresis are not disorders until after age 4 years (encopresis) or 5 years (enuresis). This is obviously an important diagnostic point to remember when a mother complains (normal finding if the child is 3 years old). Rule out physical problems (e.g., Hirschsprung disease, urinary tract infection) and then treat with behavioral therapy ("gold star for being good" charts, alarms, biofeedback). Desmopressin and imipramine are used only for refractory cases of enuresis; they are not first-line agents.

Learning Disorder

This disorder can include impairment in math, reading, writing, speech, language, or coordination, but all other skills are normal, and no mental retardation is present ("Chris just can't do math").

Mental Retardation

Most cases are idiopathic, and 85% of cases are mild (IQ range, 55–70). Patients often have a reasonable level of independence but need assistance or guidance during periods of stress. Fetal alcohol syndrome is the number one preventable cause, and Down syndrome is the number one overall cause. Fragile X syndrome (in boys) is another common cause of mental retardation.

Oppositional Defiant Disorder

This includes negative, hostile, and defiant behavior toward authority figures (parents, teachers). The child misbehaves around adults but behaves normally around peers and is not a cruel, lying criminal (as in conduct disorder).

Separation Anxiety Disorder

Look for a child who refuses to go to school. Basically, affected children think that something will happen to them or their parents if they separate; thus, they will do anything to avoid separation (stomachache, headache, temper tantrums).

Tourette Disorder

Only 10% to 30% of patients utter obscenities. Look for boys with motor tics (eye blinking, grunting, throat clearing, grimacing, barking, or shoulder shrugging) that are exacerbated by stress and remit during activity or sleep. Tourette disorder can be caused or unmasked by use of stimulants (e.g., for presumed ADHD). Antipsychotics (e.g., haloperidol) are used if the symptoms are severe. Tourette disorder tends to be a lifelong problem.

IMPORTANT POINTS

1. Depression in children often manifests as irritable mood instead of depressed mood.
2. The top three causes of adolescent deaths in order are accidents, homicide, and suicide. Together they account for about 75% of teenage deaths.

DRUGS OF ABUSE

Amphetamines

Amphetamines are classically associated with psychotic symptoms (patients may appear to be full-blown schizophrenics), but physiologic effects are similar to those of cocaine. Look for sympathomimetic stimulation on physical exam (see discussion of cocaine below). Do not restrain patients on amphetamines, cocaine, or phencyclidine (PCP) because of the risk of rhabdomyolysis.

Benzodiazepines and Barbiturates

Benzodiazepines and barbiturates cause sedation and drowsiness as well as disinhibition and a reduction of anxiety. Overdose may be fatal (respiratory depression); treat with flumazenil if needed for benzodiazepine overdose. Withdrawal also may be fatal (just as with alcohol) because of seizures or cardiovascular collapse. Treat withdrawal on an inpatient basis with a long-acting benzodiazepine; gradually taper the dose over several days. Benzodiazepines and barbiturates are especially dangerous when mixed with alcohol (all three are CNS depressants).

Cocaine

Look for sympathetic stimulation (insomnia, tachycardia, mydriasis, hypertension, sweating) with hyperalertness and possible paranoia, aggression, delirium, psychosis, or formications ("cocaine bugs"—patients think that bugs are crawling on them). Overdose can be fatal (arrhythmia, myocardial infarction, seizure, or stroke). On withdrawal, patients become sleepy, hungry (versus anorexic with intoxication), and irritable, possibly with severe depression. Withdrawal is not dangerous, but psychological cravings usually are severe. Cocaine does not appear to be directly teratogenic, but it is associated with spontaneous abortion, prematurity, abruption placentae, fetal death, and decreased fetal weights.

Inhalants

Inhalant (e.g., gasoline, glue, varnish remover) intoxication causes euphoria, dizziness, slurred speech, a feeling of floating, ataxia, or a sense of heightened power. Intoxication usually is seen in younger teenagers (11–15 years). It can be fatal in overdose (respiratory depression, cardiac arrhythmias, asphyxiation) or cause severe permanent sequelae (CNS, liver, and kidney toxicity; peripheral neuropathy). There is no known withdrawal syndrome.

LSD and Mushrooms

Symptoms of intoxication with lysergic acid diethylamide (LSD) or mushrooms include hallucinations, mydriasis, tachycardia, diaphoresis, and perception and mood disturbances. Hallucinations usually are visual rather than auditory (the opposite of schizophrenia). Overdose is not dangerous (unless the patient thinks that he or she can fly and jumps out a window). No withdrawal symptoms are noted. Patients can have flashbacks months to years later (a brief feeling of being on the drug again, although none was taken) or a bad trip (acute panic reaction or dysphoria). Treat bad trips with reassurance or benzodiazepine or antipsychotic medication (if needed).

Marijuana

Marijuana is the most commonly abused illegal drug. Look for a teenager who is withdrawn and has a decline in school performance. Other symptoms include "amotivational syndrome" (chronic use can cause laziness and lack of motivation), time distortion, and the munchies (binge eating when intoxicated). No physical withdrawal symptoms are noted, although patients can have psychological cravings. Overdose is not dangerous, but patients can have temporary dysphoria. Marijuana is not a proven teratogen.

Opioids

Heroin and other opioids cause euphoria, analgesia, drowsiness, miosis, constipation, and CNS depression. Overdose can be fatal (respiratory depression); treat with naloxone. When the drug is taken IV, there are associated morbidities and mortalities (endocarditis, hepatitis B, hepatitis C, HIV, cellulitis, talc damage). Withdrawal is not life threatening, but patients act as though they are going to die. Symptoms include gooseflesh, diarrhea, insomnia, and cramping or pain. Methadone treatment sometimes is given for addicts. Methadone or buprenorphine can be used to reduce acute withdrawal symptoms.

Phencyclidine (PCP)

PCP intoxication causes LSD or mushroom symptoms plus confusion, agitation, and aggressive behavior. Also look for vertical or horizontal nystagmus plus possible schizophrenic-like symptoms (paranoia, auditory hallucinations, disorganized behavior and speech). Overdose can be fatal (convulsions, coma, respiratory arrest). Treat with supportive care and urine acidification to hasten elimination. No withdrawal symptoms are noted.

Caffeine withdrawal can cause headaches, irritability, and fatigue.

QR CODE

The QR code includes three USMLE-style questions and answers. For more questions, redeem the PIN code on the inside cover for the Crush Step 2 question bank powered by USMLE Consult.

Please see the Introduction for instructions on how to access content using the QR codes.

Question

A 59-year-old man comes to the office asking for sleeping pills. On questioning, the patient, a Vietnam War veteran, relates a history of terrible nightmares and insomnia. He admits to daytime flashbacks and recurrent dreams about the war and memory difficulties. He is divorced, lives alone, and has no friends that he is close to currently. When asked to elaborate on his combat experience, the patient becomes angry and asks you to "keep quiet about things you don't know." The patient seems quite anxious and distracted by the smallest stimulus. What is the best course of action for this patient?

(A) Diphenhydramine at bedtime
(B) Lorazepam during waking hours and at bedtime for several months
(C) Haloperidol every morning
(D) Referral to a psychotherapist doing group work with other Vietnam War veterans
(E) Referral for electroconvulsive therapy followed by daily fluoxetine indefinitely

28 PULMONOLOGY

CHRONIC OBSTRUCTIVE PULMONARY DISEASE

In chronic obstructive pulmonary disease (COPD), the ratio of the forced expiratory volume in 1 second to the forced expiratory volume (FEV1/FEV ratio) is less than normal (<0.70), but in restrictive lung disease, the FEV1/FEV ratio is often normal. FEV1 may be low in both conditions; it is the FEV1/FEV ratio that is different. After the diagnosis of COPD has been made, the degree of FEV1 impairment is used to estimate the severity of the disease.

 A patient with COPD can live normally at a higher CO_2 and lower O_2; treat the patient, not the lab value! If the patient is asymptomatic and talking to you, the lab value should not make you panic. Conversely, the lab values may look great, but if the patient is becoming tired from increased work of breathing, intubation may be needed.

 As a rough rule, you should prepare to intubate any patient whose CO_2 is greater than 50 mm Hg or whose O_2 is less than 50 mm Hg, especially if the pH in either case is less than 7.30 while the patient is breathing room air. Usually, unless the patient is crashing rapidly, a trial of O_2 by nasal cannula (or face mask or other noninvasive means) is given first. If this approach does not work or if the patient becomes too tired (use of accessory muscles is a good clue to the work of breathing), consider intubation.

EMPHYSEMA

Emphysema almost always is caused by smoking (even if secondhand). In a young person with minimal smoke exposure (<5 years of smoking), think of α1-antitrypsin deficiency (which is also manifested by liver abnormalities).

Physical exam findings: Barrel chest (increased anteroposterior chest diameter), pursed-lip breathing, prolonged expiratory phase, clubbing of the digits, end-expiratory wheezing, decreased heart and breath sounds, and scattered rhonchi. Flattening of the diaphragms and large lung volumes may be seen on chest radiography.

Treat with smoking cessation (can't reverse emphysema but slows progression and reduces risk of death), inhaled bronchodilators (e.g., short-acting β2-agonists such as albuterol or long-acting β2-agonists such as salmeterol) and inhaled anticholinergic (e.g., short-acting anticholinergics such as ipratropium and long-acting anticholinergics such as tiotropium), antibiotics for infections, supplemental oxygen if pulse oximetry is less than 90% or arterial pCO2 is less than 60 mm Hg on room air, immunizations for influenza and pneumococcus, and as-needed corticosteroids (controversial benefit but commonly used).

ASTHMA

Look for wheezing in children, although asthma can present in adulthood as well. Treat with β2-agonists in the emergency department. As-needed β2-agonists (e.g., albuterol) are all that is needed for mild intermittent asthma. Inhaled glucocorticoids, leukotriene receptor antagonists (zafirlukast, zileuton), cromolyn, nedocromil, and long-acting β-agonists are used in asthma maintenance, not for acute attacks. Phosphodiesterase inhibitors (theophylline, aminophylline) are older, second-line agents. Use oral steroids (acutely or chronically) if asthma is severe or does not respond to β2-agonists.

Wheezing in children younger than age 2 years is often attributable to respiratory syncytial virus (RSV), especially in the winter. Look for coexisting fever.

 Do not *put patients with asthma or COPD on β-blockers, which block the $β_2$-receptors needed to open the airways.*

 Asthma is one of the top three causes of cough in the outpatient setting, the other two being gastroesophageal reflux disease and postnasal drip.

 Beware the person with acute asthmac who no longer hyperventilates or whose CO_2 is normal or rising (the patient should hyperventilate, which causes low CO_2). Do not think that patients who seem calm or sleepy are okay. They are probably crashing and need an immediate arterial blood gas analysis and possible intubation. Fatigue alone is enough reason to intubate an asthmatic patient.

PULMONARY NODULES

If a solitary pulmonary nodule (round, <3 cm) is seen on a chest radiography, the first step is to check for old radiographs. If the lesion has not changed in more than 2 years, it is likely benign. A nodule that has increased in size on serial imaging should be biopsied or excised. If there are no old radiographs, get computed tomography (CT) of chest for further characterization. If the nodule is densely calcified, it is likely benign. Many nodules remain indeterminate after this first assessment, however. Certain clues point to the etiology:

○ Immigrant: Think tuberculosis (do a skin test, acid-fast bacterial sputum cultures).
○ Southwestern United States: Think Coccidioides immitis.
○ Cave explorer, person exposed to bird droppings, or someone living in Ohio or Mississippi River valleys: Think histoplasmosis.
○ Smoker older than 40 years: Think lung cancer (positron emission tomography [PET] scan, bronchoscopy and biopsy).
○ Person younger than 40 years with none of the above: Think hamartoma.

Perform PET scan for initial noninvasive assessment of nodules that remain indeterminate after history, chest radiography, and CT scan. If PET results are positive, think biopsy. If PET results are negative, do short-interval follow-up CT scans for 2 years and think biopsy if the lesion grows.

ACUTE RESPIRATORY DISTRESS SYNDROME

The definition of acute respiratory distress syndrome (ARDS) is acute lung injury that results in noncardiogenic pulmonary edema, respiratory distress, and hypoxemia. Four criteria are required to diagnose ARDS: acute onset, bilateral infiltrates (radiographically similar to pulmonary edema), no evidence of elevated left atrial pressure (the pulmonary capillary wedge pressure is ≤18 mm Hg if measured), and a ratio of arterial oxygen tension to fraction of inspired oxygen (PaO2/FiO2) of less than 200 mm Hg.

Common causes of ARDS are sepsis, major trauma, pancreatitis, shock, near drowning, and drug over-dose. Look for ARDS to develop within 24 to 48 hours of the initial insult. Classic symptoms include mottled or cyanotic skin, intercostal retractions, rales or rhonchi, and no improvement of hypoxia with O2 administration. Radiography shows patchy pulmonary edema or air space disease, classically with a normal heart size (i.e., makes congestive heart failure much less likely). Treat with intubation, mechanical ventilation with high percentage of O2, high positive end-expiratory pressure (PEEP), and low tidal volume (permissive hypercapnia) while addressing the underlying cause (if possible). The mortality rate is high with ARDS.

PNEUMONIA

The diagnosis of pneumonia is usually based on clinical findings (rales or rhonchi, fever) plus an elevated white blood cell count and chest radiographic abnormalities. On physical exam, look to differentiate between typical (Streptococcus pneumoniae) and atypical (other organisms) pneumonia (Table 28-1), although the distinction is not always clear cut. Sputum and blood cultures usually are obtained before empiric therapy is begun.

Certain clinical clues should make you think of certain organisms:

- College student: Think *Mycoplasma* spp. (look for cold agglutinins) or *Chlamydia* spp.
- Alcoholic: Think *Klebsiella* spp. ("currant jelly" sputum), *Staphylococcus aureus*, other enteric organisms (aspiration).
- Cystic fibrosis: Think *Pseudomonas* spp. or *S. aureus*.
- Immigrant: Think tuberculosis.
- COPD: Think *Haemophilus influenzae* or *Moraxella* spp.
- Patient with known tuberculosis and pulmonary cavitation: Think *Aspergillus* spp.
- Patient with silicosis (metal, granite, pottery workers): Think tuberculosis.
- Exposure to air conditioner or aerosolized water: Think *Legionella* spp.
- HIV/AIDS: Think *Pneumocystis carinii* or cytomegalovirus (if shown a picture of koilocytosis).
- Exposure to bird droppings: Think *Chlamydia psittaci* or *Histoplasma* spp.
- Child younger than 1 year: Think RSV.
- Child 2 to 5 years: Think parainfluenza (croup) or epiglottitis.

Recurrent pediatric pneumonia in the same lung segment is classically attributable to foreign body aspiration, especially when in the right middle or lower lobe (a foreign body is more likely to go down the right mainstem bronchus). Other possibilities include reflux with aspiration, congenital lung malformation, and immunodeficiency. Patients with immunodeficiency have other signs (e.g., other types of infections, cystic fibrosis symptoms; should not always be the same lung segment involved).

A follow-up chest radiograph is routine in those older than 40 years of age who develop pneumonia to make sure the infiltrate clears after appropriate antibiotic treatment. If pneumonia does not clear by 4 to 6 weeks, suspect something other than bacterial pneumonia. The classic culprit is malignancy, specifically, bronchoalveolar carcinoma, which is a subtype of adenocarcinoma. In addition, recurrent pneumonias in the same location in an adult may be attributable to an endobronchial mass, whether benign or malignant.

TABLE 28-1 Characteristics of Typical and Atypical Pneumonia

CHARACTERISTIC	TYPICAL PNEUMONIA	ATYPICAL PNEUMONIA
Prodrome	Short (<2 days)	Long (>3 days): headache, malaise, other aches
Fever	High (>102°F)	Low (<102°F)
Age	>40 y	<40 y
Chest radiography	One distinct lobe involved	Diffuse or multilobe involvement
Infective agent	*Streptococcus pneumoniae*	Many (e.g., *Haemophilus influenzae*, *Mycoplasma* spp., *Chlamydia* spp.)
Medications*	Third-generation cephalosporin or broad-spectrum fluoroquinolone	Macrolides (e.g., azithromycin), doxycycline, or fluoroquinolone that covers atypical bugs (e.g., levofloxacin)

*Avoid the temptation to pull out the "big gun" antibiotics (very wide spectrum) unless the patient is crashing or unstable.

SINUSITIS

Sinusitis is usually viral but commonly is caused by *S. pneumoniae* or *Haemophilus* spp. infection. Look for purulent (green or yellow) nasal discharge with tenderness over the involved sinus. Associated symptoms are headache or toothache (maxillary sinusitis). You cannot transilluminate the sinuses, and radiography or CT shows opacification of the frontal or maxillary sinuses (consider ordering sinus radiography or CT to confirm the diagnosis if it has not already been done). Empiric treatment choices include amoxicillin or a second-generation cephalosporin for 10 to 14 days.

 The most common cause of epistaxis in children is nose picking (i.e., trauma). Do not assume low or defective platelets without evidence.

PLEURAL EFFUSION

Physical exam shows dull percussion note, increased tactile fremitus, and decreased breath sounds in area of effusion. Confirm with chest radiography. If you do not know the cause after chest radiography (and possibly CT scan), always consider thoracentesis to examine the fluid using Gram stain, culture and sensitivity (including tuberculosis culture), cell count with differential, cytology (to look for malignancy), glucose (low in infection), protein (high in infection), amylase (if pancreatitis is a suspected cause of effusion), triglycerides (if a chylous effusion is suspected), albumin, and lactate dehydrogenase (LDH). Albumin and LDH are used to determine whether the fluid is an exudates or transudate.

A pleural effusion is common in the setting of pneumonia and often goes away with the pneumonia, but watch for progression to empyema (infected, loculated pleural fluid), which requires chest tube drainage. Common and classic causes include infection (including tuberculosis in appropriate setting), malignancy, congestive heart failure (often bilateral), abdominal inflammation (e.g., pancreatitis, subphrenic abscess), and collagen vascular disease (e.g., rheumatoid arthritis).

 Light criteria are the most commonly used diagnostic paradigm to distinguish an exudative from a transudative pleural effusion. If at least one of the following three criteria is present, the fluid is defined as exudates:

- *Pleural fluid protein:serum protein ratio greater than 0.5*

- *Pleural fluid LDH:serum LDH ratio greater than 0.6*

- *Pleural fluid LDH greater than two-thirds the upper limits of the laboratory's normal serum LDH*

DIFFUSE PARENCHYMAL LUNG DISEASES

Diffuse parenchymal lung diseases (DPLDs), also known as interstitial lung disease (ILD), are a heterogenous group of disorders that are grouped together because of similar clinical, radiologic, and pathologic characteristics. They are most commonly related to occupational or environmental exposure, but many are also idiopathic in nature. Important diseases included in this group that may appear on Step 2 are sarcoidosis, idiopathic pulmonary fibrosis (IPF; idiopathic interstitial pneumonias), lymphangioleiomyomatosis (LAM), hypersensitivity pneumonitis, and the various pneumoconiosis.

Suspect a DPLD in patients who present with progressive dyspnea on exertion and a persistent nonproductive cough. Other less common symptoms are hemoptysis, wheezing, and pleuritic chest pain. Rales are common in most forms of ILD but are absent in some of the granulomatous diseases such as sarcoidosis. In the late stages, cor pulmonale with a loud P2 and right-sided lift may be present on cardiac exam. Clubbing may be seen peripherally. Pulmonary function tests (PFTs) usually show a restrictive pattern with decreased FEV1 but normal or increased FEV1/FVC ratio. Chest radiographs may vary depending on the disease. Early sarcoidosis classically appears with bilateral hilar fullness, and later stage sarcoidosis and idiopathic pulmonary fibrosis may appear as diffuse reticulonodular changes.

Age can help to further differentiate the conditions. Sarcoidosis, connective tissue disease–related ILD, and LAM present in younger individuals ages 20 to 40 years. IPF, on the other hand, usually occurs in individuals older than 50 years of age.

Gender is also helpful in making a diagnosis. As a whole, ILD is more common in women than men, and LAM occurs exclusively in premenopausal women.

A history of environmental exposures points to a hypersensitivity pneumonitis or one of the pneumoconiosis. Look for a history of exposure to hay (farmer's lung), birds (pigeon breeder's disease, bird fancier's lung), air conditioners, humidifiers, hot tubs, asbestos (asbestosis), beryllium (berylliosis), and silicone (silicosis).

The workup involves chest radiography, chest CT, PFTs, echocardiography, and bronchoscopic or video-assisted thoracic biopsy. Unfortunately, many of these conditions do not respond well to treatment, which usually consists of glucocorticoids.

PULMONARY FUNCTION AND SURGERY

A baseline chest radiograph is not part of the standard preoperative evaluation but is often used for patients older than age 60 years and patients with known pulmonary or cardiovascular disease. Preoperative PFT is somewhat controversial, and the question probably will not appear on Step 2. Overall, the best indicator of possible postoperative pulmonary complications is preoperative pulmonary function. The best way to reduce pulmonary complications postoperatively is to stop smoking preoperatively, especially if it is stopped at least 8 weeks before surgery. Aggressive pulmonary toilet, incentive spirometry, minimal narcotics, and early ambulation help prevent or minimize postoperative pulmonary complications. Lastly, remember that the most common cause of a postoperative fever in the first 24 hours is atelectasis.

QR CODE

The QR code includes three USMLE-style questions and answers. For more questions, redeem the PIN code on the inside cover for the Crush Step 2 question bank powered by USMLE Consult.

Please see the Introduction for instructions on how to access content using the QR codes.

Question

A 45-year-old man with a long smoking history presents with dyspnea. Vital signs are as follows:

Temperature	99.9°F
Blood pressure	168/92 mm Hg
Pulse rate	90 beats/min
Respirations	22 breaths/min

Pulse oximetry reveals an oxygen saturation of 94%. Physical examination reveals decreased breath sounds and dull percussion note in the lower right chest. Chest radiography reveals a large pleural effusion on the right with no other abnormalities. The patient denies exposure to anyone who has been sick or any change in his smoker's cough. Complete blood count and electrolytes are unremarkable. What is the best next step?

(A) Empirical coverage of tuberculosis and respiratory isolation
(B) PET scan
(C) Thoracentesis
(D) Pleural biopsy
(E) Insertion of a thoracostomy tube

29 RADIOLOGY

Table 29-1 lists radiologic screening and confirmatory tests.

TABLE 29-1 Screening and Confirmatory Radiologic Tests for Different Diseases

CONDITION	SCREENING (OR ONLY) TEST TO ORDER	CONFIRMATORY TEST	COMMENTS
Cardiovascular			
Aortic aneurysm	Abdominal US	CT with contrast	Screening US recommended for male smokers ages 65–75 y
Aortic dissection	CT with contrast	MRA or TEE	
Aortic trauma (tear)	CT with contrast	MRA or TEE	
Carotid stenosis	Duplex US	MRA	
Gastrointestinal			
Abdominal abscess	CT scan with contrast		
Abdominal trauma	FAST scan to assess for hemoperitoneum	CT with contrast	Laparotomy is the gold standard
Appendicitis	US (particularly in pregnant patients and children)	CT with contrast	Never truly confirmed until surgery
Bowel obstruction	Abdominal radiography	CT with contrast	
Bowel perforation	Upright abdominal radiography or chest white blood cell	CT with contrast	
Cholecystitis	US	Nuclear hepatobiliary study (HIDA scan)	Look for gallbladder wall thickening and pericholecystic fluid on US
Choledocholithiasis	US	ERCP or MRCP	
Cholelithiasis	US		
Diverticulitis	CT with contrast		No endoscopy acutely because there is a risk of perforation
Esophageal disease	Gastrografin or barium radiography*	CT with contrast (for rupture)	Endoscopy usually necessary as a follow-up study
GI bleeding	Endoscopy†	Tagged RBC scan if unable to visualize on endoscopy	

CT, computed tomography; ERCP, endoscopic retrograde cholangiopancreatography; FAST, focused assessment with sonography for trauma; GI, gastrointestinal; HIDA, hepato-iminodiacetic acid; MRA, magnetic resonance angiogram; MRCP, magnetic resonance cholangiopancreatography; MRI, magnetic resonance imaging; PET, positron emission tomography; RBC, red blood cell; TEE, transesophageal echocardiography; US, ultrasonography; VCUG, voiding cystourethrography; WBC, white blood cell.

(Continued)

TABLE 29-1 Screening and Confirmatory Radiologic Tests for Different Diseases—Cont'd

CONDITION	SCREENING (OR ONLY) TEST TO ORDER	CONFIRMATORY TEST	COMMENTS
Gastrointestinal			
Hematemesis	Endoscopy		
Meckel diverticulum	Meckel scan (nuclear medicine)		
Peptic ulcer disease	Endoscopy		
Pyloric stenosis	US	Barium x-ray	
Gynecologic			
Fibroids	US	MRI	
Ovarian disease	US	MRI	Laparoscopy may be needed
Pelvic mass (female)	US	MRI or CT with contrast or laparoscopy	
Pregnancy evaluation	US		Transvaginal US for early pregnancy; transabdominal for the remainder
Neurologic			
Acute stroke		Noncontrast CT	MRI
Brain tumor		CT with contrast	MRI with contrast
Head trauma		Noncontrast CT	
Intracranial hemorrhage		Noncontrast CT	
Multiple sclerosis		MRI	
Skull fracture		Noncontrast CT	
Orthopedic			
Arthritis	Radiography	MRI if more detailed evaluation is needed	
Bone metastases	Bone scan	PET scan	Plain radiographs for multiple myeloma
Fracture	Radiography	Noncontrast CT	CT can pick up many fractures not seen on x-ray
Osteomyelitis	Radiography	Bone scan or tagged WBC nuclear scan	MRI without contrast can be helpful
Pelvic trauma	Radiography	Noncontrast CT	
Scaphoid fracture	Radiography	MRI	
Respiratory			
Chest mass	Chest radiography	CT with contrast	
Chest trauma	Chest radiography	CT with contrast	
Hemoptysis	Chest radiography	Bronchoscopy or CT with contrast	
Pneumonia	Chest radiography	CT with contrast	
Pulmonary embolism	CT with contrast	Pulmonary angiography	Ventilation/perfusion nuclear scan if unable to tolerate radiation (pregnancy) or contrast
Pulmonary nodule	Chest radiography	CT with contrast	May need PET scan to assess for malignancy

TABLE 29-1 Screening and Confirmatory Radiologic Tests for Different Diseases—Cont'd

CONDITION	SCREENING (OR ONLY) TEST TO ORDER	CONFIRMATORY TEST	COMMENTS
Urologic			
Hematuria (persistent)	CT scan with contrast (without contrast if *painful* hematuria)	Cystoscopy	
Hydronephrosis	US		CT with contrast
Nephrolithiasis	Noncontrast CT		Intravenous pyelography rarely indicated or used
Ureteral reflux	VCUG		
Suspected urethral trauma	Retrograde urethrogram		

*With suspected GI perforation, do not use barium (it can cause a chemical peritonitis); use water-soluble contrast (e.g., Gastrografin).

†For brisk bleeds, endoscopy is preferred. For occult bleeding, a barium study or endoscopy may be used. An "unknown" GI bleed means that initial tests failed to localize the bleed and that the patient is still actively bleeding.

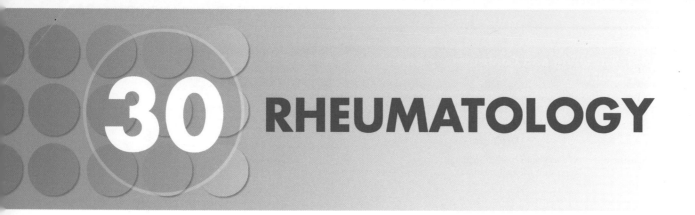

30 RHEUMATOLOGY

ARTHRITIS

The large majority of arthritis cases are attributable to osteoarthritis (OA). When in doubt or if you suspect something other than OA, perform radiography of and aspirate any fluid from the affected joint for examination. Examine the fluid for cell count and differential, glucose, bacteria (Gram stain and culture), and crystals. The characteristics of the arthritides are shown in Table 30-1.

Osteoarthritis

Osteoarthritis typically occurs in those older than 40 years of age and displays few signs of inflammation on exam (lacks hot, red, tender joints seen in all the others of this group). Symptoms include Heberden (visible and palpable distal interphalangeal [DIP] joint osteophytes) nodes (Fig. 30-1) and Bouchard (proximal interphalangeal [PIP] joint osteophytes) nodes in the fingers and worsening of symptoms in the evening and after use. Radiographs show osteophytes (bone spurs around joints), joint-space narrowing, subchondral cysts, and subchondral sclerosis. The incidence increases with age. Treat with weight reduction and nonsteroidal antiinflammatory drugs (NSAIDs or acetaminophen) as needed but beware of side effects (e.g., gastrointestinal bleeding).

Rheumatoid Arthritis

Rheumatoid arthritis (RA) often causes systemic symptoms (fever, malaise, subcutaneous nodules, pericarditis or pleural effusion, uveitis), prolonged morning stiffness, and swan neck and boutonnière deformities. The diagnosis is often made by an elevated sedimentation rate or C-reactive protein (CRP) and positive rheumatoid factor, which is present in most adults but often negative in children. Radiographs and magnetic resonance imaging can also support the diagnosis. General treatment strategies reflect the fact that the destruction of affected joints from inflammation occurs early in the course of RA. The patient should be offered treatment with disease-modifying antirheumatic drugs (DMARDs) as soon as possible after the onset of disease. Escalate the intensity of treatment until synovitis and inflammation have improved (Fig. 30-2).

Five general classes of medications are used for the treatment of RA, with DMARDs forming the backbone of treatment. Treatment options include the following: analgesics (from acetaminophen to narcotics), NSAIDs, glucocorticoids, nonbiologic DMARDs (methotrexate, sulfasalazine, leflunomide, hydroxychloroquine, and minocycline), and biologic DMARDs. Biologic DMARDs include tumor necrosis factor (TNF) inhibitors (etanercept, infliximab, and adalimumab), an interleukin-1 receptor antagonist (anakinra), a monoclonal antibody (rituximab), and biologic response modifiers (abatacept).

With juvenile RA, rheumatoid factor is often negative. Watch for uveitis as a presenting symptom, especially in the pauciarticular (few joints affected) form.

Felty syndrome is RA with splenomegaly and neutropenia.

Caplan syndrome is RA with pneumoconiosis.

TABLE 30-1 Characteristics of Arthritis

CHARACTERISTIC	OSTEOARTHRITIS	RHEUMATOID ARTHRITIS	GOUT	PSEUDOGOUT	SEPTIC ARTHRITIS
Usual age and sex	Older adults	Women 20–45 y	Older men	Older adults	Any age
Classic joints	DIP, PIP, hip, knee	PIP, MCP, wrist	Big toe	Knees, elbows	Knee
Joint fluid WBC count	<2000/µL	>2000/µL	>2000/µL	>2000/µL	>50,000
% Neutrophils	<25	>50	>50	>50	>75

DIP, distal interphalangeal; MCP, metacarpophalangeal; PIP, proximal interphalangeal; WBC, white blood cell.

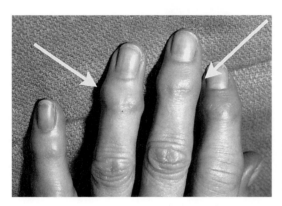

FIGURE 30-1 Patients with degenerative joint disease of the hands can present with Heberden nodes (*arrows*). These nodules represent osteophytes at the distal interphalangeal joint.

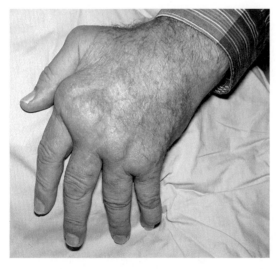

FIGURE 30-2 Classic end-stage rheumatoid hand deformity. This patient has volar subluxation of the metacarpophalangeal (MCP) joints; ulnar deviation of the digits; and hypertrophic, boggy synovium along the dorsum of the hand, particularly over the MCP joints.

Gout

Gout classically starts with podagra (gout in the big toe). Look for high uric acid levels (not always present), tophi (subcutaneous uric acid deposits, punched-out lesions on bone radiographs) (Fig. 30-3), and needle-shaped uric acid crystals (often inside leukocytes) with negative birefringence in a joint fluid sample. Gout is more common in men than women. Patients should avoid alcohol and protein-rich foods (can precipitate an attack), red meat, and thiazide diuretics. Use colchicine or NSAIDs (not aspirin, which causes decreased excretion of uric acid by the kidney) for acute attacks. Maintenance therapy includes high fluid intake, alkalinization of the urine, or probenecid or allopurinol (neither for acute attacks).

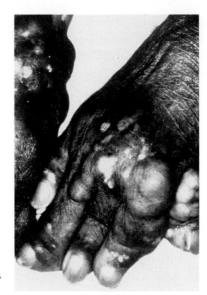

Figure 30-3 Gouty tophi. Tophaceous deposits of gout overlying digits of this patient's hand.

Pseudogout

Pseudogout is caused by calcium pyrophosphate dehydrate (CPPD) crystal deposition in the joints. Look for rhomboid-shaped crystals with weakly positive birefringence. Acute attacks are similar to those of gout clinically, thus the name, but pseudogout is a completely different disorder. When calcification of cartilage is apparent under radiographic examination of joints, the syndrome is called chondrocalcinosis.

Septic Arthritis

Synovial fluid usually shows bacteria on Gram stain. Staphylococcus aureus is the most common organism except in sexually active young adults (Neisseria gonorrhoeae is most common in this group). Do blood cultures in addition to joint cultures because the organisms usually reach the joint via the hematogenous route. Do urethral swabs and cultures in appropriate patients. Other causes of arthritis:

○ **Psoriasis:** Look for psoriatic skin lesions to make an easy diagnosis. Arthritis usually affects the hands and feet, and the arthritis resembles RA, but the rheumatoid factor is negative. NSAIDs are first-line therapy. Other treatments include methotrexate, PUVA (psoralen and ultraviolet A), retinoic acid derivatives, cyclosporine, sulfasalazine, azathioprine, and antimalarials.

○ **Lupus erythematosus or inflammatory bowel disease:** Other symptoms of the primary disease help make the diagnosis.

○ **Ankylosing spondylitis:** Associated with human leukocyte antigen (HLA)-B27. Most often occurs in 20- to 40-year-old men with a positive family history who present with back pain and morning stiffness; patients sometimes assume a bent-over posture. Sacroiliac joints are primarily affected, and radiographs might reveal a bamboo spine. Patients have other autoimmune-type symptoms, such as fever, elevated erythrocyte sedimentation rate (ESR), and anemia; some develop uveitis. Treat with NSAIDs, methotrexate, sulfasalazine, or TNF antagonists (etanercept, infliximab, adalimumab).

○ **Reactive arthritis** (previously called Reiter syndrome): Also associated with HLA-B27. The classic triad is urethritis (caused by *Chlamydia* spp. infection), conjunctivitis, and arthritis ("can't pee, can't see, can't climb a tree"). Reactive arthritis also can follow enteric bacterial infections. Superficial oral and penile ulcers are common. Diagnose and treat the sexually transmitted disease and treat the patient's sexual partners. NSAIDs are used for arthritis; methotrexate and sulfasalazine are used for treatment of more severe arthritis symptoms.

○ **Hemophilia:** Recurrent hemarthroses (bleeding into the joints) can cause debilitating arthritis. Treat with acetaminophen (avoid aspirin and other NSAIDs because of bleeding concerns).

○ **Lyme disease:** Look for tick bite or history of hiking in the woods, erythema chronicum migrans, and migratory arthritis later. Treat this *Borrelia burgdorferi*, infection, with doxycycline, amoxicillin, or cefuroxime. Use parenteral ceftriaxone for cases with carditis or other serious complications. Avoid doxycycline in children younger than the age of 8 years and in pregnant or lactating women.

○ **Rheumatic fever:** Look for previous streptococcal pharyngitis. Migratory polyarthritis is one of the major Jones criteria.
○ **Sickle cell disease:** Patients often develop arthralgias from ischemic sickle crises, but the classic cause of arthritis is avascular necrosis of the femoral or humeral head or other bone infarcts.
○ **Trauma:** Can lead to arthritis later in life
○ **Childhood orthopedic problem:** Slipped capital femoral epiphysis, congenital hip dysplasia, and Legg-Calvé-Perthes disease can cause arthritis in adulthood. Use history (age of onset) and radiographs to determine which disease the patient had as a child.
○ **Charcot joint:** Most commonly seen in diabetes mellitus; also in other neuropathies. Lack of sensation causes the patient to overuse or misuse joints, which become deformed and painful. The best treatment is prevention. After even seemingly mild trauma, patients with neuropathy in the area of the trauma need radiographs to rule out fractures.
○ **Hemochromatosis and Wilson disease:** Both may be associated with arthritis caused by deposition of iron (hemochromatosis) or copper (Wilson disease).

AUTOIMMUNE DISEASES

For board purposes, classic disease findings differentiate one condition from the other. Almost all patients have systemic signs of inflammation (elevated ESR and CRP, fever, anemia of chronic disease, fatigue, weight loss). If these symptoms are present in a woman of reproductive age, you should consider the possibility of an autoimmune disease.

Behçet Syndrome
The classic patient is a 20-something man with painful oral and genital ulcers. Patients can also have uveitis, arthritis, and other skin lesions (especially erythema nodosum). Steroids might help.

Dermatomyositis
Dermatomyositis causes polymyositis (Table 30-2) plus skin involvement (a heliotrope rash around the eyes with associated periorbital edema is classic). Patients classically have trouble rising from a chair or climbing steps because the proximal muscles are affected. Muscle enzymes are elevated, and electromyography results are irregular. Muscle biopsy establishes the diagnosis. Affected patients have an increased incidence of malignancy.

TABLE 30-2 Differential Diagnosis of Fibromyalgia, Polymyositis, and Polymyalgia Rheumatica

CHARACTERISTIC	FIBROMYALGIA	POLYMYOSITIS	POLYMYALGIA RHEUMATICA
Classic age and sex	Young adult women	Women 40–60 y	Women >50 y
Location	Various	Proximal muscles	Pectoral and pelvic girdles, neck
ESR	Normal	Elevated	Markedly elevated (often >100 mm/h)
Muscle biopsy or EMG	Normal	Abnormal	Normal
Classic findings	Anxiety, stress, insomnia, point tenderness over affected muscles, negative work-up	Elevated CPK; abnormal EMG and biopsy	Temporal arteritis, great response to steroids, very high ESR, elderly
Treatment	Antidepressants, NSAIDs, pregabalin, rest	Steroids	Steroids

CPK, creatine phosphokinase; EMG, electromyography; ESR, erythrocyte sedimentation rate; NSAID, nonsteroidal antiinflammatory drug.

Kawasaki Syndrome

Kawasaki syndrome affects children younger than 5 years old (more common in Japanese and female patients). Patients present with truncal rash, high fever (lasts >5 days), conjunctival injection, cervical lymphadenopathy, a strawberry tongue, late skin desquamation of the palms and soles, or arthritis. Patients develop coronary vessel vasculitis and subsequent aneurysms, which can thrombose and cause a myocardial infarction (suspect Kawasaki disease in any child who has a myocardial infarction). Treat during the acute stage with aspirin (one of the few pediatric diseases in which aspirin is indicated) and intravenous immunoglobulin to reduce the risk of coronary aneurysm development.

Polyarteritis Nodosa

Polyarteritis nodosa is a type of vasculitis classically associated with hepatitis B infection and cryoglobulinemia. Patients present with fever, abdominal pain, weight loss, renal disturbances, or peripheral neuropathies. Lab abnormalities include high ESR and CRP, leukocytosis, anemia, and hematuria or proteinuria. Vasculitis involves medium-sized vessels. Biopsy of an affected organ is the gold standard for diagnosis. P-ANCA (peripheral antineutrophil cytoplasmic antibodies) is associated with the microscopic polyangiitis subtype. Treatment involves steroids and immunosuppressive agents.

Scleroderma and Progressive Systemic Sclerosis

Look for CREST symptoms (calcinosis, Raynaud's phenomenon, esophageal dysmotility with dysphagia, sclerodactyly, and telangiectasia); heartburn; and masklike, leathery facies. Screening test is antinuclear antibody (ANA); confirmatory tests are anticentromere antibody (for CREST symptoms only) and antitopoisomerase (for scleroderma). Treatment depends on the symptoms but often includes corticosteroids, methotrexate, or both.

Sjögren Syndrome

Look for dry eyes (keratoconjunctivitis sicca) and a dry mouth (xerostomia); often associated with other autoimmune disease. Treat with eye drops and good oral hygiene.

Systemic Lupus Erythematosus

Malar rash, discoid rash, photosensitivity, kidney damage, arthritis, pericarditis and pleuritis, positive ANA, positive anti-ds DNA, positive anti-Smith antibody, positive Venereal Disease Research Laboratory (VDRL) or rapid plasma reagin test for syphilis, positive lupus anticoagulant, blood disorders (thrombocytopenia, leukopenia, anemia, or pancytopenia), neurologic disturbances (depression, psychosis, seizures), and oral ulcers can all be presenting symptoms. Use an ANA titer as a screening test and anti-ds. DNA or anti-Smith antibody to confirm. Treat with NSAIDs, hydroxychloroquine, and corticosteroids or other immunosuppressants (e.g., methotrexate, cyclophosphamide, azathioprine, or mycophenolate).

Remember the acronym MD SOAP BRAIN (which is useful because it includes all of the diagnostic criteria): malar rash, discoid rash, serositis (pleuritis, pericarditis), oral ulcers, arthritis, photosensitivity, blood dyscrasias (hemolytic anemia, leukopenia), renal abnormalities (proteinuria or red cell casts), ANA positive, immunologic markers (anti-Smith, anti-dsDNA, antiphospholipid antibodies), and neurologic abnormalities (seizures or psychosis).

Takayasu Arteritis

Takayasu arteritis tends to affect East Asian women between 15 and 30 years old. It is called "pulseless disease" because you might not be able to feel the patient's pulse or measure blood pressure in one or both arms. Vasculitis affects the aortic arch and the branches that arise from it. Carotid involvement can cause neurologic signs or stroke, and congestive heart failure is common. Computed tomography or magnetic resonance angiography shows the characteristic lesions. Treat with steroids.

Wegener Granulomatosis

Wegener granulomatosis resembles Goodpasture syndrome, but older patients are affected, and instead of antiglomerular basement membrane antibody seen in Goodpasture syndrome, there is a positive ANCA titer. Look for nasal (nose bleeds, nasal perforation), lung (hemoptysis, dyspnea), and kidney (hematuria, acute renal failure) involvement. Treat initially with cyclophosphamide. Methotrexate or azathioprine is used for maintenance.

FIBROMYALGIA, POLYMYOSITIS, AND POLYMYALGIA RHEUMATICA

The differential diagnosis of fibromyalgia, polymyositis, and polymyalgia rheumatica is given in Table 30-2.

PAGET DISEASE

Paget disease is a disease of bone in which bone is broken down and regenerated, often simultaneously. It is usually seen in patients older than 40 years of age and is more common in men. It is often discovered in an asymptomatic patient via radiography. Classic sites of involvement are the pelvis (Fig. 30-4) and skull.

Watch for a person who has had to buy larger-size hats. Patients might complain of bone pain; arthritis; or, rarely, nerve deafness or paraplegia. Alkaline phosphatase is markedly elevated in the presence of normal calcium and phosphorus. The risk of osteosarcoma is increased in affected bones.

The main treatment is antiresorptive agents (e.g., zoledronic acid, alendronate, risedronate, pamidronate).

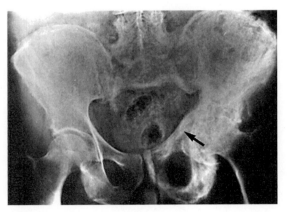

FIGURE 30-4 Paget disease of the pelvis. The entire left hemipelvis is involved, and there are arthritic changes of the left hip. Note the classic thickening of the iliopectineal line (arrow).

QR CODE

The QR code includes three USMLE-style questions and answers. For more questions, redeem the PIN code on the inside cover for the Crush Step 2 question bank powered by USMLE Consult. Please see the Introduction for instructions on how to access content using the QR codes.

Question

A 34-year-old woman complains of gradually worsening weakness and fatigue over the past 2 months. She notes that she especially has trouble getting out of a chair. When asked about depression, the patient shrugs her shoulders and says she's tired more than anything else. Her medical history is insignificant. Vital signs are within normal limits. Physical examination reveals marked symmetric weakness of the shoulder muscles and hip flexors. These muscles are also tender to palpation. There is mild periorbital edema with a slight purple color in the upper eyelids. Laboratory tests reveal the following:

Hemoglobin	10 g/dL
Mean corpuscular volume	86 μm/cell volume
Platelets	450,000/μL
Creatine kinase	1500 U/L (reference range, 10–80 U/L)

Which of the following is true regarding the most likely cause of the woman's symptoms?
(A) The cause is most likely a subclinical depression.
(B) An electrocardiogram should be done immediately to rule out a silent myocardial infarction.
(C) Muscle biopsy most likely would be normal.
(D) Electromyography would be expected to show spontaneous fibrillations and irritability.
(E) The woman has about a 95% chance of developing a malignancy during her lifetime.

31 UROLOGY

KIDNEYS

Nephrolithiasis

Signs and symptoms include severe flank pain, which often radiates to the groin and is colicky; hematuria; and stones on abdominal radiographs (85% of stones are radiopaque) or computed tomography (CT) (Fig. 31-1). Symptoms occur after the stone leaves the kidney and gets stuck in or irritates the renal pelvis or ureter, which can cause unilateral urinary obstruction and hydronephrosis and can lead to infection or kidney damage if not treated or if the stone doesn't pass.

○ **Composition:** About 75% to 85% of stones are composed of calcium (look for hypercalcemia and hyperparathyroidism; small bowel bypass also increases oxalate absorption and thus calcium stone formation), 15% are struvite or magnesium–ammonium–phosphate stones (think of infection with *Proteus* species, the cause of staghorn calculi), 7% are uric acid stones (look for history of gout or leukemia), and 2% are cystine stones (think of cystinuria).

○ **Diagnosis:** Noncontrast CT is the gold standard for diagnosis and is therefore the test of choice. Intravenous pyelography (IVP) was previously the diagnostic procedure of choice, but because of contrast reactions, lower sensitivity, and higher radiation exposure, it has been replaced by noncontrast CT as the test of choice. Ultrasonography is useful in the evaluation of pregnant women with suspected nephrolithiasis.

○ Treat stones with lots of hydration, narcotics for pain, and observation. Most stones pass by themselves. Stone passage can be facilitated with the use of α-blockers (usually tamsulosin) and calcium channel blockers (usually nifedipine). Treat uric acid stones and cystine stones with potassium citrate to alkalinize the urine and treat struvite stones with antibiotics to eradicate the underlying infection. Stones larger than 10 mm aren't likely to pass spontaneously. If a stone does not pass spontaneously or if the stone is larger than 10 mm, do lithotripsy, ureteroscopy with stone retrieval, or surgery as a last resort (laparoscopic is more common than open nowadays).

○ Watch out for complications such as acute kidney injury and urosepsis.

Urinary Obstruction

In addition to stones that obstruct the ureter, tumors are another potential cause of urinary obstruction. Either situation can lead to hydronephrosis and permanent damage if not addressed. Surgical intervention is indicated to relieve obstruction, whether via stone retrieval or lithotripsy, cancer surgery, or placement of a percutaneous nephrostomy tube (through the kidney into the renal collecting system to allow urine drainage), ureteral stent, or Foley or suprapubic catheter (for bladder outlet obstruction). In the setting of coexisting infection, prompt intravenous (IV) antibiotics are needed and emergent drainage is indicated.

Renal Cell Carcinoma

Painless hematuria (gross or microscopic) is the most typical presenting sign of renal cell carcinoma. Patients rarely present with the classic triad of hematuria, flank pain, and a palpable flank mass. CT scan (preferred over IVP) is a good initial diagnostic test. Treatment for disease confined to the kidney or with extension limited to renal vein invasion (classic) is surgical resection. With other organ invasion or distant metastatic disease (usually to lung or bone), immunotherapy (e.g., interleukin-2 [IL-2]) is the preferred treatment.

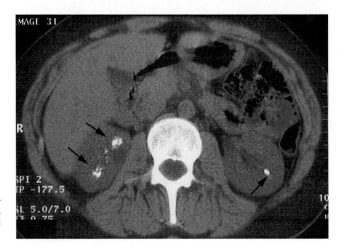

FIGURE 31-1 Unenhanced computed tomography image demonstrates high-density areas in both kidneys (*arrows*), which represent renal calculi.

Renal Transplant

Transplant is an option for patients with end-stage renal disease unless they have active infections or other life-threatening conditions (e.g., AIDS, malignancy). Lupus and diabetes mellitus are not contraindications to transplant. Living related donors are best (siblings or parents), especially when they are human leukocyte antigen (HLA) similar, but cadaveric kidneys are more common because of availability. Before the transplant, perform ABO and lymphocytotoxic (HLA) cross-matching.

○ A transplanted kidney is placed in the iliac fossa (for easy biopsy access in case of problems as well as for technical reasons); usually the recipient's kidneys are left in place to reduce morbidity.

○ Unacceptable kidney donors include newborns, persons older than 60 years, history of generalized or intraabdominal sepsis, history of disease with possible renal involvement (e.g., diabetes mellitus, hypertension, lupus), and history of malignancy. Types of renal rejection:

  ○ **Hyperacute rejection:** Preformed cytotoxic antibodies (considered a type II hypersensitivity reaction) against donor kidney (happens with ABO mismatch as well as other preformed antibodies). Classic description: The surgery is complete and the vascular clamps are released and the kidney quickly turns bluish-black. Treat by removing the kidney.

  ○ **Acute rejection:** T-cell–mediated rejection that manifests during first several months with fever, oliguria, weight gain, tenderness and enlargement of the graft, hypertension, or renal function lab derangement. Treatment involves pulse corticosteroids, anti–T-cell antibody therapies (polyclonal antibodies, OKT3), other antibody therapies (basiliximab, daclizumab), and other immunosuppressants (tacrolimus, mycophenolate, cyclosporine). Accelerated rejection occurs over the first few days and is thought to reflect reactivation of previously sensitized T cells.

  ○ **Chronic rejection:** Mediated by T cells or antibodies. This is a late cause of renal deterioration manifesting with gradual decline in kidney function, proteinuria, and hypertension. Treatment is supportive and not effective, but the graft can last several years before it gives out completely. The patient may receive a new kidney transplant.

  ○ **Asymptomatic rejection:** Follow creatinine to assess (more reliable than blood urea nitrogen).

  Immunosuppressive medications used in transplant medicine:

○ **Antithymocyte globulin** is an antibody against T cells.

○ **Azathioprine** is an antineoplastic that is cleaved into mercaptopurine and inhibits DNA and RNA synthesis, which decreases B-cell and T-cell production.

○ **Basiliximab** is a monoclonal antibody against the IL-2 receptor.

○ **Cyclosporine** inhibits IL-2 production.

○ **Daclizumab** is a monoclonal antibody against the IL-2 receptor.

○ **Hydroxychloroquine** interferes with antigen presentation.

○ **Methotrexate** is a folic acid antagonist, but its precise mechanism in immunosuppression is unclear.

○ **Mycophenolate** prevents T-cell activation.

○ **OKT3** is an antibody to the CD3 receptor on T cells.

○ **Steroids** inhibit IL-1 production.

○ **Tacrolimus** inhibits signaling through the T-cell receptor.

○ **Thalidomide's** mechanism of action is not known.

Cyclosporine causes nephrotoxicity, which can be difficult to clinically distinguish from graft rejection. When in doubt, do a percutaneous needle biopsy of the graft because histologic differentiation is usually possible. Renal ultrasonography can also help to distinguish between nephrotoxicity and graft rejection. Practically speaking, if you increase the immunosuppressive dose, acute rejection should decrease, but cyclosporine toxicity stays the same or worsens.

Immunosuppression carries the risk of infection (with common as well as the strange organisms that infect patients with AIDS) and increased risk of cancer (especially lymphomas and epithelial cell cancers).

Prostate

Prostatitis tends to occur in young and middle-aged men. Common symptoms include fever, chills, malaise, cloudy urine, pain (in the perineum, testicles, penis, or lower abdomen), bladder irritation, and urinary obstructive symptoms (dribbling, hesitancy). A digital rectal examination typically reveals a tender, boggy prostate gland. Urinalysis and urine culture should be performed to guide therapy. Broad-spectrum antibiotic therapy should be started as empiric therapy, and hospitalization may be required for IV antibiotic therapy. Typical oral agents that may be used include trimethoprim–sulfamethoxazole, fluoroquinolones (typically ciprofloxacin or levofloxacin), tetracyclines, and nitrofurantoin. An aminoglycoside (e.g., gentamicin) may be combined with a fluoroquinolone if IV therapy is indicated.

Symptoms of benign prostatic hyperplasia (BPH) include urinary hesitancy, intermittency, terminal dribbling, decreased size and force of stream, sensation of incomplete emptying, nocturia, urgency, dysuria, and frequency.

○ BPH can result in urinary retention, urinary tract infections (UTIs), hydronephrosis, and even kidney damage or failure in severe cases.

○ Other causes of lower urinary tract symptoms (LUTS) that can mimic BPH include UTI; prostatitis; and some urologic tumors, including prostate cancer. When evaluating LUTS, consider diagnostic steps such as digital rectal exam, urinalysis or urine culture, prostate specific antigen PSA, measurement of postvoid residual, and urinary flow studies (depending on the clinical scenario presented on the exam question).

○ Drug therapy is started when the patient becomes symptomatic and after other causes of LUTS have been ruled out. Options include $\alpha1$-blockade (prazosin, terazosin, doxazosin), 5-α-reductase inhibitors (finasteride, dutasteride), antiandrogens, and gonadotropin-releasing hormone analogs.

○ Transurethral resection of the prostate (TURP) is used for more advanced cases, especially with repeated UTIs, urinary retention, and hydronephrosis or kidney damage caused by reflux. Prostatectomy also may be used but is a more complicated operation.

Urinary Retention

Acute urinary retention occurs frequently in men older than the age of 60 years and is most commonly associated with BPH. Other causes of acute urinary retention include constipation, prostate cancer, urethral stricture, neurologic disorders, medications, postoperative status, UTI, and urolithiasis. Medications are a common and frequently tested cause of urinary retention. Common culprits include antihistamines (e.g., diphenhydramine, fexofenadine), anticholinergics (e.g., oxybutynin), antispasmodic agents (e.g., tolterodine), opiates, and tricyclic antidepressants (e.g., imipramine, amitriptyline, nortriptyline, doxepin).

With acute urinary retention (pain, palpation of full bladder on abdominal exam, history of BPH, no urination in past 24 hours), the first step is to empty the bladder. If you cannot pass a regular Foley catheter, consider the use of a large catheter with a firm Coudé tip or alternatively do a suprapubic tap. Then address the underlying cause (surgery [TURP] is usually recommended for BPH in this setting).

Scrotum and Testes
Cryptorchidism

Cryptorchidism is arrest of descent of the testicle(s) somewhere between the renal area and the scrotum. The more premature the infant, the greater the likelihood of cryptorchidism. Many arrested testes eventually descend on their own within the first year of life. Intramuscular human chorionic gonadotropin (hCG) may be used to induce testicular descent. After 1 year, surgical intervention (orchiopexy) is warranted to attempt to preserve fertility as well as facilitate future testicular exams (because of increased cancer risk). Cryptorchidism is a major risk factor for testicular cancer (40-fold increased risk), and bringing the testis into the scrotum does not alter the increased risk of testicular cancer. The higher the testicle is found (the farther away from the scrotum), the higher the risk of developing testicular cancer and the lower the likelihood of retaining fertility.

Hydrocele and Varicocele

Hydrocele represents a remnant of the processus vaginalis (remember embryology?) and transilluminates. It generally causes no symptoms and does not require treatment. A varicocele is a dilation of the pampiniform venous plexus ("bag of worms," usually on the left). It does not transilluminate, disappears in the supine position, and becomes prominent with standing or the Valsalva maneuver. Varicoceles may cause male infertility or pain (in which case it is surgically treated).

 Whereas the right testicular or ovarian vein drains into the inferior vena cava, the left ovarian or testicular vein drains into the left renal vein.

Orchitis

Remember mumps as a cause of orchitis (painful, swollen testis, usually unilateral, in a postpubertal male patient). The best treatment is prophylactic (immunization). Mumps rarely causes sterility because it is usually unilateral. Epididymo-orchitis is more common and typically caused by spread from adjacent bacterial epididymitis.

Priapism

Priapism is a persistent erection not associated with sexual stimulation or desire. Ischemic priapism results from failure of detumescence and is a urologic emergency. Nonischemic priapism usually results from a fistula between the cavernosal artery and corpus cavernosum. The diagnosis of priapism generally is straightforward (pun intended) and should be obvious from the vignette on the USMLE. Priapism is treated with pain medication and intracavernosal injection of a sympathomimetic agent (often phenylephrine).

Testicular Cancer

Testicular cancer usually manifests as a painless mass in a young man (ages 20–40 years). The main risk factor is cryptorchidism. Roughly 90% are germ cell tumors, the most common being seminoma. Ultrasonography is the first step in evaluating a testicular mass. Treatment generally consists of orchiectomy and radiation. Chest radiographs and CT of the abdomen and pelvis are used to evaluate for metastatic disease. If disease is widespread, use chemotherapy. Alpha fetoprotein is a tumor marker for yolk sac tumors, and hCG is a marker for choriocarcinoma. Leydig cell tumors can secrete androgens and cause precocious puberty.

Testicular Torsion and Epididymitis

Testicular torsion and epididymitis are compared in Table 31-1.

TABLE 31-1 Differential Diagnosis of Testicular Torsion and Epididymitis		
FEATURE	**TESTICULAR TORSION**	**EPIDIDYMITIS**
Age (y)	<30 (usually prepubertal)	>30
Appearance	Testes may be elevated into the inguinal canal; swelling	Swollen testis, overlying erythema, positive urinalysis results, urethral discharge, urethritis, prostatitis
Prehn sign	Pain stays the same or worsens with testicular elevation	Pain decreases with testicular elevation
Treatment	Immediate surgery to salvage testis; orchiopexy of both testes	Antibiotics*

*In men younger than 40 years of age, epididymitis is commonly caused by a sexually transmitted disease (chlamydial infection, gonorrhea); treat accordingly. In men older than 40 years of age, it is commonly caused by urinary tract infection organisms; treat with trimethoprim–sulfamethoxazole or ciprofloxacin.

PENIS

Impotence

Impotence is most commonly caused by vascular or neurologic problems. Medications are also a common culprit (especially antihypertensives and antidepressants). Diabetes mellitus may be a vascular (increased atherosclerosis) or neurogenic cause of impotence. Remember "point and shoot": Parasympathetics mediate erection, and sympathetics mediate ejaculation. Patients undergoing dialysis also are commonly impotent.

The history often gives you a clue if the cause of impotence is psychogenic. Look for a normal pattern of nocturnal erections; selective dysfunction (a patient who has normal erections when masturbating but not with a partner); and stress, anxiety, or fear when the cause is psychological.

Penile Anomalies

Hypospadias occurs when the urethra opens on the ventral side (undersurface when flaccid) of the penis; epispadias occurs when the urethra opens on the dorsal side (top) of the penis (associated with extrophy of the bladder). Treat both surgically. Chordee is a bending of the penis most evident during erection that can occur in either condition but is classic in hypospadias (when it is a downward bending). Peyronie disease is an acquired localized fibrotic disorder resulting in penile deformity, pain, and sometimes erectile dysfunction. Urologic consultation is indicated for medical management (e.g., pentoxifylline), intralesional drug injection, or surgery.

MISCELLANEOUS

Trauma

In patients with trauma, especially when pelvic fractures are present, look for signs of urethral injury (a high-riding, ballottable prostate; blood at the urethral meatus; ecchymosis of the scrotum or perineum) before trying to pass a Foley catheter. If any of these signs are present or pelvic fractures are severe, do not try to pass a Foley catheter until you have gotten a retrograde urethrogram to rule out urethral injury. Urethral injury is a contraindication to a Foley catheter.

Hematuria

Worry about cancer on the boards (kidney > bladder > ureteral > urethral) when hematuria is painless. Hematuria is classically caused by urolithiasis when painful. Get a CT scan without contrast for suspected urinary tract stones and get a CT with and without contrast for painless hematuria to assess for malignancy (i.e., CT urography) or with trauma. CT urography has replaced IVP as the initial imaging modality. If the imaging workup results are negative, endoscopy via a urethral approach is generally indicated in adults. If red blood cell casts are present, think glomerulonephritis. In reproductive-age women, watch for false-positive test results from menstrual bleeding caused by improper specimen collection. Ultrasonography should be used instead of CT in pregnant women.

Urinary Incontinence

Urge incontinence is the involuntary leakage of urine. Urinary incontinence can be divided into subtypes, which helps in diagnosis and treatment. These subtypes include stress, urge, mixed, and overflow. Each of these subtypes is outlined in Table 31-2. Remember that symptoms of incontinence may be related to an underlying neurologic disease (e.g., multiple sclerosis) or malignancy (e.g., spinal cord compression). The diagnostic evaluation generally begins with urinalysis, urine culture, and assessment of renal function. Voiding diaries and urodynamic testing sometimes are helpful. Treatment options are outlined in Table 31-2.

TABLE 31-2 Types of Urinary Incontinence

TYPE	HISTORY	MECHANISM	KEY POINTS	TREATMENT
Urge	Involuntary leakage of urine accompanied by a sense of urgency; may range from drops of urine to soaking; precipitants may include running water or washing hands	Uninhibited bladder contractions	May be caused by interstitial cystitis in younger women; commonly idiopathic	Bladder training or biofeedback; antimuscarinics (e.g., oxybutynin, tolterodine)
Stress	Involuntary leakage of urine with exertion, sneezing, coughing, or laughing	Leakage occurs when increases in intraabdominal pressure overcome sphincter closure mechanisms in the absence of bladder contraction	Common in multiparous women and after pelvic surgery	Weight loss; Kegel exercises; pessaries; surgical sling procedures or injection of urethral bulking agents
Mixed	Involuntary leakage of urine associated with urgency and with exertion, sneezing, coughing, or laughing	The mechanisms in urge and stress incontinence overlap, resulting in both bladder overactivity and impaired urethral sphincter function	The most common type of urinary incontinence in women	Bladder training or biofeedback; antimuscarinics (e.g., oxybutynin, tolterodine)
Overflow	Continuous leakage of urine associated with incomplete bladder emptying; symptoms include a weak urinary stream, dribbling, hesitancy, frequency, and nocturia	Impaired bladder contractility or bladder outlet obstruction	Bladder outlet obstruction is uncommon in women; the most common causes in men are BPH, prostate cancer, and urethral stricture; common causes in women include pelvic organ prolapse and prior surgery for prolapse; suprasacral spinal cord injury can result in overflow incontinence in both sexes	Indwelling catheter (associated with high morbidity; timed voiding; treatment of underlying disease; treatment of BPH in men

BPH, benign prostatic hyperplasia.

QR CODE

The QR code includes three USMLE-style questions and answers. For more questions, redeem the PIN code on the inside cover for the Crush Step 2 question bank powered by USMLE Consult.

Please see the Introduction for instructions on how to access content using the QR codes.

Question

An 18-year-old man presents to the office with a chief complaint of severe testicular pain that started suddenly 2 hours ago after lifting weights. He says the pain is a 10 out of 10 and is constant; he also reports nausea. The patient has no significant medical history and is on no medications. He reports no recent urinary symptoms or illnesses and is not sexually active. On examination, the patient has some scrotal wall edema and erythema as well as marked testicular tenderness to palpation. The testicular pain is not decreased by manual testicular elevation. There is no evidence of direct or indirect hernia. Which of the following is true?

(A) The patient requires immediate referral to a urologist.

(B) The patient requires antibiotics to cover possible chlamydial infection and follow-up in 2 weeks.

(C) The patient requires an exploratory laparotomy.

(D) The patient should use scrotal ice packs and nonsteroidal antiinflammatory drugs and follow-up in 48 hours.

(E) The patient probably has mumps.

32 VASCULAR SURGERY

ATHEROSCLEROSIS

Abdominal Aortic Aneurysm

Look for a pulsatile abdominal mass that can cause abdominal pain. If pain is present, suspect possible rupture of abdominal aortic aneurysm (AAA), although even an unruptured AAA may cause some pain. Computed tomography (CT) scan with intravenous (IV) contrast usually is used for initial evaluation in symptomatic patients (can use ultrasonography in asymptomatic patients with a pulsatile mass and suspected AAA). If the AAA is smaller than 5 cm and not leaking or ruptured, follow it with serial ultrasonography to make sure that it is not enlarging. If the AAA is larger than 5 cm (or you are told that it is rapidly enlarging) or there is evidence of leak or rupture, open or endovascular surgical correction should be done.

A pulsatile abdominal mass + hypotension = emergent laparotomy (means ruptured AAA, which has a mortality rate of roughly 90%). If there is time while the operating room staff is setting up, you can get CT or ultrasonography, but don't delay laparotomy if imaging is not immediately available.

Acute Bowel Infarction

Look for a patient with a history of extensive atherosclerosis or multiple atherosclerosis risk factors who presents with abdominal pain or tenderness, bloody diarrhea, and possibly peritoneal signs (e.g., rebound tenderness, guarding). Watch for "thumbprinting" (thickened bowel walls that resemble thumbprints) on abdominal radiographs. Patients also may have tachycardia, hypotension, or shock.

Carotid Stenosis

The classic presentation of carotid stenosis is a transient ischemic attack (TIA), especially amaurosis fugax, which is characterized by the sudden onset of transient unilateral blindness, sometimes described as a "shade pulled over one eye." Patients classically have a carotid bruit on exam. If a bruit is heard or the patient has a TIA, ultrasonography or CT angiogram or magnetic resonance (MR) angiogram of the carotid arteries (Fig. 32-1) should be done to determine the degree of stenosis.

Decisions regarding the management of carotid stenosis begin with consideration of whether the patient is symptomatic (defined as TIA or stroke within the past 6 months) or asymptomatic.

○ **Symptomatic patients**: If stenosis is greater than 70% to 99%, perform carotid endarterectomy (CEA). If stenosis is 50% to 69%, the data are less clear, and patient factors affect the decision. CEA is generally indicated for men, patients ages 75 or older, patients with recent stroke (not TIA), and patients with hemispheric symptoms rather than transient monocular blindness (amaurosis fugax). Female patients, patients younger than 75 years, and those with mild symptoms generally do better with medical management if stenosis is 50% to 69%. If stenosis is less than 50%, medical management is indicated.

  ○ Patients should not undergo CEA after a stroke that leaves them severely disabled (too late to make a difference), nor should they undergo CEA during a TIA or stroke in evolution. CEA is an elective, not emergent, procedure.

○ **Asymptomatic patients:** If stenosis is 60% to 99%, CEA is indicated. If stenosis is less than 60%, medical management is indicated.

  ○ Medical management includes antihypertensive agents, statins, and antiplatelet therapy.

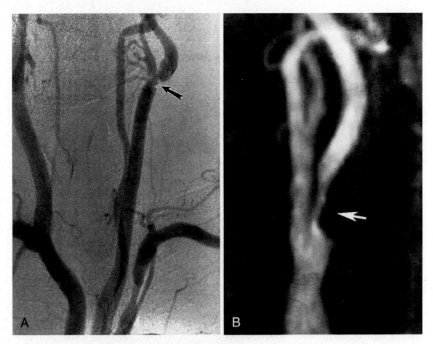

FIGURE 32-1 Atherosclerotic plaque involving the posterolateral wall of the left carotid bulb (*arrows*) on a conventional angiogram (**A**) and a magnetic resonance angiogram (**B**).

○ Carotid stenosis is a generalized marker for atherosclerosis. Virtually all patients have significant coronary artery disease; perioperative myocardial infarction (MI) is the most common cause of death in patients undergoing vascular surgery. Be sure to evaluate risk factors for atherosclerosis (cholesterol, hypertension, smoking, diabetes).

Claudication

Claudication is pain in the lower extremity brought on by exercise and relieved by rest. Claudication is an indicator of severe atherosclerotic disease and is the peripheral vascular equivalent of angina. Associated physical findings include cyanosis (with dependent rubor), atrophic changes (thickened nails, loss of hair, shiny skin), decreased temperature, and decreased (or absent) distal pulses.

Neurogenic pain can present in a similar fashion to claudication, so the next step after a history and physical exam should be an ankle-brachial index (ABI). The ABI is the ratio of the blood pressure in the lower legs to the arms. A lower blood pressure in the leg is an indication of peripheral arterial disease. Know how to interpret an ABI:

○ 0.9 to 1.2 is considered normal.
○ 0.8 to 0.9 indicates mild disease.
○ 0.5 to 0.8 indicates moderate disease and may be accompanied by claudication.
○ <0.5 indicates severe disease. After the ABI is less than 0.3, the patient may have rest pain, arterial ulcerations, or gangrene.

The best treatment is conservative, including smoking cessation; exercise; and control of cholesterol, diabetes mellitus, and hypertension. Antiplatelet agents are warranted in patients with claudication. Aspirin is preferred, but clopidogrel may be used for patients who cannot tolerate aspirin. Cilostazol may be used for the treatment of intermittent claudication. β-Blockers may worsen claudication (as a result of β_2 receptor blockade), but benefits may outweigh the risks in some patients (e.g., prior MI).

If the patient progresses to rest pain in the forefoot that generally occurs at night and is relieved by hanging the foot over the edge of the bed or if the patient cannot continue current lifestyle or work obligations, consider a revascularization procedure. Contrast angiography is the gold standard for evaluating a patient with claudication symptoms preparing to undergo revascularization.

○ Severe pain in the foot that has a sudden onset without previous history, trauma, or any associated chronic physical findings is generally more serious and might represent an embolus (Fig. 32-2) (look for atrial fibrillation) or compartment syndrome (commonly occurs after revascularization procedures).

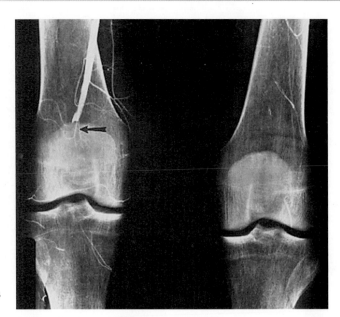

FIGURE 32-2 Right popliteal artery embolus (arrow).

○ Claudication and peripheral vascular disease are generalized markers for atherosclerosis. Check patients for other atherosclerosis risk factors.
○ Ischemic (arterial) ulcers form at pressure points; venous stasis ulcers form superior to the medial ankle.

Leriche Syndrome

Leriche syndrome consists of claudication in the buttocks, buttock atrophy, and impotence in men. It is a classic marker for aortoiliac occlusive disease. Patients usually need an aortoiliac bypass graft or a stent or endograft.

Mesenteric Ischemia

The classic patient with chronic mesenteric ischemia has a long history of postprandial abdominal pain (caused by intestinal angina, similar to cardiac angina after exercising), which causes a fear of food and thus leads to extensive weight loss. This diagnosis is difficult because, similar to all atherosclerotic disease, it occurs in patients older than 40 years who might have other disorders that cause the problem (e.g., peptic ulcer disease, pancreatic cancer, stomach cancer). Look for a history of extensive atherosclerosis (previous MIs, cerebrovascular accidents, known coronary artery disease, peripheral vascular disease, or several risk factors), possible abdominal bruit, and a lack of jaundice (the presence of which would steer you toward pancreatic cancer). CT scan results may be normal or show bowel wall thickening and atherosclerosis of the mesenteric arteries. Diagnose with CT, MR, or conventional angiography and treat surgically with revascularization because of the risks of bowel infarction and malnutrition.

Acute mesenteric ischemia may result from thrombosis, emboli (e.g., atrial fibrillation), or low-flow states (nonocclusive mesenteric ischemia [NOMI]). Acute mesenteric ischemia presents with severe, sudden pain out of proportion to the exam findings and can progress to peritonitis as a result of ischemia and eventual gangrene of the bowel wall. CT and MR angiography are useful in diagnosing acute mesenteric ischemia. Interventional radiology procedures and laparotomy are the cornerstones of treatment.

Subclavian Steal Syndrome

Subclavian steal syndrome is usually caused by left subclavian artery obstruction proximal to the origin of the vertebral artery. To get blood to an exercising arm, blood is "stolen" from the vertebrobasilar system; it flows backward into the distal subclavian artery instead of forward into the brainstem. As a result, the patient develops central nervous system (CNS) symptoms (syncope, vertigo, confusion, ataxia, dysarthria) and upper extremity claudication during exercise. Treat with angioplasty or stent placement or, less commonly, surgical bypass.

MISCELLANEOUS

Aortic Dissection

Aortic dissection consists of aortic wall splits and blood dissecting in between layers of the media in the arterial wall. It classically causes a tearing or ripping type of chest pain that can radiate to the back and is generally seen in the setting of hypertension (whether essential or induced by cocaine) or Marfan syndrome. When aortic dissection is suspected clinically, a CT scan of the chest (and possibly abdomen and pelvis) with IV contrast should be ordered.

Treatment depends on the type. A dissection involving the ascending aorta (Stanford type A and DeBakey types I and II) is treated with immediate surgery (5% of patients survive 1 year without surgery). A dissection that spares the ascending aorta (typically beginning just beyond the origin of the left subclavian artery in the isthmus of the aorta or proximal descending thoracic aorta and extending over a variable distance) is managed medically with antihypertensives (>70% of patients survive longer than 1 year without surgery), assuming there are no signs of impending rupture or end-organ ischemia from vascular compromise.

An aortic dissection might or might not be associated with an aneurysm (the term *dissecting aneurysm* is not a good one).

Superficial Thrombophlebitis

Patients with varicose veins, localized leg pain with superficial cordlike induration or palpable clot, reddish discoloration, and mild fever have superficial thrombophlebitis (not deep vein thrombosis), which rarely leads to pulmonary embolism. Patients do not need anticoagulation. Treatment is usually conservative, including nonsteroidal antiinflammatory drugs and warm compresses. The condition generally subsides on its own within a few days. A thrombectomy under local anesthesia can be done for severe or nonresolving symptoms.

Thoracic Outlet Syndrome

Thoracic outlet obstruction refers to symptoms caused by obstruction of the nerves or blood vessels serving the arm as the neurovascular bundle passes from the thoracocervical region to the axilla. Affected patients have upper extremity paresthesias (nerve impingement), weakness, cold temperature (arterial compromise), edema, or venous distension (venous compromise). The absence of CNS symptoms helps to differentiate this condition from subclavian steal syndrome. Causes include cervical ribs (ribs arising from a cervical vertebrae that are usually asymptomatic but may compromise subclavian blood flow), anomalous ligaments, cervical trauma, or muscular hypertrophy (classic in young male weight lifters). Treat with surgical intervention (e.g., cervical rib resection).

Venous Insufficiency

The term *venous insufficiency* generally refers to the lower extremities. Patients might have a history of deep vein thrombosis; swelling in the extremity with pain, fatigability, and heaviness, which are relieved by elevating the extremity; or varicose veins. Skin pigmentation can increase around the ankles, with possible skin breakdown and ulceration (Fig. 32-3). Initial treatment is conservative and includes elastic compression stockings; elevation with minimal standing; and treatment of any ulcers with cleaning, wet-to-dry dressings, and antibiotics (if cellulitis is present).

Note *After a penetrating trauma in an extremity (or iatrogenic catheter damage), an arteriovenous fistula or pseudoaneurysm can result. Look for bruits over the area or a palpable pulsatile mass. Such fistulas or pseudoaneurysms are generally treated with open or endovascular surgery.*

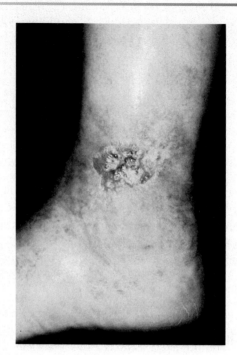

FIGURE 32-3 Venous stasis ulcer.

QR CODE

The QR code includes two USMLE-style questions and answers. For more questions, redeem the PIN code on the inside cover for the Crush Step 2 question bank powered by USMLE Consult.

Please see the Introduction for instructions on how to access content using the QR codes.

Question

A 63-year-old man presents to the office with a chief complaint of pain in the calf when walking. He claims that the farther he walks, the more likely he is to get pain in his left calf, and the worse the pain is likely to get. When he stops to rest, the pain goes away. The pattern had been stable over a few months because the patient just avoided walking long distances, but he says it is now slowly getting worse, and shorter distances are bringing on the pain. Medical history is significant for a myocardial infarction 4 years ago, hypertension, hypercholesterolemia, gout, and tobacco use of 2 packs per day for the past 20 years. Medications include carvedilol, enalapril, pravastatin, aspirin, and allopurinol.

Vital signs are within normal limits. Extremity examination reveals shiny skin without hair on both legs below the knee and thickened, somewhat distorted toenails. Temperature is decreased on the surface of both feet compared with the rest of the body. Pedal and popliteal pulses are not palpable bilaterally, but femoral pulses are normal bilaterally. Which of the following should be the next step in the management of this patient?

(A) Encourage the patient to quit smoking.
(B) Start heparin.
(C) Refer for an urgent revascularization procedure.
(D) Increase the dose of carvedilol.
(E) Stop the aspirin.

The most common images that show up on Step 2 are electrocardiograms, radiology images (radiographs, computed tomography scans, magnetic resonance imaging scans), clinical images (dermatology photos, funduscopic images), and charts (fetal tracings, karyotypes, milestones). Also, audio clips of heart murmurs are common on Step 2. Although some questions with photos can be answered without looking at the photo, this is not always the case. The entities listed below are fair game for Step 2. Remember that you may be asked for more information than simple identification of the image, including pathophysiology, treatment, or complications of the disease.

In the following lists, the higher yield images are listed first. Images for the highest yield topics are provided in this book. Lower yield images can be accessed through the QR codes provided. The sections beginning with Blood Smears include topics that may appear as images on the USMLE but are lower yield topics.

ELECTROCARDIOGRAMS

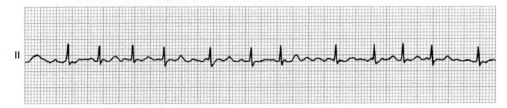

FIGURE 33-1 **Atrial fibrillation.** There are no true P waves, and the ventricular rate is irregular. *(From Goldberger AL: Clinical Electrocardiography: A Simplified Approach, 7th ed. Philadelphia, Mosby, 2006, Figure 15-4.)*

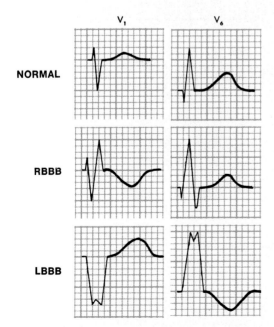

FIGURE 33-2 **Bundle branch block (RBB), right and left.** RBBB shows rSR′ complex in lead V1 and qRS complex in lead V6. Left bundle branch block shows a wide QS complex in lead V1 and wide R wave in lead V6. *(From Goldberger AL: Clinical Electrocardiography: A Simplified Approach, 7th ed. Philadelphia, Mosby, 2006, Figure 7-6.)*

Third-Degree (Complete) AV Block

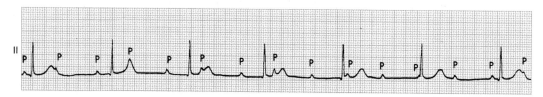

FIGURE 33-3 **Complete third degree heart block.** Independent P and QRS activity. *(From Goldberger AL: Clinical Electrocardiography: A Simplified Approach, 7th ed. Philadelphia, Mosby, 2006, Figure 17-5.)*

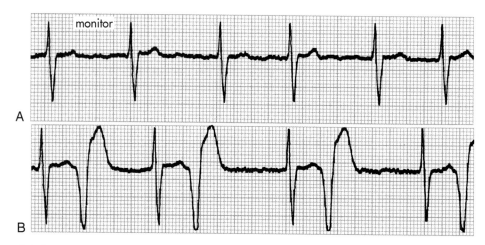

FIGURE 33-4 **Digitalis toxicity. A,** Underlying atrial fibrillation. **B,** Ventricular bigeminy with each normal QRS followed by a ventricular premature beat. *(From Goldberger AL: Clinical Electrocardiography: A Simplified Approach, 7th ed. Philadelphia, Mosby, 2006, Figure 18-1.)*

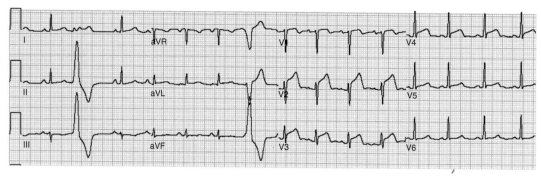

FIGURE 33-5 **Anterior wall MI.** ST-segment elevation in leads V1 to V4. *(From Marx J, Hockberger R, Walls R: Rosens's Emergency Medicine, 7th ed. Philadelphia, Mosby, 2010, Figure 76-5.)*

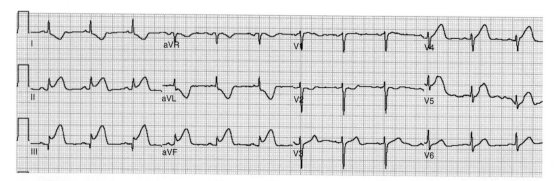

FIGURE 33-6 **Inferior wall myocardial infarction.** ST-segment elevation in leads II, III, and aVF and ST-segment depression in leads I and aVL. *(From Marx J, Hockberger R, Walls R: Rosen's Emergency Medicine, 7th ed. Philadelphia, Mosby, 2010, Figure 76-7.)*

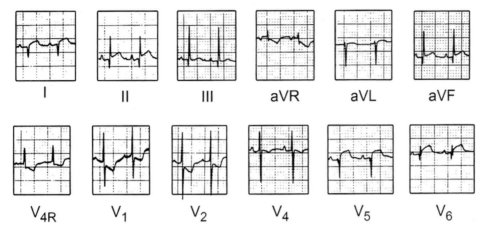

FIGURE 33-7 **Lateral wall myocardial infarction.** – ST-segment elevation in leads I, aVL, V5, and V6. *(From Keane JF, Fyler DC, Lock JE: Nadas' Pediatric Cardiology, 2nd ed. Philadelphia, Saunders, 2006, Figure 12-50. From Fyler DC. Nadas' Pediatric Cardiology. Philadelphia: Hanley & Belfus, 1992.)*

RIGHT PRECORDIAL LEADS

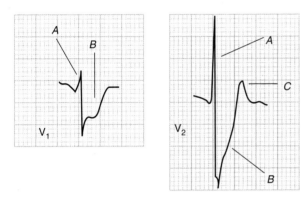

FIGURE 33-8 **Posterior wall myocardial infarction.** – ST-segment elevation in leads V8 and V9 and ST-segment depression in leads V1, V2, and V3. *(From Marx J, Hockberger R, Walls R: Rosen's Emergency Medicine, 7th ed. Philadelphia, Mosby, 2010, Figure 76-8.)*

POSTERIOR LEADS

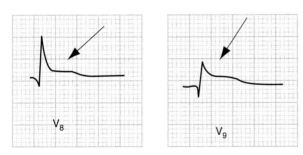

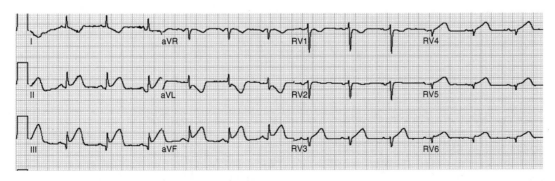

FIGURE 33-9 **Right ventricle myocardial infarction (MI).** – ST-segment elevation in right-sided precordial leads RV3 to RV6. Also note the features of inferior wall MI. *(From Marx J, Hockberger R, Walls R: Rosen's Emergency Medicine, 7th ed. Philadelphia, Mosby, 2010, Figure 76-9.)*

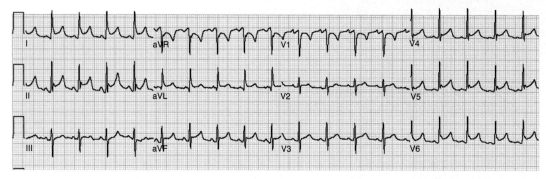

FIGURE 33-10 **Pericarditis**. Diffuse upward ST-segment elevation, PR depression in lead II, and PR elevation in lead aVR. *(From Marx J, Hockberger R, Walls R: Rosen's Emergency Medicine, 7th ed. Philadelphia, Mosby, 2010, Figure 76-12.)*

Torsades de Pointes: Sustained

Monitor lead

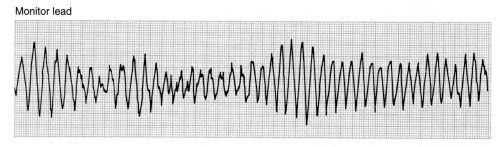

FIGURE 33-11 **Torsades de pointes.** Ventricular tachycardia with QRS axis that appears to rotate in a systematic way. *(From Goldberger AL: Clinical Electrocardiography: A Simplified Approach, 7th ed. Philadelphia, Mosby, 2006, Figure 16-18.)*

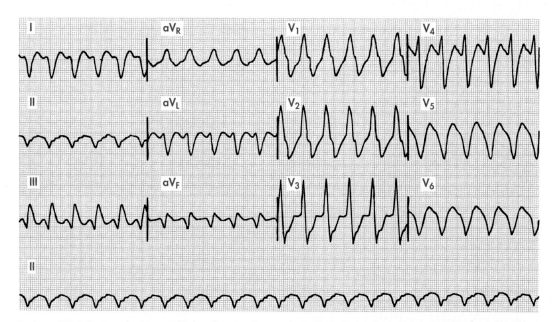

FIGURE 33-12 **Ventricular tachycardia.** Wide complex QRS tachycardia. *(From Goldberger AL: Clinical Electrocardiography: A Simplified Approach, 7th ed. Philadelphia, Mosby, 2006, Part 4, Case 3.)*

Ventricular Fibrillation

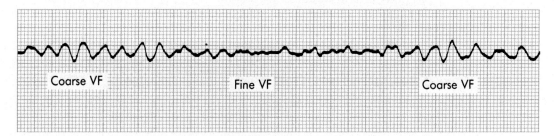

FIGURE 33-13 **Ventricular fibrillation.** Fibrillatory waves in an irregular pattern. *(From Goldberger AL: Clinical Electrocardiography: A Simplified Approach, 7th ed. Philadelphia, Mosby, 2006, Figure 16-13.)*

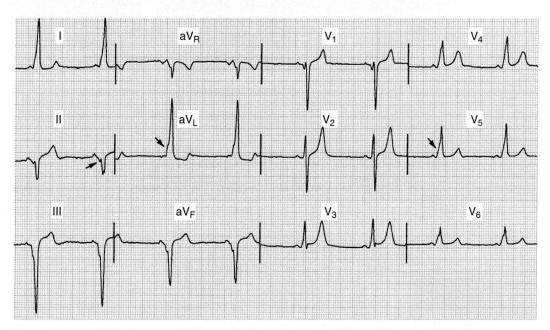

FIGURE 33-14 **Wolff-Parkinson-White pattern.** Triad of a wide QRS complex, a short PR interval, and delta waves *(arrows). (From Goldberger AL: Clinical Electrocardiography: A Simplified Approach, 7th ed. Philadelphia, Mosby, 2006, Figure 12-3.)*

RADIOLOGIC FINDINGS

Cardiopulmonary

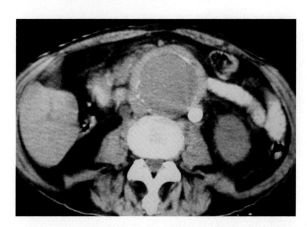

FIGURE 33-15 **Abdominal aortic aneurysm (AAA).** Computed tomography scan with contrast shows a large AAA with thick outer wall. *(From Adam A, Dixon AK, Grainger RG, Allison DJ (eds): Grainger & Allison's Diagnostic Radiology, 5th ed. London, Churchill Livingstone, 2008, Figure 27.34.)*

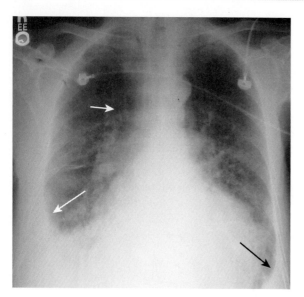

FIGURE 33-16 Congestive heart failure. Chest radiography with cardiomegaly, pleural effusions, and central interstitial thickenings (including Kerley A lines). *(Courtesy of Michael B. Gotway, MD, Scottsdale Medical Imaging and the Department of Radiology, University of California, San Francisco.)*

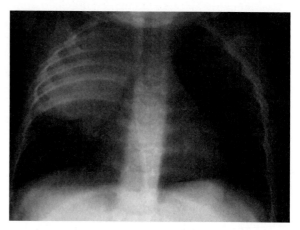

FIGURE 33-17 Lobar pneumonia. Note the bulging of the horizontal fissure. *(From Long SS, Pickering LK, Prober CG: Principles and Practice of Pediatric Infectious Diseases, 3rd ed. Philadelphia, Saunders, 2008, Figure 134-5.)*

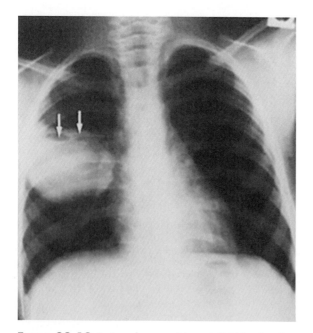

FIGURE 33-18 Lung abscess. Note air-fluid levels, often caused by anaerobic organisms. *(From Brook I: Lung abscess and pulmonary infections due to anaerobic bacteria. In Chernick V, Boat TF, Wilmott RW, Bush A [eds]: Kendig's Disorders of the Respiratory Tract in Children, 7th ed. Philadelphia, Saunders, 2006, p 482.)*

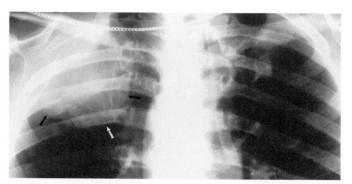

FIGURE 33-19 Lung cancer. Pancoast tumor, an upper lobe mass that can cause Horner syndrome. *(From Mercier L: Practical Orthopedics, 6th ed. Philadelphia, Mosby, 2008, Figure 5-52.)*

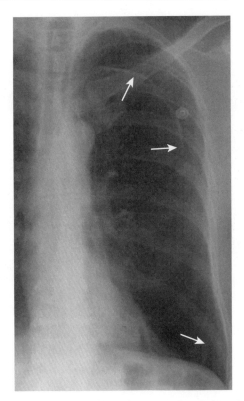

FIGURE 33-20 **Pneumothorax.** Pleural line has lucency on either side. *(Courtesy of Michael B. Gotway, MD, Scottsdale Medical Imaging and the Department of Radiology, University of California, San Francisco.)*

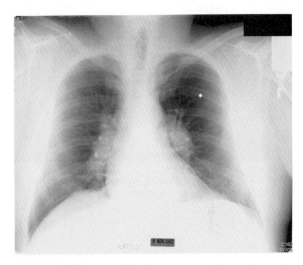

FIGURE 33-21 **Sarcoidosis.** Prominent hilar adenopathy with normal-appearing lungs. *(From Mason RJ, Broaddus VC, Martin T, et al: Murray and Nadel's Textbook of Respiratory Medicine, 5th ed. Philadelphia, Saunders, 2010, Figure 59-1.)*

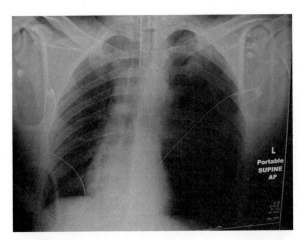

FIGURE 33-22 **Tension pneumothorax.** Note the mediastinal shift. *(From Marx J, Hockberger R, Walls R: Rosen's Emergency Medicine, 7th ed. Philadelphia, Mosby, 2010, Figure 42-7.)*

Severe carotid artery stenosis on angiogram

Abdominal and Gastrointestinal

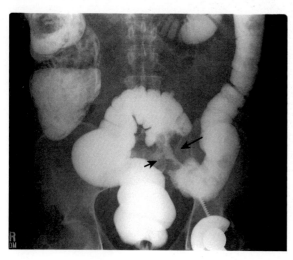

FIGURE 33-23 **Colon cancer.** Apple core lesion on barium enema. *(Courtesy Dr. Perry Pernicano.)*

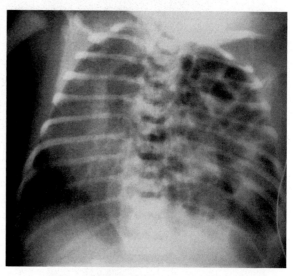

FIGURE 33-24 **Congenital diaphragmatic hernia.** Bowel extending into the left hemithorax with shift of the mediastinum to the right side. *(From Adam A, Dixon AK, Grainger RG, Allison DJ (eds): Grainger & Allison's Diagnostic Radiology, 5th ed. London, Churchill Livingstone, 2008, Figure 64.13.)*

FIGURE 33-25 **Sigmoid volvulus.** Air-filled, dilated sigmoid colon with a point of apparent termination. *(From Duthie E: Practice of Geriatrics, 4th ed. Philadelphia, Saunders, 2007, Figure 41.3.)*

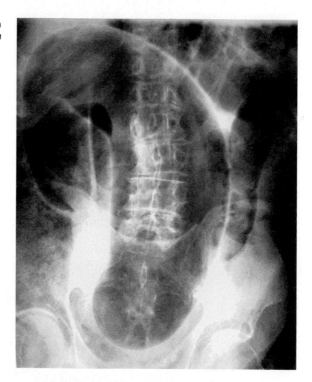

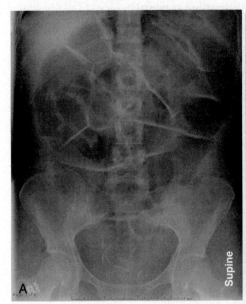
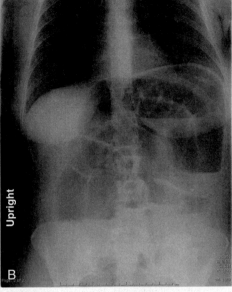

FIGURE 33-26 **Small bowel obstruction. A,** Supine radiograph showing dilated loops of small bowel. **B,** Upright radiograph showing multiple air-fluid levels. *(From Marx J, Hockberger R, Walls R: Rosen's Emergency Medicine, 7th ed. Philadelphia, Mosby, 2010, Figure 90-1.)*

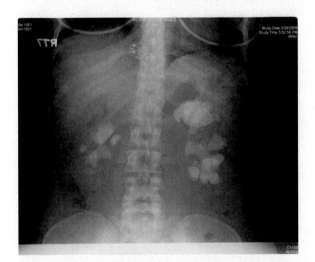

FIGURE **33-27 Staghorn calculus.** Bilateral struvite calculi.*(From McDougal WS, Wein AJ, Kavoussi LR, et al: Campbell-Walsh Urology, 9th ed. Philadelphia, Saunders, 2007, Figure 43-9.)*

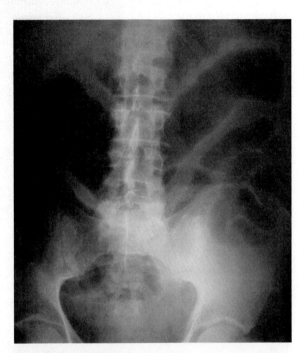

FIGURE **33-28 Toxic megacolon.** The colon appears gas-filled and dilated with a thickened wall. *(From Adam A, Dixon AK, Grainger RG, Allison DJ (eds): Grainger & Allison's Diagnostic Radiology, 5th ed. London, Churchill Livingstone, 2008, Figure 29.23.)*

Achalasia. Esophagus on barium swallow radiograph, bird's beak appearance.

Duodenal atresia. The "double-bubble" sign.

Esophageal atresia. Barium radiograph or nasogastric tube coiled in neck on chest radiograph.

Liver tumor on computed tomography scan. Metastasis 20 times more likely than a primary tumor.

Head and Neck

FIGURE **33-29 Acute and chronic sinusitis.** Air-fluid level on the right (*arrow*) diagnostic of acute sinusitis. Secretions and peripheral ring of enhancing inflamed mucosa on the left typical of chronic sinusitis. *(From Flint PW, Haughey BH, Lund VJ, et al: Cummings Otolaryngology: Head & Neck Surgery, 5th ed. Philadelphia, Mosby, 2010, Figure 11-62.)*

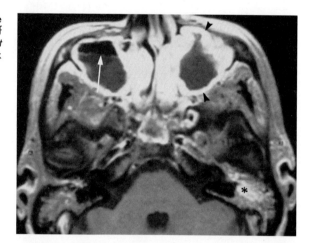

Neurology

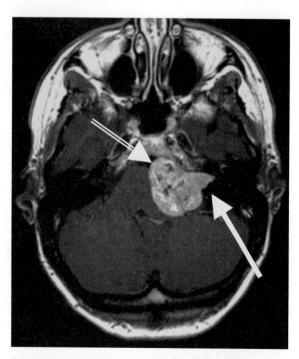

FIGURE **33-30 Acoustic neuroma.** T1-weighted magnetic resonance image showing a mass within the internal auditory canal. *(From Goldman L, Ausiello D: Cecil Medicine, 23rd ed. Philadelphia, Saunders, 2008, Figure 419-9.)*

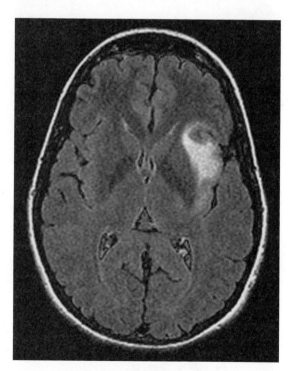

FIGURE **33-31 Astrocytoma.** Fluid attenuated inversion recovery magnetic resonance image showing a mass without ring enhancement. *(From Bope E, Rakel R, Kellerman R: Conn's Current Therapy 2010. Philadelphia, Saunders, 2010, Section 14, Figure 1, page 979.)*

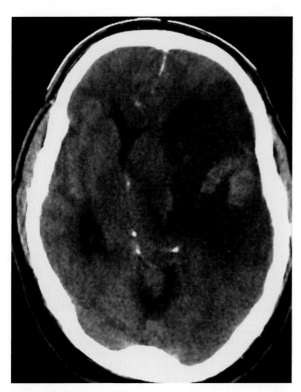

FIGURE 33-32 Large middle cerebral artery infarct on computed tomography - Three days after the infarct, there is edema and hemorrhagic transformation (higher density areas). *(From Adam A, Dixon AK, Grainger RG, Allison DJ (eds): Grainger & Allison's Diagnostic Radiology, 5th ed. London, Churchill Livingstone, 2008, Figure 57.1 C.)*

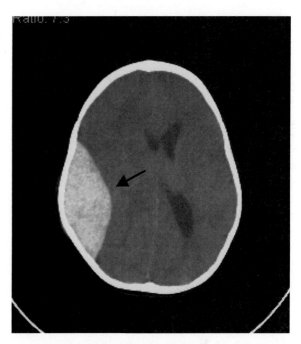

FIGURE 33-33 Epidural hematoma. Computed tomography scan showing a lens-shaped appearance and smooth inner border. *(From Bradley WG: Neurology in Clinical Practice, 5th ed. Philadelphia, PA Butterworth-Heinemann, 2008, Figure 54B-4).*

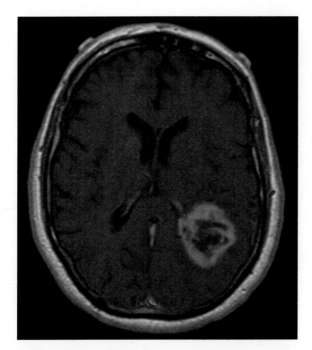

FIGURE 33-34 Glioblastoma multiforme. Magnetic resonance image with a ring-enhancing mass with central necrosis. *(From Bope E, Rakel R, Kellerman R: Conn's Current Therapy 2010. Philadelphia, Saunders, 2010, Section 14, Figure 2, page 980.)*

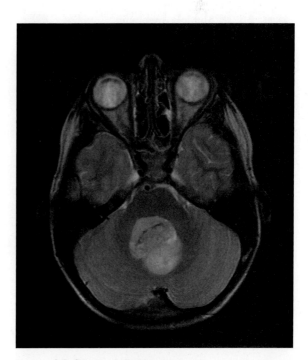

FIGURE 33-35 Medulloblastoma. T2-weighted magnetic resonance image showing a heterogeneous mass typically in the posterior fossa or cerebellum. *(Courtesy of Dr R. Gunny.)*

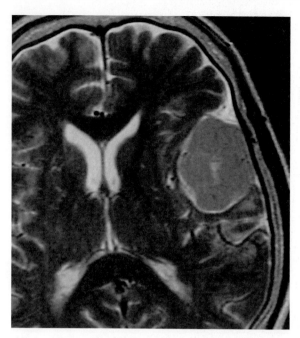

FIGURE 33-36 Meningioma. T2-weighted magnetic resonance image showing an isointense mass arising from the meninges. *(From Adam A, Dixon AK, Grainger RG, Allison DJ (eds): Grainger & Allison's Diagnostic Radiology, 5th ed. London, Churchill Livingstone, 2008, Figure 56.19A.)*

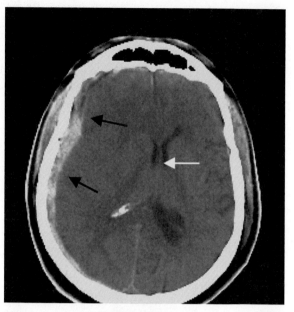

FIGURE 33-37 Subdural hematoma. Computed tomography scan showing spread over the entire surface of the hemisphere with associated swelling. *(From Bradley WG: Neurology in Clinical Practice, 5th ed. Philadelphia, PA Butterworth-Heinemann, 2008, Figure 54B-3.)*

Orthopedics

FIGURE 33-38 Multiple myeloma. Osteolytic skull lesions. *(From Abeloff MD: Abeloff's Clinical Oncology, 4th ed. Philadelphia, Churchill Livingstone, 2008, Figure 110-2.)*

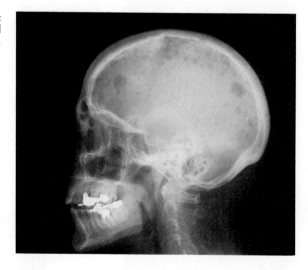

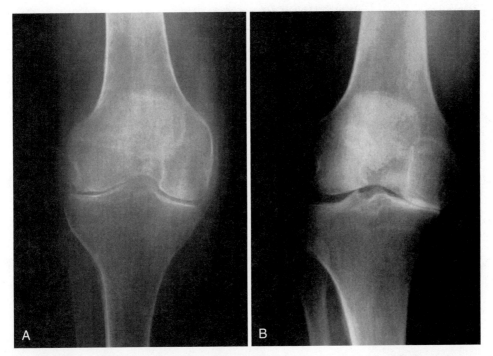

FIGURE 33-39 Rheumatoid arthritis (A) and osteoarthritis (B). Complete symmetrical loss of joint space in A and asymmetric loss of joint space and subchondral sclerosis in osteoarthritis in B. *(From Goldman L, Ausiello D: Cecil Medicine, 23rd ed. Philadelphia, Saunders, 2008, Figure 285-6.)*

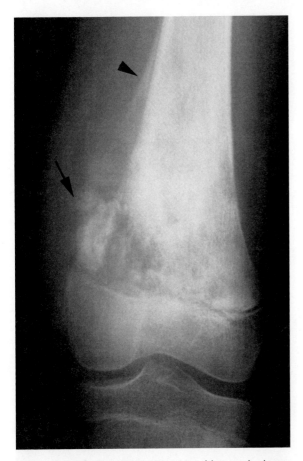

FIGURE 33-40 Osteosarcoma. Mixed lytic and sclerotic areas, tumor bone formation in extraosseous mass and proximal Codman triangle. *(From Adam A, Dixon AK, Grainger RG, Allison DJ (eds): Grainger & Allison's Diagnostic Radiology, 5th ed. London, Churchill Livingstone, 2008, Figure 48.15.)*

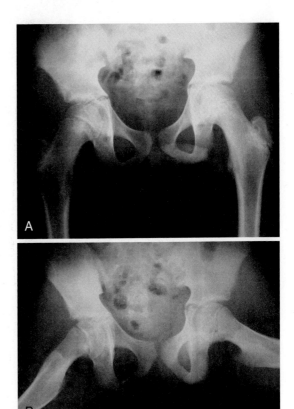

FIGURE 33-41 Slipped capital femoral epiphysis. Note widening of the epiphysis on the right compared with the left. *(Courtesy of Marianne Gausche-Hill, MD.)*

Lytic lesions of bone on radiography (consider possible malignancy).

Osteoarthritis (osteophytes, interphalangeal joint changes).

Shoulder dislocation on radiography.

Pulmonary

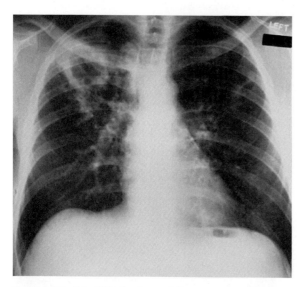

FIGURE 33-42 **Classic chest radiograph of tuberculosis.** Chest radiograph showing a right upper lobe cavitary lesion in a patient with reactivation tuberculosis. *(From Mason RJ, Broaddus VC, Martin T, et al: Murray and Nadel's Textbook of Respiratory Medicine, 5th ed. Philadelphia, Saunders, 2010, Figure 34-7.)*

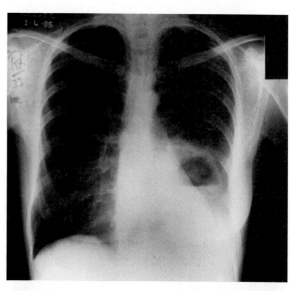

FIGURE 33-43 **Lung abscess on chest radiograph.** Lung abscess associated with lower lobe pneumonia. *(From Albert RK, Spiro SG, Jett JR: Clinical Respiratory Medicine, 3rd ed. Philadelphia, Mosby, 2008, Figure 27-2A.)*

FIGURE 33-44 **Pleural effusion.** On the posteroanterior radiograph, the effusion simulates a high hemidiaphragm. *(From Adam A, Dixon AK, Grainger RG, Allison DJ (eds): Grainger & Allison's Diagnostic Radiology, 5th ed. London, Churchill Livingstone, 2008, Figure 13.20A.)*

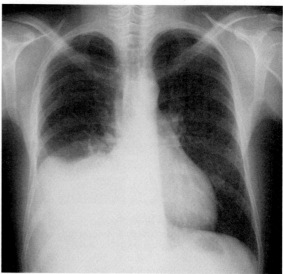

Pulmonary embolism.

Pancoast tumor on chest radiograph.
Large upper lobe lung cancer or mass;
can cause Horner syndrome.

Sarcoidosis (bilateral
hilar adenopathy).

DERMATOLOGY AND SKIN FINDINGS

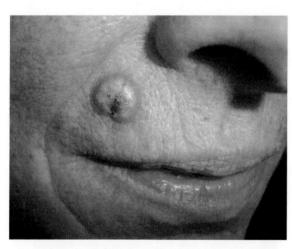

FIGURE 33-45 **Basal cell carcinoma.** Typical nodular variant with central ulceration. (*From Pfenninger JL, Fowler GC: Pfenninger and Fowler's Procedures for Primary Care, 3rd ed. Philadelphia, Saunders, 2011, Figure 12-5B.*)

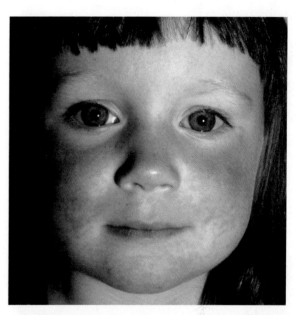

FIGURE 33-46 **Erythema infectiosum.** "Slapped cheek." The red plaque covers the cheek and spares the nasolabial fold and the circumoral region. (*From Habif TP: Clinical Dermatology, 5th ed. Philadelphia, Mosby, 2010, Figure 14-17.*)

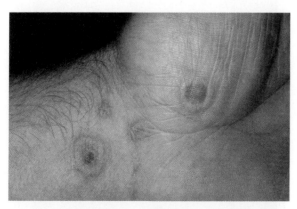

FIGURE 33-47 **Erythema multiforme.** Target or "bull's-eye" annular lesions with central vesicles and bullae. (*From Goldman L, Ausiello D: Cecil Medicine, 23rd ed. Philadelphia, Saunders, 2008, Figure 465-10.*)

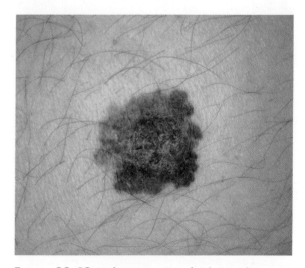

FIGURE 33-48 **Melanoma.** Superficial spreading type, irregular pigmentation and borders. (*From Townsend CM, Beauchamp D, Evers M, Mattox KL: Sabiston Textbook of Surgery, 18th ed. Philadelphia, Saunders, 2008, Figure 30-3.*)

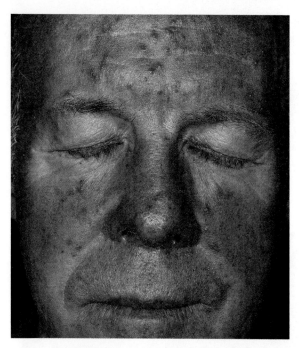

FIGURE 33-49 Rosacea. Pustules and erythema occur on the forehead, cheeks, and nose. *(From Habif TP: Clinical Dermatology, 5th ed. Philadelphia, Mosby, 2010, Figure 7-55.)*

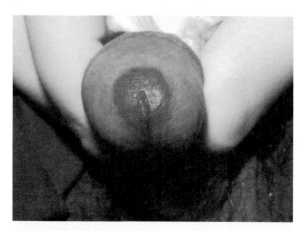

FIGURE 33-50 Squamous cell carcinoma in situ. Erythroplasia of Queyrat of the glans penis surrounding the urethral meatus. *(From McDougal WS, Wein AJ, Kavoussi LR, et al: Campbell-Walsh Urology, 9th ed. Philadelphia, Saunders, 2007, Figure 32-29.)*

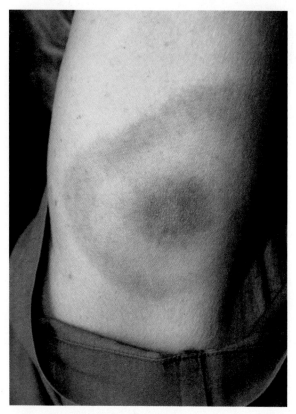

FIGURE 33-51 Erythema migrans. Skin lesion of Lyme disease with a broad oval area of erythema that has slowly migrated from the central area. *(From Habif TP: Clinical Dermatology, 5th ed. Philadelphia, Mosby, 2010, Figure 15-30.)*

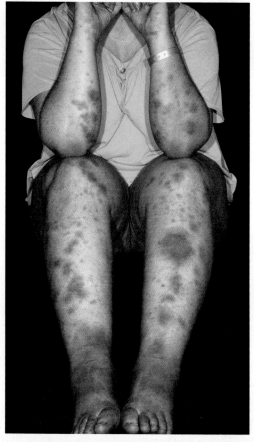

FIGURE 33-52 Erythema nodosum. Red, nodelike swelling in the characteristic distribution. *(From Habif TP: Clinical Dermatology, 5th ed. Philadelphia, Mosby, 2010, Figure 18-11.)*

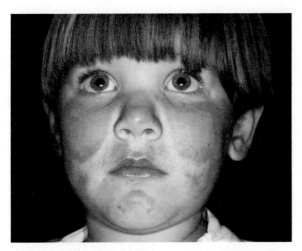

FIGURE **33-53 Systemic lupus erythematous** - Malar rash with sparing of the nasolabial folds. Typically acute in onset, frequently after exposure to sun. *(From Kliegman RM, et al: Nelson Textbook of Pediatrics, 18th ed. Philadelphia, Saunders, 2007, Figure 644-1.)*

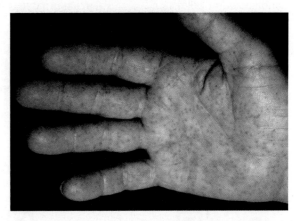

FIGURE **33-54** Rocky Mountain Spotted Fever - Classic distribution of rash on the palms (shown) and soles occurs relatively late in the course. *(From Habif TP: Clinical Dermatology, 5th ed. Philadelphia, Mosby, 2010, Figure 15-36.)*

Acne.

Actinic keratosis.

Allergic contact dermatitis.

Cavernous hemangioma.
In children, most lesions resolve on their own.

Condyloma acuminata (genital warts).

Heliotrope rash (dermatomyositis).

Henoch-Schönlein purpura (rash).

Impetigo (honey-colored crusts).

Keloid (usually in blacks).

Molluscum contagiosum (umbilicated papule).

Pityriasis rosea (herald patch).

Psoriasis (skin findings and nail pitting).

Scabies.

Temporal arteritis. The patient's face reveals a tortuous-looking temporal artery.

Tinea capitis.

Tinea corporis.

Tinea cruris.

Vitiligo (associated with pernicious anemia and hypothyroidism).

Abdominal striae in Cushing syndrome.

Acanthosis nigricans. This is a marker for insulin resistance and visceral malignancy.

Adenoma sebaceum (i.e., angiofibromas, a marker for tuberous sclerosis).

Arterial insufficiency (skin changes).

Café-au-lait patches. Neurofibromatosis in patients with a normal IQ and McCune-Albright syndrome with mental retardation.

Cheilitis or stomatitis (think of B vitamin deficiencies).

Clubbing of the fingers.

Cullen sign. A blue periumbilical area, marker for retroperitoneal hemorrhage).

Diabetic foot ulcers. These are similar in appearance to arterial insufficiency ulcers but usually painless.

Erythema marginatum (rheumatic fever).

Grey Turner sign. Blue flank, a marker for retroperitoneal hemorrhage.

Herpes (1 and 2).

Hirsutism (know conditions associated with it).

Janeway lesions and Osler nodes (endocarditis).

Oral hairy leukoplakia (caused by Epstein-Barr virus; seen in HIV-positive patients).

Periorbital myxedema (Graves disease).

Pyoderma gangrenosum (think of inflammatory bowel disease).

Raynaud phenomenon (finger autoamputation; often seen in scleroderma).

Stasis dermatitis or venous insufficiency (skin changes, ulcers).

Sturge-Weber syndrome. Hemangioma, a port-wine stain on one side of face.

Secondary Syphilis.

Toxic shock syndrome, scalded skin syndrome. Blisters and skin peeling off in large sheets.

Varicella zoster virus. Herpes zoster involving the ophthalmic nerve.

OPHTHALMOLOGY

Ophthalmologic Problems

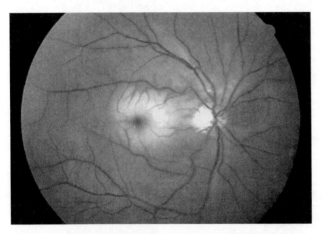

FIGURE **33-55 Central retinal artery occlusion.** Note the cherry-red spot (fovea). *(Image courtesy of www.tedmontgomery.com.)*

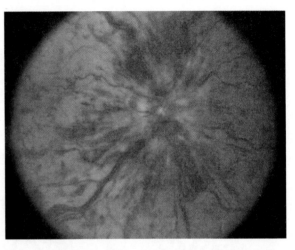

FIGURE **33-56 Central retinal vein occlusion.** Diffuse intraretinal hemorrhages in all four quadrants. *(From Goldman L, Ausiello D: Cecil Medicine, 23rd ed. Philadelphia, Saunders, 2008, Figure 449-19.)*

Bacterial conjunctivitis (especially in neonates).

Cataracts (bad enough to notice with the naked eye).

Herpes zoster keratitis (dendritic ulcer seen with fluorescein; avoid steroids).

Orbital cellulitis (proptosis).

Retinoblastoma (leukocoria; white reflex instead of red).

Ophthalmologic Signs of Other Problems

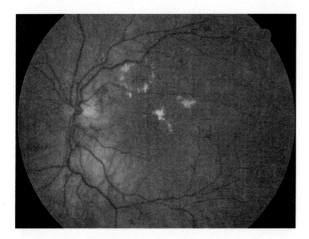

Figure 33-57 Diabetic retinopathy. Scattered dot and blot intraretinal hemorrhages and retinal exudates with a circinate exudate surrounding a microaneurysm. *(From Goldman L, Ausiello D: Cecil Medicine, 23rd ed. Philadelphia, Saunders, 2008, Figure 449-15.)*

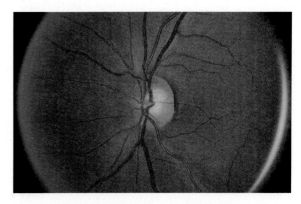

Figure 33-58 Hypertensive retinopathy. Note the color change in the retinal arterioles and the early arteriovenous crossing changes. *(From Yanoff M, Duker JS: Ophthalmology, 3rd ed. Philadelphia, Mosby, 2009, Figure 6-15-1.)*

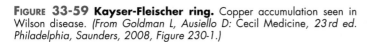

Figure 33-59 Kayser-Fleischer ring. Copper accumulation seen in Wilson disease. *(From Goldman L, Ausiello D: Cecil Medicine, 23rd ed. Philadelphia, Saunders, 2008, Figure 230-1.)*

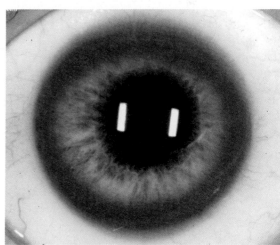

Graves disease (exophthalmos).

Papilledema.

Roth spots (think of endocarditis).

Xanthelasma.

CHARTS

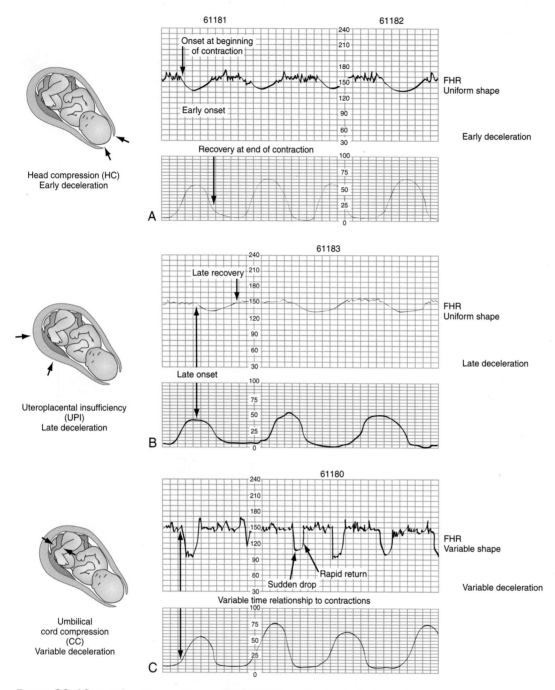

FIGURE 33-60 **Deceleration patterns of the fetal heart rate. A,** Early deceleration caused by head compression. **B,** Late deceleration caused by uteroplacental insufficiency. **C,** Variable deceleration caused by cord compression. *(Modified from Lowdermilk DL, et al: Maternity and Women's Health Care, 6th ed. St. Louis, Mosby, 1997.)*

KARYOTYPES

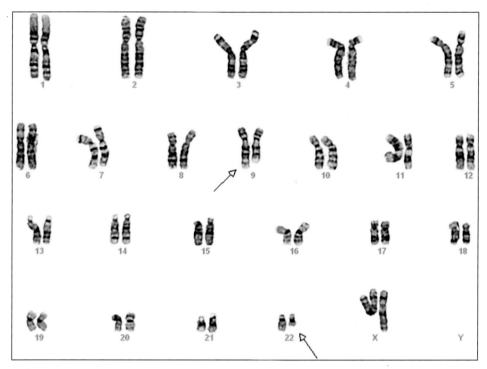

FIGURE 33-61 Chronic myeloid leukemia. Karyotype illustrates t(9;22) BCR/ABL rearrangement. *(From Abeloff MD: Abeloff's Clinical Oncology, 4th ed. Philadelphia, Churchill Livingstone, 2008, Figure 18-1.)*

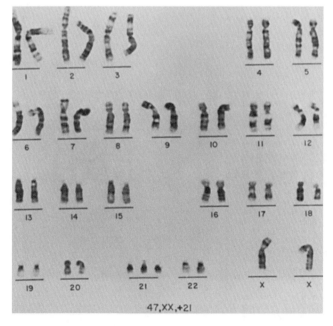

FIGURE 33-62 Down syndrome. Karyotype of a trisomy 21 cell. *(From Simpson JL, Elias S: Genetics in Obstetrics and Gynecology, 3rd ed. Philadelphia, WB Saunders Company, with permission.)*

BLOOD SMEARS

Anemia

Folate or vitamin B$_{12}$ anemia (macrocytic, hypersegmented neutrophils).

Iron-deficiency anemia (microcytic, hypochromic erythrocytes).

Sideroblastic anemia (ringed sideroblasts).

Cancer

Acute lymphoblastic leukemia.

Acute myeloid leukemia (Auer rods).

Acute promyelocytic anemia.

Chronic lymphocytic leukemia (smudge cell).

Chronic myelogenous leukemia.

Hairy cell leukemia

Multiple myeloma (Rouleaux formation).

Reed-Sternberg cell (Hodgkin lymphoma).

Other

Acanthocytes (abetalipoproteinemia).

Basophilic stippling (lead poisoning, thalassemia).

Döhle bodies (toxic lymphocytes; for the boards, think of Epstein-Barr virus).

Heinz bodies and "bite cells" (glucose-6-phosphate dehydrogenase deficiency).

Howell-Jolly bodies (asplenia or splenic dysfunction).

Malaria.

Schistocytes and helmet cells. Disseminated intravascular coagulation, thrombotic thrombocytopenic purpura, and microangiopathic hemolysis.

Sickle cell disease.

Spherocytosis.

Target cells (thalassemia, severe liver disease).

Teardrop cells (myelofibrosis, myelodysplasia).

MICROSCOPIC FINDINGS

Caseating granuloma (tuberculosis, fungi).

Clue cells (*Gardnerella* spp. vaginitis).

Cryptococcus neoformans.

Giardia **spp**.

Goodpasture disease (linear immunofluorescence in the kidney).

Gout (needle-shaped crystals from a joint with no birefringence).

Gram stain (gram-negative = red; gram-positive = blue) plus morphology and clustering tendencies.

Koilocytosis (think of human papillomavirus or cytomegalovirus).

Noncaseating granulomas (sarcoidosis).

Positive India ink preparation for *Cryptococcus* meningitis.

Pseudogout (rhomboid-shaped crystals with weakly positive birefringence).

***Trichomonas* spp.**

GENERAL CLINICAL PHOTOS AND FIGURES

Face

Bell palsy (facial asymmetry).

Congenital syphilis (Hutchinson teeth, saddle nose deformity).

Fetal alcohol syndrome (facies).

Gross Appearance

Graves disease (exophthalmos).

Horner syndrome (unilateral ptosis and miosis and history of hemianhydrosis).

Peutz-Jeghers syndrome (freckling pattern on the face).

Scleroderma (late-stage facies).

Achondroplasia (overall appearance; usually autosomal dominant).

Acute pharyngitis (viral or streptococcal).

Acute tonsillitis (*Streptococcus* spp. or Epstein-Barr virus; rarely diphtheria in unimmunized patient).

Candidal infection (vaginal, thrush).

Dactylitis (sickle cell disease; psoriatic arthritis).

Decubitus ulcers (best prevention is frequent turning of the patient).

Dilated cardiomyopathy (gross specimen; severe disease).

Down syndrome (facies, simian crease).

Erb palsy (waiter's tip).

Gonorrhea (yellowish discharge).

Gynecomastia (normal finding in pubertal boys; think liver disease in a man).

Herpes simplex.

Lichen planus.

Lichen sclerosus et atrophicus.

Lichen simplex chronicus.

Pseudohermaphroditism (picture of ambiguous genitalia; look for 21-hydroxylase deficiency).

Osteoarthritis (Heberden and Bouchard nodes).

Polycystic kidneys (gross pathologic specimen appearance).

Rheumatoid arthritis (swan-neck deformity, boutonnière deformity, ulnar deviation, rheumatoid nodules).

Spina bifida (gross appearance; encephalocele, meningocele, meningomyelocele, patch of hair in spina bifida occulta).

Strawberry tongue (scarlet fever and Kawasaki disease).

Tophaceous gout.

Turner syndrome (body habitus, widely spaced nipples, webbed neck, cubitus valgus).

Varicose veins.

SIGNS, SYMPTOMS, AND SYNDROMES

SIGNS AND SYNDROMES

○ **Babinski sign:** Stroking the foot yields extension of the big toe and fanning of other toes in patients with upper motor neuron disease.

○ **Beck triad:** Jugular vein distension, muffled heart sounds, and hypotension in cardiac tamponade; do pericardiocentesis.

○ **Behçet syndrome:** Oral ulcers, genital ulcers, anterior uveitis, erythema nodosum.

○ **Brudzinski sign:** Pain on neck flexion with meningeal irritation.

○ **Carcinoid syndrome:** Flushing, valvular heart disease, diarrhea; tumor secreting serotonin or 5-HIAA.

○ **Cauda equina syndrome:** Bladder atony, bilateral sciatica, saddle anesthesia, loss of anal sphincter tone caused by nerve root problem (a surgical emergency).

○ **Charcot triad:** Fever and chills, jaundice, and right upper quadrant pain in patients with cholangitis.

○ **Courvoisier sign:** A painless, palpable gallbladder should make you think of pancreatic cancer.

○ **Chvostek sign:** Tapping on the facial nerve elicits tetany in hypocalcemia.

○ **Cullen sign:** Bluish discoloration of periumbilical area caused by retroperitoneal hemorrhage (pancreatitis).

○ **Cushing reflex:** Hypertension, bradycardia, and irregular respirations with very high intracranial pressure.

○ **Gower sign:** A patient uses the hands to "walk up" from a squatting position, indicating proximal muscle weakness of the lower limbs; associated with muscular dystrophy.

○ **Grey Turner sign:** Bluish discoloration of the flank from retroperitoneal hemorrhage (think of pancreatitis).

○ **Homan sign:** Calf pain on forced dorsiflexion of the foot in patients with deep vein thrombosis (insensitive and unreliable but classic).

○ **Horner syndrome:** Ptosis, miosis, and anhydrosis; associated with Pancoast tumor.

○ **Kehr sign:** Pain referred to the left shoulder with a ruptured spleen.

○ **Leriche syndrome:** Claudication and atrophy of the buttocks with impotence (seen with aortoiliac occlusive disease).

○ **McBurney sign:** Tenderness at McBurney point with appendicitis.

○ **Metabolic syndrome:** Hypertension, impaired fasting glucose, abdominal obesity, elevated triglycerides, and decreased high density lipoprotein.

○ **Murphy sign:** Arrest of inspiration when palpating right upper quadrant under the rib cage in patients with cholecystitis.

○ **Ortolani sign/test:** A palpable or audible click with abduction of an infant's flexed hip means congenital hip dysplasia.

○ **Prehn sign:** Elevation of a painful testicle relieves pain in epididymitis (vs. torsion).

○ **Rovsing sign:** Pushing on the left lower quadrant produces pain at McBurney point in patients with appendicitis.

○ **Tinel sign:** Tapping on the volar surface of the wrist elicits paresthesias in carpal tunnel syndrome.

○ **Trousseau sign:** Pumping up a blood pressure cuff causes carpopedal spasm (tetany) in hypocalcemia.

○ **Trousseau syndrome:** Migratory thrombophlebitis (i.e., pops up in one site, goes away, and then appears in a different part of the body) as a sign of visceral malignancy.

○ **Verner-Morrison syndrome:** Watery diarrhea, achlorhydria, and hypokalemia caused by a pancreatic islet cell tumor oversecreting vasoactive intestinal peptide (i.e., VIPoma).
○ **Virchow triad:** Stasis, endothelial damage, and hypercoagulability (three broad categories of risk factors for deep vein thrombosis).

WORD ASSOCIATIONS

Word associations are not 100% accurate, but they are useful in board exam emergencies.
○ **Abdominal striae:** Cushing syndrome (or possible pregnancy)
○ **Acanthosis nigricans:** Diabetes or gastrointestinal malignancy
○ **Ambiguous genitalia and hypotension:** Female patient with 21-hydroxylase deficiency (give corticosteroids and intravenous fluids)
○ **Anaphylaxis from immunoglobulin therapy:** Immunoglobulin A (IgA) deficiency
○ **Baby weighing >10 lb:** Maternal diabetes
○ **Bilateral hilar adenopathy in a black female patient:** Sarcoidosis
○ **Blueberry muffin rash in a baby:** Congenital rubella
○ **Bitot spots:** Vitamin A deficiency
○ **Bronze (skin) diabetes:** Hemochromatosis (look also for cardiac and liver dysfunction)
○ **Catlike cry in children:** Cri-du-chat syndrome
○ **Café-au-lait spots:** Neurofibromatosis (if mental retardation is present, think of McCune-Albright syndrome or tuberous sclerosis)
○ **Cherry-red spot on the macula:** Tay-Sachs disease (no hepatosplenomegaly) or Niemann–Pick disease (hepatosplenomegaly)
○ **Children who torture animals:** Conduct disorder (may be antisocial as adults)
○ **Clue cells:** *Gardnerella* spp. infection
○ **Constant clearing of the throat (children):** Tourette syndrome
○ **Currant jelly stools in children:** Intussusception
○ **Daytime sleepiness and occasional falling down (cataplexy):** Narcolepsy
○ **Decreased breath sounds in a trauma patient:** Pneumothorax
○ **Dendritic corneal ulcers:** Herpes keratitis (seen best with fluorescein; avoid steroids)
○ **Fractures or bruises in different stages of healing (children):** Child abuse
○ **Friction rub:** Pericarditis (Fig. 34-1)
○ **Heavy young woman with papilledema and negative radiologic evaluation results:** Pseudotumor cerebri
○ **Heliotrope rash:** Dermatomyositis
○ **Honey or home-canned goods:** Infant botulism
○ **Hot potato voice:** Epiglottitis
○ **Howell-Jolly bodies:** Sickle cell anemia; indicative of a nonfunctioning spleen
○ **Increased hemoglobin A2 and anemia:** Thalassemia
○ **Intermittent bursts of swearing or repetitive grunting:** Tourette syndrome
○ **Kayser-Fleischer ring:** Wilson disease
○ **Koilocytosis:** Human papillomavirus or cytomegalovirus
○ **Kussmaul breathing:** Deep, rapid breathing seen in metabolic acidosis (think of diabetic ketoacidosis)
○ **Left lower quadrant tenderness or rebound:** Diverticulitis
○ **Low-grade fever in first 24 hours after surgery:** Atelectasis
○ **Malar rash:** Lupus erythematosus
○ **Meconium ileus:** Cystic fibrosis
○ **Pear-shaped motile organisms on Pap smear:** Trichomonas
○ **Postpartum fever unresponsive to broad-spectrum antibiotics:** Septic pelvic thrombophlebitis (give heparin for a cure and retrospective diagnosis)
○ **Rash after ampicillin or amoxicillin for a sore throat:** Epstein-Barr virus infection
○ **Rectal prolapse:** Cystic fibrosis
○ **Rouleaux formation:** Multiple myeloma
○ **Salty-tasting baby:** Cystic fibrosis
○ **Self-mutilating child:** Lesch-Nyhan syndrome

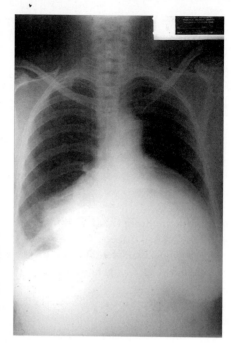

FIGURE 34-1 An enlarged globular cardiac silhouette is statistically more likely to be related to chronic cardiomegaly from heart disease but keep in mind that an enlarged cardiac silhouette on chest radiography can be attributable to cardiomegaly, pericardial effusion, or a cardiac or paracardiac mass. The globular "water bottle" configuration is suggestive, and if a friction rub is heard in the chest or if a recent prior chest radiography showed a normal cardiac size, the chest radiographic findings would be highly suggestive. In this case, the patient had a large pericardial effusion.

- ○ **Shopping sprees:** Mania
- ○ **Sudden death in a young athlete:** Hypertrophic obstructive cardiomyopathy
- ○ **Vietnam or Iraq war veteran:** Posttraumatic stress disorder
- ○ **Worst headache of patient's life:** Subarachnoid hemorrhage

QR CODE

The QR code includes three USMLE-style questions and answers. For more questions, redeem the PIN code on the inside cover for the Crush Step 2 question bank powered by USMLE Consult.

Please see the Introduction for instructions on how to access content using the QR codes.

Question

In which condition is a nontender, palpable gallbladder most likely?
(A) Pancreatic cancer
(B) Chronic cholecystitis
(C) Cholelithiasis
(D) Acute cholecystitis
(E) Cholangitis

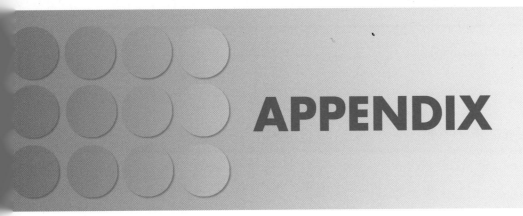

APPENDIX

Abbreviations

- ○ AAA abdominal aortic aneurysm
- ○ Ab antibody
- ○ ABC, ABCD, ABCDE airway, breathing, circulation, disability, exposure (trauma protocol)
- ○ ABG arterial blood gas
- ○ ABO blood types (A, B, AB or O)
- ○ ACE angiotensin-converting enzyme
- ○ ACEI angiotensin-converting enzyme inhibitor
- ○ ACL anterior cruciate ligament
- ○ ACTH adrenocorticotropic hormone
- ○ ADH antidiuretic hormone
- ○ ADHD attention-deficit/hyperactivity disorder
- ○ AFP alpha fetoprotein
- ○ AIDS acquired immunodeficiency syndrome
- ○ ALL acute lymphoblastic leukemia
- ○ ALS amyotrophic lateral sclerosis (aka Lou Gehrig's disease)
- ○ ALT alanine aminotransferase
- ○ AML acute myeloid leukemia
- ○ ANA antinuclear antibody
- ○ ANCA antineutrophil cytoplasmic antibody
- ○ ANOVA analysis of variance
- ○ ARB angiotensin receptor blocker
- ○ ARDS acute respiratory distress syndrome
- ○ ARF acute renal failure
- ○ ASA acetylsalicylic acid (aspirin)
- ○ ASD atrial septal defect
- ○ AST aspartate aminotransferase
- ○ ATG antithymocyte globulin
- ○ AVM arteriovenous malformation
- ○ AXR abdominal x-ray
- ○ AZT azidothymidine (zidovudine)
- ○ B, β beta
- ○ BP blood pressure
- ○ BPH benign prostatic hyperplasia, benign prostatic hypertrophy
- ○ BPP biophysical profile
- ○ BT bleeding time
- ○ BUN blood urea nitrogen
- ○ C Celsius, centigrade (e.g., 37° C); complement (e.g., C1, C3, C4); cervical (e.g., C5 vertebral body)
- ○ c-section cesarean section
- ○ CA cancer antigen (e.g., CA-125)
- ○ CAD coronary artery disease
- ○ CBC complete blood count
- ○ CD cluster of differentiation (e.g., CD4, CD8)
- ○ CEA carcinoembryonic antigen

- CHD coronary heart disease; congenital hip dysplasia
- CHF congestive heart failure
- CK creatine kinase
- CLL chronic lymphocytic leukemia
- cm centimeter
- CML chronic myelocytic (or myelogenous) leukemia
- CMV cytomegalovirus
- CN cranial nerve
- CNS central nervous system
- CO carbon monoxide or cardiac output
- CO_2 carbon dioxide
- COPD chronic obstructive pulmonary disease
- COX cyclooxygenase
- CPD cephalopelvic disproportion
- CPK creatine phosphokinase
- Cr creatinine
- CRF chronic renal failure
- CSF cerebrospinal fluid
- CT computed tomography scan
- CVA cerebrovascular accident (stroke)
- CXR chest x-ray
- D5W 5% dextrose in water
- D&C dilation and curettage
- DDI dideoxyinosine (antiretroviral medication)
- DES diethylstilbestrol
- DI diabetes insipidus
- DIC disseminated intravascular coagulation
- DIP distal interphalangeal (joint)
- DKA diabetic ketoacidosis
- dL deciliter
- DM diabetes mellitus
- DMSA 2,3-dimercaptosuccinic acid, succimer
- DNA deoxyribonucleic acid
- DTP diphtheria, tetanus, pertussis (trivalent vaccine)
- DUB dysfunctional uterine bleeding
- DVT deep venous thrombosis
- EBV Epstein–Barr virus
- ECG electrocardiogram
- EDTA edetate (ethylenediaminetetraacetic acid)
- EEG electroencephalogram
- EKG electrocardiogram
- ELISA enzyme-linked immunosorbent assay
- EMG electromyogram
- ERCP endoscopic retrograde cholangiopancreatography
- ESR erythrocyte sedimentation rate
- FDP fibrin degradation product
- Fe iron
- FEV forced expiratory volume
- FEV1 forced expiratory volume in 1 second
- FFP fresh frozen plasma
- FSH follicle-stimulating hormone
- FTA-ABS fluorescent treponemal antibody-absorption test (for syphilis)
- FVC forced vital capacity
- g gram
- G6PD glucose-6-phosphate dehydrogenase
- GERD gastroesophageal reflux disease
- GGT γ-glutamyltranspeptidase

○ GI gastrointestinal
○ GnRH gonadotropin-releasing hormone
○ GU genitourinary
○ GYN gynecology or gynecologic
○ H2 histamine type 2 receptor
○ H&P history and physical examination
○ HAV hepatitis A virus
○ HbA1c glycosylated hemoglobin
○ HBcAb/Ag hepatitis B core antibody/antigen
○ HBeAb/Ag hepatitis B e antibody/antigen
○ HBsAb/Ag hepatitis B surface antibody/antigen
○ HBV hepatitis B virus
○ HC head circumference
○ hCG human chorionic gonadotropin
○ HCV hepatitis C virus
○ HDL high-density lipoprotein
○ HELLP **h**emolysis, **e**levated **l**iver enzymes, **l**ow **p**latelets (syndrome)
○ 5-HIAA 5-hydroxyindoleacetic acid
○ HIV human immunodeficiency virus
○ HLA human leukocyte antigen
○ HPV human papillomavirus
○ h hour(s)
○ HRT hormone replacement therapy
○ HSP Henoch–Schönlein purpura
○ HSV herpes simplex virus
○ HTN hypertension
○ HUS hemolytic uremic syndrome
○ IBD inflammatory bowel disease
○ IBS irritable bowel syndrome
○ ICP intracranial pressure
○ ICU intensive care unit
○ Ig immunoglobulin (e.g., IgA, IgM, IgG, IgE)
○ IL interleukin (e.g., IL-2)
○ IM intramuscular
○ IPV inactivated poliovirus vaccine
○ IQ intelligence quotient
○ IU international units
○ IUD intrauterine device
○ IUGR intrauterine growth retardation, intrauterine growth restriction
○ ITP idiopathic thrombocytopenic purpura
○ IV intravenous
○ IVC inferior vena cava
○ IVDA intravenous drug abuse
○ IVF intravenous fluids; in vitro fertilization
○ IVP intravenous pyelogram
○ K potassium
○ kg kilogram
○ KOH potassium hydroxide
○ L liter or lumbar (e.g., L5 nerve root)
○ LA left atrium
○ LAE left atrial enlargement
○ lb pound
○ LCP Legg–Calvé–Perthes disease
○ LDH lactate dehydrogenase
○ LDL low-density lipoproteins
○ LES lower esophageal sphincter
○ LFT(s) liver function test(s)

○ LGI lower gastrointestinal (below the ligament of Treitz)
○ LH luteinizing hormone
○ LLQ left lower quadrant
○ LMN lower motor neuron
○ LMP last menstrual period
○ LR lactated Ringer's solution
○ L/S lecithin/sphingomyelin ratio
○ LSD lysergic acid diethylamide
○ LUQ left upper quadrant
○ LV left ventricle
○ LVH left ventricular hypertrophy
○ MAI *Mycobacterium avium–intracellulare* complex
○ MAOI monoamine oxidase inhibitor
○ MCHC mean corpuscular hemoglobin concentration
○ MCL medial collateral ligament
○ MCP metacarpophalangeal (hand joint)
○ MCV mean corpuscular volume
○ MEN multiple endocrine neoplasia
○ mg milligram
○ MG myasthenia gravis
○ $MgSO_4$ magnesium sulfate
○ MHA-TP microhemagglutination assay for antibodies to *Treponema pallidum* (for syphilis)
○ MI myocardial infarction
○ mL milliliter
○ mm millimeter
○ MMR measles, mumps, rubella (vaccine)
○ mo month(s)
○ MRA magnetic resonance angiogram
○ MRCP magnetic resonance cholangiopancreatography
○ MRI magnetic resonance imaging scan
○ MRSA methicillin-resistant *Staphylococcus aureus*
○ Na sodium
○ NPH isophane insulin suspension (neutral protamine Hagedorn)
○ NPO nothing by mouth
○ NPV negative predictive value
○ NS normal saline
○ NSAID nonsteroidal antiinflammatory drug
○ O_2 oxygen
○ OA osteoarthritis
○ OCP oral contraceptive pill
○ OPV oral poliovirus vaccine
○ P1, P2 heart sounds made by the pulmonary valve
○ PCN penicillin
○ PCOS polycystic ovary syndrome
○ PCP phencyclidine; *Pneumocystis* pneumonia
○ PCWP pulmonary capillary wedge pressure
○ PDA patent ductus arteriosus
○ PE pulmonary embolus
○ PEEP positive end-expiratory pressure
○ PG prostaglandin (e.g., PGE2, PGF); phosphatidylglycerol
○ pH hydrogen ion concentration scale (measures acidity)
○ PH pulmonary hypertension
○ PID pelvic inflammatory disease
○ PIP proximal interphalangeal (joint)
○ PMN polymorphonuclear leukocyte
○ PMS premenstrual syndrome
○ PO_4 phosphate

- PPD purified protein derivative (tuberculosis skin test)
- PPV positive predictive value
- prn as needed (pro re nata)
- PPROM preterm premature rupture of the membranes
- PROM premature rupture of the membranes
- PSA prostate-specific antigen
- PT prothrombin time
- PTH parathyroid hormone
- PTT partial thromboplastin time
- PUD peptic ulcer disease
- PVC premature ventricular contraction
- PVD peripheral vascular disease
- RA right atrium; rheumatoid arthritis
- RAE right atrial enlargement
- RAI radioactive iodine
- RBC red blood cell
- RDW red blood cell distribution width
- REM rapid eye movement (dream sleep)
- RF rheumatic fever
- Rh Rhesus blood group antigen
- RI reticulocyte index
- RLQ right lower quadrant
- RNA ribonucleic acid
- RPR rapid plasma reagin test (for syphilis)
- RSV respiratory syncytial virus
- RUQ right upper quadrant
- RV right ventricle
- RVH right ventricular hypertrophy
- S sacral (e.g., S1 nerve root)
- S1, S2, S3, S4 heart sounds 1 to 4
- SBO small bowel obstruction
- SCD sickle cell disease
- SCFE slipped capital femoral epiphysis
- SD standard deviation
- SIADH syndrome of inappropriate antidiuretic hormone secretion
- SIDS sudden infant death syndrome
- spp. species
- SSRI selective serotonin reuptake inhibitors
- STD sexually transmitted disease
- SVC superior vena cava
- Svo2 systemic venous oxygen saturation
- SVR systemic vascular resistance
- T1DM type 1 diabetes mellitus
- T2DM type 2 diabetes mellitus
- T3 triiodothyronine
- T4 thyroxine
- TB tuberculosis
- TCA tricyclic antidepressant
- Td tetanus–diphtheria booster vaccine
- TE tracheoesophageal
- TIA transient ischemic attack
- TIBC total iron-binding capacity
- TIPS transjugular intrahepatic portosystemic shunt
- TMP-SMX trimethoprim–sulfamethoxazole
- TOF tetralogy of Fallot
- TORCH **t**oxoplasmosis, **o**ther infections, **r**ubella, **c**ytomegalovirus, **h**erpes simplex
- tPA tissue plasminogen activator

- ○ TRH thyroid-releasing hormone
- ○ TSH thyroid-stimulating hormone
- ○ TTP thrombotic thrombocytopenic purpura
- ○ TURP **t**rans**u**rethral **r**esection of the **p**rostate
- ○ UGI upper gastrointestinal (proximal to the ligament of Treitz)
- ○ UMN upper motor neuron
- ○ URI upper respiratory infection
- ○ US ultrasound
- ○ UTI urinary tract infection
- ○ VACTERL **v**ertebral, **a**nal, **c**ardiac, **t**rach**e**oesophageal, **r**enal, **l**imb (malformations)
- ○ VDRL **V**enereal **D**isease **R**esearch **L**aboratory test (for syphilis)
- ○ VFib, Vfib ventricular fibrillation
- ○ VIPoma pancreatic tumor that secretes vasoactive intestinal peptide
- ○ VMA vanillylmandelic acid
- ○ V/Q ventilation–perfusion (ratio)
- ○ VSD ventricular septal defect
- ○ VTach, Vtach ventricular tachycardia
- ○ vWF von Willebrand's factor
- ○ WBC white blood cells
- ○ WPW Wolff–Parkinson–White syndrome
- ○ yr year(s)

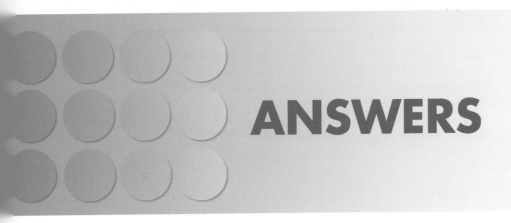

ANSWERS

CHAPTER 1

B. This patient most likely has viral pericarditis, which is usually caused by coxsackievirus or echovirus. This is the most likely diagnosis in a young person with a history of a recent upper respiratory infection, low-grade fever, pleuritic-type chest pain that changes with position, and a pericardial friction rub (the scratchy sound). Electrocardiography classically shows diffusely elevated ST segments in the precordial and limb leads, not Q waves. Myocardial infarction (MI) is extremely unlikely in this patient given the age, lack of mentioned risk factors, and lack of *significant* family history (MI in first-degree male relative younger than 55 years old or female relative younger than 65 years old). A stress test is not indicated at this time. Although endocarditis cannot be excluded entirely, there is little in the history to suggest a risk for endocarditis (e.g., dental surgery, intravenous drug abuse), and it is less likely given the friction rub. There is no reason to suspect a previously damaged heart valve, although abnormal valves are more likely to be affected by subacute endocarditis.

CHAPTER 2

B. The white patches shown are most characteristic of tinea versicolor, also called pityriasis versicolor, a fungal infection. This condition often is noticed in whites after sun exposure because the lesions fail to tan and become more noticeable. Treatment with selenium sulfide lotion or topical antifungals often is effective. The other choices all tend to cause pigmented lesions.

CHAPTER 3

A. Although the other choices can cause hearing loss, presbycusis, the normal sensorineural hearing loss that occurs with age, is the most common. Although there is a wide range of severity, the highest frequencies generally are affected first, and lower frequencies become involved gradually. Meningitis is probably the most common cause of acquired sensorineural hearing loss in children. Otosclerosis is fairly common but usually causes conductive hearing loss rather than sensorineural hearing loss. In this condition, the otic bones become stiffened and fused. Drug-induced causes of hearing loss are important to be aware of but are relatively uncommon. It can be frustrating when question ask for the most common etiology or condition, but this is often how a differential diagnosis is formed (i.e., from the most common or most likely to the least common or least likely). It is part of the transition from the books to the wards to learn that 95% of patients with hypertension have plain old boring essential hypertension and that you may never get to see an actual case of pheochromocytoma in your career.

CHAPTER 4

A. This patient has developed neuroleptic malignant syndrome, a potentially fatal side effect of antipsychotic medication. Autonomic instability with high fevers, fluctuating hypertension, tachycardia, and tachypnea normally is present along with muscular rigidity ("lead pipe") and markedly elevated creatine kinase secondary to muscle necrosis. The mainstay of therapy is to first stop the antipsychotic and then provide supportive care, including intravenous hydration, antipyretics, and cooling blankets. This syndrome is thought to be related to malignant hyperthermia, and some have used dantrolene with success, although many patients do well with supportive care alone. Sodium bicarbonate may be needed to prevent renal shutdown from myoglobinuria. The mortality rate is said to be 10%, and this syndrome is not dose dependent and may occur at any time during antipsychotic treatment, although classically it occurs when a patient has been recently started on antipsychotics.

CHAPTER 5

D. This woman most likely has Graves disease with atrial fibrillation and pretibial myxedema, a specific finding of hyperthyroidism caused by Graves disease (not seen with other causes of hyperthyroidism). Radioactive ablation, antithyroid medications, and surgery may be used to treat this condition, although medications are not curative and are typically used as temporizing therapies only. Although viral thyroiditis is a potential cause of hyperthyroidism, it does not cause pretibial myxedema and is not as common as Graves disease. Thymectomy often is a part of myasthenia gravis treatment, and markedly elevated catecholamine breakdown products in the urine suggest a pheochromocytoma. Alprazolam sometimes is used in generalized anxiety disorder, which this woman probably does not have.

CHAPTER 6

C. A living will should be respected even in the face of family members or others who disagree with it. A competent adult patient can make his or her own decisions, and the question doesn't give you enough information to question the patient's competence when the will was drafted. The woman is understandably upset because she does not want to lose her husband. She needs calm reassurance, comforting, and understanding, but the patient's wishes must be respected. It is not necessary to contact an attorney or schedule a family meeting because the living will clearly states the patient's wishes. Being short or refusing to deal with the woman is the easy way out but is not appropriate in this setting. Avoid being rude, short, nasty or condescending to patients or their family members—especially when taking the USMLE!

CHAPTER 7

D. This patient has Wilson disease, an autosomal recessive disorder characterized by excessive copper accumulation in the body. Penicillamine is a copper chelator used to treat patients with the disorder. The diagnosis should be suspected because of the findings of liver disease, neurologic and psychiatric abnormalities, and a low level of ceruloplasmin. This patient undoubtedly has a Kayser-Fleischer ring around her corneas, which is virtually pathognomonic of Wilson disease. Iron therapy is not used, although zinc therapy may be helpful in patients who cannot tolerate penicillamine. It is unlikely that this patient has chronic viral hepatitis (she would not benefit from antiviral therapy), although with a positive surface antibody, she may have been vaccinated in the past (further serology would be needed to determine). In Wilson disease, the serum copper level may be high, low, or normal and is not a reliable test. A low ceruloplasmin level (main condition for which this test is useful, so if it is mentioned, think Wilson disease) is fairly sensitive, however, and a liver biopsy (the confirmatory diagnostic test) should reveal increased levels of hepatic copper stores.

CHAPTER 8

E. The patient most likely has a pneumothorax that is turning into a tension pneumothorax, which occurs when any injury to lung parenchyma acts as a one-way valve, allowing air to enter but not exit the pleural cavity. In the setting of blunt trauma to the chest, decreased breath sounds with a hyperresonant percussion note on the affected side equals pneumothorax. The development of neck vein distension and worsening shortness of breath most likely indicates the development of a tension pneumothorax, and a trachea deviated away from the affected side and subcutaneous air (crepitus) would further confirm the diagnosis. A hemothorax causes decreased breath sounds with a dull percussion note. Cardiac tamponade usually occurs after penetrating trauma to the left chest in the area of the heart and normally does not affect breath sounds, although it can result in neck vein distension (treated with pericardiocentesis, choice B). Intubation with positive-pressure ventilation (choice D) often is used with an open pneumothorax, in which a chest wall opening allows air into the thoracic cavity, and with significant pulmonary contusion or "flail" chest (multiple contiguous complex rib fractures that result in a section of the chest moving paradoxically during respiration). Positive-pressure ventilation, in this case, would worsen the tension pneumothorax.

Sending this patient for imaging studies in the radiology department (choices A and C) would be dangerous because deterioration already has begun (and radiologists rarely carry stethoscopes). A tension pneumothorax should always be diagnosed clinically rather than radiographically because compression of the ipsilateral lung and vena cava can rapidly lead to decreased preload, shock, and death without timely treatment. Tube thoracostomy is the treatment of choice, but in an unstable patient, one should proceed immediately to needle thoracentesis, which involves placing a needle through the second intercostal space at the midclavicular line. This should cause an audible rush of air that indicates the tension pneumothorax has been converted into a simple pneumothorax. A tube thoracostomy (chest tube) should then be placed.

CHAPTER 9

D. This is straight memorization and regurgitation, which is less prevalent on USMLE exams than it used to be but can never completely disappear given the vast amount of ever-increasing knowledge medical school graduates must accumulate.

CHAPTER 10

B. In 2000, there were an estimated 35 million persons age 65 years or older in the United States, accounting for almost 13% of the total population, and this number is increasing. Approximately 5% live in nursing homes. About 15% of people older than 65 have some form of dementia; this percentage increases with increasing age (e.g., <5% from 65–69 years of age but closer to 30% in those older than age 85 years). People in this age group are more likely to commit suicide than younger persons. Sundowning, or confusion or worsening delirium or dementia at night, is not normal in healthy persons of any age.

CHAPTER 11

C. Oral contraceptive pills (OCPs) have many effects besides preventing pregnancy of which you need to be aware. They decrease the incidence of ovarian and endometrial cancers, dysmenorrhea, menorrhagia, functional ovarian cysts, and benign breast disease. OCPs are a frequent cause of secondary hypertension in women, are contraindicated in the presence of active liver disease, and may cause liver tumors (benign adenomas). OCPs commonly cause weight gain, edema, and bloating and increase the risk of thromboembolic disease, especially in women older than 35 years who smoke (these women should not be offered OCPs). OCPs may worsen or cause migraines, seizures, dyslipidemia, and gallbladder disease.

CHAPTER 12

D. The lupus anticoagulant causes a prolonged partial thromboplastin time test but paradoxically causes an increased tendency for thrombosis. It also is associated with a false-positive Venereal Disease Research Laboratory syphilis test and recurrent first-trimester abortions. Given the presence of all of these things in the history, this is the most likely cause.

CHAPTER 13

C. Immunoglobulin therapy should be avoided in individuals with immunoglobulin A (IgA) deficiency because anti-IgA antibodies may be present, causing an allergic reaction. IgA deficiency is the most common immunodeficiency, affecting roughly one in 500 people. It commonly leads to recurrent upper respiratory and gastrointestinal infections because IgA normally is secreted to prevent these infections. Although anaphylaxis can occur in anyone for various reasons, there is no reason to suspect any of the other conditions in this situation without a suggestive history.

CHAPTER 14

B. This patient most likely has infectious mononucleosis caused by the Epstein-Barr virus (EBV), which always should be in the differential diagnosis with upper respiratory infection symptoms of fever and pharyngitis, especially in a young adult. When these patients are given amoxicillin or ampicillin, 90% or more develop a generalized rash, usually maculopapular. This rash does not indicate sensitivity to β-lactam antibiotics in the future and usually subsides after the inciting antibiotic is discontinued. *Streptococcus pyogenes* is probably more common than EBV infection but should have improved with antibiotics. In addition to fever, pharyngitis, and fatigue, the patient with EBV can present with generalized lymphadenopathy, tonsillar exudates, and eyelid edema. EBV also may result in splenomegaly; lymphocytosis with toxic lymphocytes seen on peripheral smear; anemia, thrombocytopenia, or both; and hepatitis. Diagnosis is normally with a disposable heterophil-antibody agglutination test (monospot test), although serum heterophil or EBV-specific antibody titers can be used in cases of high clinical suspicion and negative Monospot test results (the Monospot test result can be negative for several weeks after symptom onset). Treatment is supportive, and contact sports should be avoided during the first month because of the rare complication of splenic rupture when splenomegaly is present. Although an amoxicillin allergy is possible, it is not the best answer for two reasons: It does not explain the patient's persistent symptoms, and she did not have a problem when she took penicillin in the past.

CHAPTER 15

B. The patient shows symptoms and signs of hypocalcemia, which in adults often is from inadvertent surgical removal of the parathyroid glands during thyroid surgery. Trousseau sign (carpopedal spasm with inflation of a blood pressure cuff) is present, and Chvostek sign (facial muscle tetany from tapping on the facial nerve) probably could be elicited in this patient. Electrocardiography normally shows QT interval prolongation in hypocalcemia versus QT interval shortening in hypercalcemia. By causing a respiratory alkalosis, hyperventilation shifts calcium to the intracellular space and may worsen or cause hypocalcemia symptoms and signs. There is little reason to suspect Graves disease from the history, and corticosteroids are not indicated for hypocalcemia.

CHAPTER 16

C. There was probably hemolysis of the blood sample, resulting in an elevated potassium level, a common laboratory problem. The patient does not appear to have renal or adrenal problems because blood urea nitrogen, creatinine, electrolytes, acid–base status, and electrocardiography (EKG) findings are normal. There is no reason to suspect multiple myeloma. Whenever an elevated potassium level does not make sense clinically, consider hemolysis. For example, it is highly unlikely that a potassium level this high would not cause symptoms or EKG findings. Also, in the absence of symptoms or EKG findings, urgent treatment is not needed. Remember the old clinical adage: "Treat the patient, not the lab value or x-ray result."

CHAPTER 17

D. Thiazide diuretics absorb calcium, preventing more of it from going into the urine, where it may precipitate out and form a calcium stone. Anything that increases calcium or oxalate excretion into the urine increases the risk of calcium stones. Hyperoxaluria is an uncommon condition usually caused by small bowel disease (e.g., Crohn disease) or resection.

CHAPTER 18

D. This patient most likely had a transient ischemic attack secondary to a small cholesterol plaque embolus. He should have a carotid ultrasound (duplex) study to look for carotid artery stenosis; however, the decision whether or not to do a carotid endarterectomy (CEA) should be withheld pending the results of the study. CEA is an elective procedure generally reserved for stable patients and is contraindicated In patients with recent myocardial infarction (within 6 months); additionally, the patient may not have a lesion amenable to surgery.

The patient would benefit from being put on aspirin (after a computed tomography scan is done to rule out an intracranial hemorrhage in this setting), a β-blocker (to reduce the incidence of a second heart attack and improve survival), and an angiotensin-converting enzyme inhibitor (to slow progression of nephropathy and neuropathy) if they can be tolerated. This patient needs a fasting lipid profile to determine the need for cholesterol-lowering therapy and should quit smoking. With his multiple atherosclerosis risk factors and clinical evidence of atherosclerosis, this patient needs aggressive medical management (and possible surgical intervention if testing reveals any surgically correctable lesions in the coronary or carotid arteries) to prevent further morbidity and death.

CHAPTER 19

C. This patient is displaying the **Cushing reflex**, which occurs with markedly increased intracranial pressure (ICP) secondary to head trauma and probable delayed cerebral edema, hemorrhage, or both. The reflex consists of a triad including elevated blood pressure, bradycardia, and irregular respirations and indicates life-threatening levels of intracranial hypertension. There is no reason to suspect infection because the patient had a closed head injury and is afebrile. Hypoxia always is a possibility with acute delirium, but you would expect the patient to be breathing hard and fast consistently to improve oxygenation, and hypoxia would not explain the marked increase in blood pressure. Acute cocaine withdrawal, although it may cause delirium, does not present in this fashion. Intensive care unit delirium is a well-known phenomenon but is not enough to explain the blood pressure and irregular respirations. This patient needs prompt intubation and neurosurgical evaluation. Forced hyperventilation can lessen ICP temporarily; mannitol or furosemide can be used as well. A craniotomy may be required in severe cases.

CHAPTER 20

D. Maternal serum alpha-fetoprotein determinations ideally are done at 16 to 18 weeks' gestation. A low alpha-fetoprotein level may mean Down syndrome, trisomy 18, fetal demise, or inaccurate dates (the fetus is younger than estimated). A high alpha-fetoprotein level may mean neural tube defects (e.g., anencephaly, spina bifida), ventral wall defects (e.g., omphalocele, gastroschisis), multiple gestation, fetal demise, or inaccurate dates (the fetus is older than estimated).

CHAPTER 21

C. Human chorionic gonadotropin is commonly followed during choriocarcinoma treatment. Liver and certain testicular tumors may be followed with alpha-fetoprotein, and epithelial ovarian cancer is most commonly associated with CA-125 antigen, although other tumor markers may be used with ovarian germ cell tumors. Pancreatic cancer most commonly is followed with CA 19-9 and carcinoembryonic antigen (CEA) antigens. Breast cancer may be followed with CA 15-3 or CA 27.29.

TUMOR MARKER	CANCER(S)
Alpha-fetoprotein	Liver, testicular (yolk sac)
Bladder tumor antigen, NMP 22	Bladder
CA 15-3, CA 27.29	Breast
CA 19-9	Pancreas, lung
CA-125	Ovarian
CEA	Colon, pancreas, other GI tumors
Chromogranin A	Carcinoid tumors, neuroblastoma
Human chorionic gonadotropin	Hydatiform moles, choriocarcinoma
β2-Microglobulin	Multiple myeloma, chronic lymphocytic leukemia
Prostate-specific antigen	Prostate (early)
S-100	Melanoma, CNS tumors, nerve tumors
Thyroglobulin	Thyroid

CEA, carcinoembryonic antigen; CNS, central nervous system; GI, gastrointestinal.

CHAPTER 22

A. This patient has developed a right central retinal artery occlusion, causing blindness secondary to temporal arteritis with probable coexisting polymyalgia rheumatica (50% of patients with temporal arteritis have polymyalgia rheumatica). Immediate corticosteroid therapy is indicated with suspicion of temporal arteritis to preserve vision (in this case, to preserve vision in the left eye because when blindness develops, it is usually irreversible). Treatment should be started even before the diagnosis is confirmed with a temporal artery biopsy, the gold standard for diagnosis. Again, more than one answer, but the single best answer for "what to do next" is an important distinction because this is an ophthalmologic emergency. An antinuclear antibody titer is not helpful (low sensitivity and non-specific), and muscle biopsy (as well as electromyography) is normal in polymyalgia rheumatica. The patient's low-grade fever is most likely secondary to the active arteritis, and cultures are not indicated with the given description. Things in the vignette that should raise suspicion of temporal arteritis include age older than 50 years, jaw claudication, scalp tenderness, fever with a normal white blood cell count, and a markedly elevated sedimentation rate.

CHAPTER 23

A. The epidemiology of slipped capital femoral epiphysis is important to increase your suspicion of the condition. It tends to affect overweight boys between the ages of 9 and 13 years and frequently causes a limp with pain in the ipsilateral knee, thigh, or groin (referred pain). Plain radiographs are the initial diagnostic study of choice and are generally all that is needed to confirm the diagnosis. Early surgical pinning generally is used to prevent further slippage of the femoral epiphysis with resultant abnormalities of the hip joint. Legg-Calvé-Perthes disease, or idiopathic avascular necrosis of the femoral head, can cause similar symptoms but tends to affect children between the ages of 4 and 9 years and is not associated with obesity.

CHAPTER 24

E. Although fertility is reduced (roughly 50% fertility rate) in women with cystic fibrosis (CF) and pregnancy can be hazardous to maternal health, many women with CF have delivered healthy offspring. The infants would be expected to be healthy (unless the father is a carrier for CF), although all offspring would be carriers for CF. Of men with CF, 98% are infertile. CF is an autosomal recessive condition (choices A and B are incorrect); both the mother and father usually are carriers if a child gets the disease. After an affected child from two healthy adults, there is roughly a 25% chance (not 50%) that the next child would have CF. The diagnosis is made presumptively by elevated sodium or chloride (not potassium) in the sweat. Genetic studies can be done to confirm the diagnosis and specific mutation type.

CHAPTER 25

C. Barbiturates, antiepileptics, and rifampin are the classic liver enzyme inducers, and cimetidine and ketoconazole are the classic liver enzyme inhibitors; this is important to remember because of drug–drug interactions. Penicillin, lansoprazole, and fluoxetine have little effect on liver enzymes.

CHAPTER 26

C. People who take more pills tend to have more diseases or more severe disease and probably die of their diseases, not the medications. Disease would be the confounding variable in this case. If a researcher measures the number of ashtrays owned and mortality and concludes that ashtrays cause death, smoking would be the confounding factor. Interviewer bias is not likely when the outcome is death and the measurement is so objective (i.e., number of pills). The large number of subjects in the study makes a type II error much less likely.

CHAPTER 27

D. This patient has a history consistent with posttraumatic stress disorder, which affects a large number of Vietnam veterans. In the history, look for a severely traumatic event (e.g., war, rape, natural disaster) with reexperiencing of the event (e.g., nightmares, flashbacks, illusions) and an attempt to avoid things that trigger a memory of the event. These patients often have chronic anxiety, hyperalertness, and a feeling of detachment from others. Treatment with sedatives, such as diphenhydramine and lorazepam, although a possible adjunct to other treatment modalities, is inappropriate in isolation and not the cornerstone of management. Many of these patients are prone to developing alcoholism and drug addiction to diminish their emotional pain.

Haloperidol is not indicated in this disorder unless frank psychosis develops (not present in this case), and electroconvulsive therapy is a second-line treatment for depression, usually used after a trial of medication is unsuccessful. Fluoxetine and other selective serotonin reuptake inhibitors (SSRIs), however, have been shown to be beneficial in patients with this condition. The best answer is D because group therapy with others who are experiencing similar problems is an effective therapy and may provide a support group, which many of these patients lack. Adjunctive medications, such as the SSRIs, are also commonly prescribed.

CHAPTER 28

C. A thoracentesis probably would relieve the patient's symptoms as well as provide important diagnostic information. The other options are premature, other than respiratory isolation, which is a reasonable precaution in many cases. Empirical tuberculosis therapy is not given—a diagnosis should be secured first. The causes of a pleural effusion are many, ranging from those causing transudative effusions (congestive heart failure, cirrhosis) to exudative effusions (infection, cancer, autoimmune disorders). Evaluation of the pleural fluid can help narrow the differential diagnosis and guide further therapy. It also may reveal the underlying process, which can be obscured by the fluid on radiographs. Right and left decubitus views of the chest also would be helpful to evaluate the underlying lung parenchyma and to determine if the effusion is free flowing or loculated. A computed tomography scan of the chest may be of benefit after thoracentesis as well, but a positron emission tomography scan is not indicated for workup of a pleural effusion.

CHAPTER 30

D. This woman has dermatomyositis, a fairly uncommon connective tissue disease that classically causes proximal muscle weakness and tenderness; elevated creatine kinase levels resulting from muscle destruction; and a rash classically around the eyelids (i.e., heliotrope rash), hands, and elbows (Gottron sign). Patients are at an increased risk for malignancy, although fewer than 10% of patients develop one.

This patient also has anemia, which is likely anemia of chronic disease. Muscle biopsy is an important part of making the diagnosis because it is almost uniformly abnormal, with degeneration of muscle fibers, inflammation, centralization of nuclei, and interstitial fibrosis. Electromyography results are usually abnormal as well and classically show spontaneous fibrillations with sharp waves; bizarre, high-frequency discharges; and small-amplitude, short-duration polyphasic motor unit potentials. A silent myocardial infarction and depression are unlikely as the cause of this woman's symptoms (and wouldn't explain the anemia or eyelid changes), although coexisting depression may worsen fatigue and should be asked about in more detail.

CHAPTER 31

A. This patient most likely has a testicular torsion, a surgical emergency. In this condition, the sooner surgery is performed, the more likely it is that the testicle can be salvaged. A delay in surgery could result in testicular infarction. Prehn sign is mentioned in the question, which entails elevating the testicle to see if pain is relieved. Pain often is relieved (positive sign) if the patient has epididymitis, the primary differential diagnosis in a case such as this, but the pain does not improve after this maneuver in patients with testicular torsion. Other important signs include a swollen, retracted testicle and absent cremasteric reflex on the affected side in testicular torsion. Scrotal ultrasonography, when readily available, is used to confirm the diagnosis before surgical intervention and usually shows decreased to absent blood flow. Ultrasonography can also make the diagnosis of epididymitis and orchitis, the two primary differential considerations (both more common than torsion)

Epididymitis has a more gradual in onset and often is associated with urinary tract or urethritis symptoms. It also tends to be more common in men older than age 30 years, but torsion is more common in men younger than age 20 years. Laparotomy is not indicated; rather, local scrotal exploration with orchiopexy of *both* testicles to reduce the chance of a further episode of torsion is indicated if torsion is confirmed by ultrasonography (or ultrasonography is not available). Although mumps can cause orchitis, there is no suggestive history, and this condition is rare in the United States because of mandatory vaccination.

CHAPTER 32

A. This patient has claudication, the peripheral vascular disease equivalent of angina. The best initial management is conservative, including cessation of smoking, initiation of an exercise program, and control of other atherosclerosis risk factors (cholesterol, hypertension, and diabetes). Revascularization may be required eventually but carries a significant morbidity and mortality because of the presence of widespread atherosclerosis and should be reserved for severe, disabling symptoms or failure of conservative management. Urgent referral is inappropriate, although consulting a vascular surgeon would be appropriate. Heparin is not needed in this instance. This patient needs to be on aspirin to prevent a second heart attack and to reduce the risk of stroke. The patient also needs to be on carvedilol to decrease the risk of a second heart attack and control his hypertension. Because the patient is currently normotensive, increasing the dose of carvedilol is not needed at this time. Additionally, such a dose increase may theoretically worsen his claudication because β_2-receptors stimulate vasodilation of the vessels that supply muscle beds and increase blood flow to muscles.

CHAPTER 34

A. Courvoisier sign describes a nontender, palpable gallbladder, usually caused by pancreatic cancer. Courvoisier postulated that a fibrotic gallbladder wall, which would be expected with cholelithiasis and chronic cholecystitis owing to chronic inflammation, would not be able to distend readily and would not be palpable. If a malignancy, such as pancreatic cancer or a bile duct malignancy, occluded the cystic duct of a healthy gallbladder (acutely or subacutely), the gallbladder would be more likely to distend to the point of being palpable. Acute cholecystitis and cholangitis cause tenderness in the region of the gallbladder, although the gallbladder usually is not palpable.

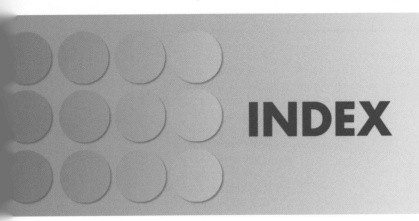

INDEX

Note: Page numbers followed by *b* indicate boxes, *f* indicate figures and *t* indicate tables.

Tanner stages, 225
Tardive dyskinesia, due to antipsychotic medications, 244
Target cells, 307*f*
TBG (thyroid-binding globulin), 36*b*
TCAs (tricyclic antidepressants)
  antidote for overdose with, 233*t*
  for depression, 247
Teardrop cells, 308*f*
Temporal arteritis, 201–202, 300*f*
TEN (toxic epidermal necrolysis), 16
Tensilon (edrophonium) test, 148–149
Tension headache, 148
Tension pneumothorax, 68, 69*f*
  imaging of, 289*f*
Teratogenic agents, 168, 169*t*
Teratoma, ovarian, 190
Term pregnancy, 163*t*
Testes, 273
  cancer of, 274
  cryptorchidism of, 273
  epididymitis of, 274, 274*t*
  orchitis of, 274
  torsion of, 274, 274*t*
Testicular cancer, 195, 274
Testicular torsion, 274, 274*t*
Testicular veins, drainage of, 274*b*
Tetanus immunization, for adults, 238*t*
Tetany, due to hypocalcemia, 128
Tetracyclines, side effects of, 232*t*
Tetralogy of Fallot, 216*t*
Thalassemia, 91
Thalidomide, with transplant, 272
Thematic Apperception Test, 250
Thermal burns, 30–31
Thiamine, for alcoholism, 124
Thiamine deficiency, 131*t*
  neurologic signs and symptoms of, 154
Thiazide diuretics
  for hypertension, 115*t*
  side effects of, 231
Thioridazine, side effects of, 232*t*
Third degree heart block, 9*t*
Third trimester bleeding, 174–175, 175*f*
Thoracic outlet syndrome, 281
Thoracic trauma, 67–69
  airway obstruction due to, 67
  aortic rupture due to, 69
  cardiac tamponade due to, 68
  diaphragm rupture due to, 69
  flail chest due to, 69
  imaging of, 261*t*
  liver lacerations and contusions due to, 69
  massive hemothorax due to, 68–69
  pneumothorax due to
    open, 68
    tension, 68, 69*f*
  pulmonary contusion due to, 69
  pulsus paradoxus due to, 68
Throat, peritonsillar and retropharyngeal abscess of, 27–28

Throat clearing, 313
Thrombocythemia, primary, 183*t*
Thrombocytopenia
  causes of, 96
  heparin-induced, 6, 96*b*, 96*t*
  platelets with, 96*b*
Thrombocytopenic purpura
  idiopathic, 96*t*
    in children, 222*t*
  thrombotic, 96*b*, 96*t*
    in children, 222*t*
Thromboembolism, oral contraceptives and, 80
Thrombolysis, for myocardial infarction, 2
Thrombophlebitis
  postpartum pelvic, 180
  superficial, 6, 281
Thromboplastin time, partial, 6, 96*t*
Thrombosis
  deep vein. *See* Deep vein thrombosis (DVT).
  venous sinus, 158
Thrombotic thrombocytopenic purpura (TTP), 96*b*, 96*t*
  in children, 222*t*
Thrush, with HIV, 100
"Thumb sign," 226, 227*f*
Thyroglobulin, as tumor marker, 185*t*
Thyroglossal duct cysts, 27
Thyroid cancer, 196
  risk factors for, 184*t*
Thyroid function tests
  for hyperthyroidism, 35
  for hypothyroidism, 34
  during pregnancy, 164
Thyroid nodules, 36, 36*f*, 196
Thyroid-binding globulin (TBG), 36*b*
Thyroiditis
  Hashimoto, 34
  hyperthyroidism due to, 35
  subacute granulomatous, 34
Thyroid-stimulating hormone (TSH), in amenorrhea, 79
Thyrotoxicosis, neonatal, 39
TIA (transient ischemic attack), 144, 145*t*
  due to carotid stenosis, 278
TIBC (total iron-binding capacity), in iron-deficiency anemia, 90
Tic douloureux, 145
Tinea
  capitis, 17, 17*f*, 300*f*
  corporis, 17, 300*f*
  cruris, 17, 300*f*
  pedis, 17
  unguium, 17
  versicolor, 21–22, 22*f*
Tinel sign, 312
Tissue plasminogen activator (t-PA), for ischemic stroke, 143–144, 145*t*
Tongue, strawberry, 311*f*
Tonic-clonic seizures, 151

Tonsillitis, acute, 309*f*
Tooth avulsion, 33
Tophi, 265, 266*f*, 311*f*
Topiramate, for seizures, 152*t*
TORCH infections, 168–169
  hearing loss due to, 24
Torsades de points, EKG of, 286*f*
Total cholesterol, 120, 121
Total iron-binding capacity (TIBC), in iron-deficiency anemia, 90
Tourette syndrome, 252
Toxic adenoma, hyperthyroidism due to, 35
Toxic epidermal necrolysis (TEN), 16
Toxic megacolon, 49, 50*f*
  imaging of, 291*f*
Toxic multinodular goiter, 35
Toxic shock syndrome, 111, 133, 302*f*
Toxicology, 32
  poisonings and antidotes in, 32
  toxidromes in, 32
Toxidromes, 32
Toxins
  acute renal failure due to, 138
  vision loss due to, 199
Toxoplasmosis *(Toxoplasma gondii)*
  with HIV, 100, 100*f*
  during pregnancy, 103, 168
  seizures due to, 103
t-PA (tissue plasminogen activator), for ischemic stroke, 143–144, 145*t*
Tracheoesophageal fistula, 217*t*, 229
  in children, 217*t*, 229
Transferrin, in iron-deficiency anemia, 90
Transfusion(s), 94–95
Transfusion reactions, 95
Transient ischemic attack (TIA), 144, 145*t*
  due to carotid stenosis, 278
Transplant rejection
  acute, 272
  asymptomatic, 272
  chronic, 272
  hyperacute, 98, 272
Transposition of great vessels, 216*t*
Transurethral resection of prostate (TURP), 273
Transvaginal ultrasonography, 168
Trastuzumab, for breast cancer, 188
Trauma, 66–70, 67*b*
  ABCDE of, 66
  abdominal
    blunt, 67
    imaging of, 261*t*
    penetrating, 67
  aortic, 261*t*
  arthritis due to, 267
  blood and fluid loss with, 68*t*
  chest, 261*t*
  decreased breath sounds in, 313
  Glasgow Coma Scale for, 68*t*